Religion, Spirituality and Health: A Social Scientific Approach

Volume 1

The relationship between religious/spiritual belief or behaviour and health behaviour has been explored over several decades and across various disciplines. Religious variables have consistently been found to have a direct relationship to physical and mental health. At the same time - research has also indicated potential societal tensions that can exist between religion and health – we have seen this in relation to family planning, HIV/AIDS, and reproduction. This book series aims to uncover the impact of religion on individual health behaviours and outcomes but also the influence of religion on health practices at the community level. This book series uncovers the impact of religion on individual health behaviors and outcomes, as well as the influence of religion on health practices at the community level. It consists of volumes that are based on multi-methodological approaches, provide quantitative and qualitative forms of analysis, and advance the understanding of the intersection between religion and health beyond the correlation of religious belief and health outcomes. Building on earlier research, the series explores the direct relationship between religious variables and physical and mental health, as well as the potential societal tensions that have been shown to exist between religion and health – for example in relation to family planning, HIV/AIDS, and reproduction. Spoken values are often shared within religious communities; however, religious influence can at times be extended outside of the community in instances of service provisions such as hospital ownership, various research active think tanks, political action, and the development of community mores.

More information about this series at http://www.springer.com/series/13437

Kevin J. Flannelly

Religious Beliefs, Evolutionary Psychiatry, and Mental Health in America

Evolutionary Threat Assessment Systems Theory

Springer

Kevin J. Flannelly
Center for Psychosocial Research
Massapequa, NY, USA

Religion, Spirituality and Health: A Social Scientific Approach
ISBN 978-3-319-52487-0   ISBN 978-3-319-52488-7 (eBook)
DOI 10.1007/978-3-319-52488-7

Library of Congress Control Number: 2017935569

Printed on acid-free paper

This Springer imprint is published by Springer Nature
The registered company is Springer International Publishing AG
The registered company address is: Gewerbestrasse 11, 6330 Cham, Switzerland

Acknowledgments

I am deeply indebted to the late Dr. Eugene B. Brody, the longtime Editor-in-Chief of *The Journal of Nervous and Mental Disease*, for affording me and my colleagues a forum to publish our original theoretical paper on "Beliefs, Mental Health, and Evolutionary Threat Assessment Systems in the Brain" and an earlier study about belief in life after death and mental health that led directly to the development of ETAS theory. I am also indebted to Professor Paul Gilbert of the University of Derby, whose insights and guidance enabled us to publish the original theoretical article and two subsequent articles about ETAS theory.

I thank my friend and colleague Chris Ellison (Dr. Christopher G. Ellison) for spurring my interest in studying the connection between religious beliefs and mental health, encouraging me to write this book, and providing me the opportunity to publish the book in the Springer Series *Religion, Spirituality and Health: A Social Scientific Approach*, on which he is an editor. I thank my wife Laura (Dr. Laura T. Flannelly), who is also my colleague and friend, for her support while writing the book and for editing all the book chapters.

The studies in this book by my colleagues and me that were published between 2005 and 2010 were partly supported by a grant from the John Templeton Foundation to HealthCare Chaplaincy in New York City for a 3-year "postdoctoral research fellowship on religion and health" and subsequent Templeton funding of that program. The studies by my colleagues and me that were published between 2011 and 2015 were funded, in part, by Templeton Grant # 21296, "Spiritual Beliefs as Predictors of Mental Health: A Test of ETAS Theory" (Kevin J. Flannelly, Ph.D., and Kathleen Galek, Ph.D., coprincipal investigators). I am grateful to Dr. Jackson Kytle for his advocacy of theory development and basic research at HealthCare Chaplaincy during his tenure there as the Vice President of Academic Affairs.

Contents

Chapter 1
Introduction

Abstract It is often said that religious faith consists of three dimensions (belonging, behaving, and believing). Yet, beliefs have long been neglected in research on physical and mental health. This chapter provides basic information about the history of research on religion and health in the U.S. and the extent of this neglect, with respect to research on mental health, as background for understanding the book's focus. It also explains the importance of the book's historical perspective on the development of theories of organic evolution, religious and secular reactions to them, and the development of Evolutionary Psychiatry, which is based on Charles Darwin's theories of evolution. This is followed by a discussion of the reasons for the author's interest in religious beliefs and mental health (more specifically, psychiatric symptoms), the purpose of different parts of the book, and the religious beliefs examined in the book. A brief summary of the basic tenets of Evolutionary Threat Assessment Systems Theory is then presented, including the central premise that instinctive, emotional, and cognitive brain systems evolved at different points in our evolutionary heritage to assess the potential threats of harm posed by a dangerous world, and that psychiatric symptoms are the product of these brain systems. Finally, the chapter divides research on ETAS Theory into four different levels of analysis related to its propositions about behavior, the neural correlates of psychiatric symptoms, the specific neural organization and functioning of ETAS, and the evolutionary origins of psychiatric symptoms.

Keywords Dimensions of religion • ETAS Theory • Evolutionary psychiatry • Levels of analysis • Religious beliefs • Threat assessment

1.1 Religious Belonging, Behaving, and Believing

It has often been said that religious faith consists of three dimensions: belonging, behaving, and believing [1–4]. Early U.S. research on the relationship between religion and health mainly focused on belonging; that is, the degree to which health was associated with belonging to different religious faiths, especially Judaism, Mormonism (Latter Day Saints), and Seventh-Day Adventism [5].

K.J. Flannelly, *Religious Beliefs, Evolutionary Psychiatry, and Mental Health in America*, Religion, Spirituality and Health: A Social Scientific Approach 1,
DOI 10.1007/978-3-319-52488-7_1

U.S. research in the 1960s began to examine the association between health and religious behavior, particularly how often adults in the general population attended church or other religious services [6]. This was usually measured by simply asking "How often do you attend Sunday worship services?" [7]. Since then, religious attendance has continued to be one of the most commonly used measures of religious faith in research on physical and mental health in the U.S., according to the comprehensive *Handbook of Religion and Health* [8].

Although researchers have developed many other measures of religion over the years, an analysis of studies in the *Handbook of Religion and Health* conducted by psychologists Kathleen Galek and Matthew Porter [9] found that belonging to a religion (religious affiliation) and religious behavior, in the form of attending services, were major measures of religion in more than two-thirds of U.S. studies of mental health. In contrast, they found that religious beliefs were measured in less than 10% of the studies. Perhaps, this discrepancy may be attributed to the fact that researchers find it difficult to measure beliefs for some reason. Indeed, Dr. Neal Krause, who did sociological and psychological research on religion and health for decades, once said: "The difficulty in studying religious beliefs in research on religion and health arises from the fact that there are so many of them" (p. 268) [10]. On the other hand, Crystal L. Park [11], a psychology professor at the University of Connecticut, observed that even when researchers attempt to measure religious beliefs they often confound beliefs with other aspects of religious faith. The purpose of this book is to summarize what U.S. research has found about the relationship between religious beliefs and mental health, and to put those findings into a theoretical context that explains how and why religious beliefs affect mental health, especially psychiatric symptoms. I think research on beliefs is essential for understanding the relationship between religion and mental health because beliefs are stored and processed in the brain; therefore, they can directly affect other brain processes.

1.2 Personal Perspective and the Book's Organization

My own involvement in research on religious beliefs and mental health began in 2004, leading to the publication of a 2006 study on belief in life-after-death and psychiatric symptoms in the U.S. general public [12], which I co-authored with Dr. Neal Krause, a professor at the University of Michigan School of Public Health, Dr. Christopher G. Ellison, then a sociology professor at The University of Texas at Austin, Dr. Harold G. Koenig, a professor of psychiatry at Duke University, and Dr. Kathleen Galek, who was then a clinical researcher at The HealthCare Chaplaincy in New York City. The study found a strong salubrious[1] association between belief in life-after-death and several classes of psychiatric symptoms.

[1] I use the words salubrious and salutary interchangeably throughout out the book when referring to the beneficial or advantageous effects of belief s or other variables on mental health.

I was so struck by the findings of the study that I felt driven to determine how belief in life-after-death could affect psychiatric symptoms. Having been trained as a physiological psychologist, I was particularly determined to find a plausible biological mechanism through which religious and other beliefs could affect psychiatric symptoms. Some readers may ask why I wanted to investigate the relationship between religious beliefs and psychiatric symptoms at all, since psychiatric disorders form the extreme end of the spectrum of mental health. The answer to this question is two-fold: the first answer addresses my interest in psychiatric symptoms and the second answer addresses my interest in the relationship between religious beliefs and psychiatric symptoms.

First, I have been intrigued with psychiatry since I read Sigmund Freud's *Psychopathology of Everyday Life* [13] in the 1960s. Contrary to what one might think, psychiatric symptoms are not the extreme end of a continuum of mental health, they are an everyday experience. Part III explains the reasons why all of us experience psychiatric symptoms in our daily lives as a result of our evolutionary heritage. Clinical psychologists and psychiatrists since the 1980s have written books and articles proposing that psychiatric symptoms are the by-product of brain mechanisms that have evolved to protect us from harm. Their ideas formed the foundation of Evolutionary Psychiatry or Darwinian Psychiatry, which should not be confused with Evolutionary Psychology. Because psychiatric symptoms are rooted in our evolutionary history, all of us exhibit psychiatric symptoms to some degree; however, most of us do not have symptoms that are so severe that we need psychiatric help to deal with them.

Second, as I mentioned earlier, although researchers have studied the relationship between various aspects of religion and mental health, few have studied the relationship between religious beliefs and mental health. This seemed to me to be an important gap in the research because I thought one had to show that religion is represented in the brain to be able to make a causal connection between religion and mental health. Unlike religious practices, religious affiliation, and various other measures of religion, I felt sure that religious beliefs must be located somewhere in the brain, and therefore, that they could affect psychiatric symptoms. As discussed in Part III, some of the same clinical psychologists who have proposed that psychiatric symptoms are the result of brain mechanism that evolved to protect us from harm also have proposed that psychiatric symptoms are related to beliefs about the dangerousness of the world. Thus, I thought religious beliefs might alter one's perception about the dangerousness of the world.

A 2007 theoretical article by me and my colleagues titled, "Beliefs, Mental Health and Evolutionary Threat Assessment Systems in the Brain," described how different parts of the brain, which assess threats of personal harm, cause psychiatric symptoms, and how beliefs influence psychiatric symptoms through their effects on threat assessments [14], which is the central premise of this book. Part III gives a much more detailed description of these notions than the original theoretical paper did and briefly describes the proposed evolutionary origins of causal beliefs. In doing so, Part III lays the foundation for interpreting the results described in Part IV, which indicates how different religious beliefs can ameliorate or exacerbate psychiatric symptoms, according to ETAS Theory. Since the publication of the 2007 article, I have come to think that ETAS may be the embodiment of Aaron Beck's concept of "modes." Beck, an American psychologist who was one of the founders of cognitive behavior therapy, said in a 1996 article that: (a) a mode is "a network of cognitive, affective, motivational, and behavioral components," (b) modes "are derivatives of ancient organizations that evolved in prehistoric circumstances and are manifested in survival reactions," and (c) some modes are expressed "in an exaggerated way in psychiatric disorders" (p. 2) [15]. Beck initially described the concept of modes in his 1985 book about anxiety disorders and phobias [16].

Part IV of the book provides comprehensive coverage of U.S. studies on the relationship religious beliefs and mental health, many of which were published by Chris Ellison, Neal Krause, and Harold Koenig. I focus on U.S. research in Part IV because the vast majority of studies on religious beliefs and mental health have been conducted in the U.S. Research findings from outside the U.S. are presented when they fill in important gaps in American research. Most of the research results are primarily based on Christian samples because the vast majority of Americans are Christians. I originally tried to integrate findings from other counties with those from the U.S., but I found that my descriptions of research from outside the U.S. sounded more like the sidebars of newspaper and magazine articles, which did not fit in well with the main topics that I wanted to cover.

As the claim of ETAS Theory that religious beliefs affect mental health is based on evolutionary psychiatry, and evolutionary psychiatry is based on Darwin's evolutionary theories, I thought it would be helpful to devote a small portion of the book (Part II) to Darwin's three books about evolution and science's and society's reactions to them. Since the concept of evolution is controversial, if not an anathema to many religious individuals, and this book is predicated on the theory that religious beliefs affect evolved brain systems that govern mental health, I thought it was reasonable to place the conflict between evolutionary theory and religious faith in a historical context in Part I of the book. The current conflict is briefly discussed in Part II.

The Chaps. 25 through 30 of Part V summarize the key points made in each of the chapters in Parts I–III and summarize and discuss the major results presented in Part IV in relation to ETAS Theory. Hence, if you are not particularly interested in some topic, you are in a hurry, or you find a chapter to be tedious, you can skip a chapter or an entire section of the book, and read one or more of the summaries provided in Part V. For other readers, Part V is a helpful review of all the major topics and research findings. The final chapter of Part V offers suggestions for future research on ETAS Theory.

In all, then, the book consists of five sections or parts. Part I describes the intellectual and religious environment preceding the development of theories of organic evolution and the contemporaneous context in which early ideas about evolution emerged. Part II focuses on Charles Darwin's theories of evolution and scientific and social reactions to them. Part III describes the empirical and theoretical foundations of evolutionary psychiatry and ETAS Theory, and Part IV describes research findings on the relationship between religious beliefs and mental health, which I interpret in light of ETAS Theory. The chapters in Part V summarize the major points made in Parts I through IV and describe possible avenues of further research related to ETAS Theory. Before describing the basic elements of ETAS Theory, I will briefly enumerate the religious beliefs discussed in Part IV of the book.

1.3 Religious Beliefs Examined in This Book

As already mentioned, Part IV, which is the heart of the book, describes the results of primarily U.S. studies on religious beliefs and mental health. Chapter 15 on American beliefs about life-after-death and God is the lead chapter in Part IV because I thought it was necessary to summarize research on these topics as many of the studies described in Part IV are about the association of mental hea (Chaps. 16, 17 and 18) and belief in God (Chaps. 19, 20 and 21). Chapter 18 examines the effects of various beliefs about the afterlife on mental health and Chap. 19 examines the effects of various beliefs about God on mental health. Chapters 20 and 21 focus on different beliefs about one's relationship with God.

Research on individuals' beliefs about their relationship with God led to the development of the concept of "spiritual struggles," which originally encompassed beliefs about having a poor relationship with God. The use of the term has since been expanded to include having conflicts with members of one's religious congregation and having doubts about one's religious faith [17–19]. My own search of Google Scholar identified close to 100 articles with "spiritual struggles" in their title. Research results about mental health and beliefs about one's relationship with God are presented in Chap. 20 and results about mental health and religious doubt are presented in Chap. 23.

The subsequent chapters of Part IV report the results of local, regional, and national studies on the relationship between other religious beliefs and mental health. Specifically, Chaps. 22 and 24 summarize study results demonstrating empirical relationships between mental health and: (a) believing life has meaning and purpose; (b) believing that one has been forgiven by God; (c) belief in human an supernatural evil; and (d) believing that the Bible is literally true. Chapter 24 also presents evidence that believing the Bible is literally true encourages people to seek help for mental-health problems from clergy and discourages people from seeking help from mental-health professionals.

1.4 Brief Summary of ETAS Theory

Evolutionary Threat Assessment Systems Theory (ETAS Theory) proposes that some areas of the vertebrate brain have evolved at different points in time, partly to assess potential threats of harm, including portions of the brain stem, the basal ganglia, the limbic system, and the prefrontal area of the cortex (the PFC) (see Chaps.

9, 10 and 14), Potential threats of harm include dangerous situations, predators, and members of one's own species. The evolution of these successive brain structures increased the flexibility of reactions to threats, including the ability to assess a wider range of threats and to initiate a wider range of responses to threats. Because of their evolutionary origins, these four areas of the brain process information about potential threats differently: the PFC assesses threats using cognitive processing; areas of the limbic system, notably the amygdala, use affective processing; and areas of the basal ganglia and the brain stem use instinctive processing.

Threat assessment systems underlie certain types of psychiatric symptoms, as explained in Chaps. 11 and 12. Most of these symptoms involve fear, which is produced by the amygdala – a small limbic structure (see Chap. 10). Specifically, psychiatric symptomology reflects the action of different kinds of proximate mechanisms that evolved to assess different kinds of threats of harm (see Chaps. 11 and 12). As such, psychiatric symptoms represent evolutionary adaptations that once were essential for survival.

Areas of the PFC involved in threat assessments (particularly the ventromedial PFC) can moderate threat assessments from subcortical structures and can reduce the activity of the amygdala, and therefore, fear (see Chap. 14). Threat assessments made by the PFC are influenced by stimuli that promote a sense of security and safety. As the PFC (especially the vmPFC) also is involved in the processing of beliefs, beliefs can affect threat assessments, and hence, psychiatric symptoms (see Chap. 14). These beliefs include basic beliefs about the nature of the world at large (e.g., the world is a dangerous place), the nature of people (e.g., human nature is basically evil or basically good), and beliefs that offer a sense security and safety (e.g., a caring and loving God). Extensive evidence of the link between beliefs and psychiatric symptoms is presented in Chap. 13; the role of security and safety on threat assessment is described in Chap. 14.

Beliefs interact with each other to moderate threat assessments and psychiatric symptoms. For example, believing in guardian angels (which provide a sense of safety) may offset the pernicious[2] effect of believing in supernatural demons (which pose a threat of harm) on anxiety. Finally, anxiety-related symptoms affect other aspects of mental health, including psychological well-being and positive emotions.

1.5 Levels of Analysis of ETAS Theory

ETAS Theory can be viewed from four different perspectives or levels, each of which is associated with its own methodological approach: (I) psychological and sociological research to test behavioral predictions from ETAS Theory; (II) research

[2] I use the word pernicious throughout the book to refer to the harmful, injurious, or deleterious effects of beliefs or other variables on mental health.

in cognitive-affective neuroscience to confirm the association between psychiatric symptoms and brain structures implicated by ETAS Theory; (III) detailed neuro-anatomical and neuro-physiological research to define specific ETAS and to determine their operation at the neural level; and (IV) comparative anatomical and comparative behavioral research to examine the evolutionary origin of psychiatric symptoms, as proposed by ETAS Theory.

Level I falls squarely within the realm of this Springer series, "Religion, Spirituality and Health: A Social Scientific Approach," in that it provides a theoretical framework within which to understand the relationship between behavior and health (particularly mental health), just as Identity Theory and Attachment Theory do. The fundamental tenets of Level I are that: (a) perceptions of threat underlie psychiatric symptoms; (b) a sense of safety can ameliorate psychiatric symptoms; (c) beliefs about the world (including religious beliefs) moderate psychiatric symptoms; and (d) anxiety-related symptoms affect other aspects of psychological well-being and positive emotions. Level I encompasses common psychological and sociological concepts, such as self-esteem, self-efficacy, social support, and different types of social relationships. Analysis at this level does not require that one accept ETAS Theory's propositions about the brain or evolution. However, ETAS Theory's evolutionary perspective offers valuable insights into the nature of psychiatric symptoms, just as the evolutionary assumptions of Attachment Theory, which is described in detail in Chap. 21, provide insight into the nature of human relationships that are widely applied in social science research, including research on religion.

Level II is a cognitive neuroscience perspective (more properly called cognitive-affective neuroscience in this context), which is another necessary element of research to achieve the goal of understanding the relationship between religion, spirituality and health. I expect some other books in this series also will take this perspective, which is becoming increasingly common in studies that attempt to integrate knowledge and research methodology from psychology and neuroscience. This perspective examines the role of brain processes and brain structures on behavior, in this case, measures of mental health (such as positive emotions and psychological well-being) and mental illness (particularly psychiatric symptoms). This is the level of analysis needed to determine the associations among brain structure, brain function, psychiatric symptoms, and beliefs predicted by ETAS Theory. The interpretation of research findings from Level II (like those from Level I) do not require one to accept ETAS Theory's assumptions about the evolutionary origins of cognitive, affective, and instinctive processing, or the evolutionary origins of the neural structures associated with them. However, this level of analysis is predicated on a recognition of the importance of neuro-affective brain systems, which have been the stepchild of neuroscience research.

Level III is the neuro-operational level of analysis, which is needed to understand the detailed neural organization and neural functioning of ETAS. This level of analysis requires a much finer analysis of the neural circuits comprising individual ETAS underlying specific psychiatric disorders and research on how the neural circuits operate. Level IV is the evolutionary level of analysis to understand the evolution of ETAS. This level of analysis entails comparative research on the anatomy and behavior of different classes of vertebrates, orders of mammals, and families of primates to establish the points in geological time in which the proximate mechanisms underlying different psychiatric symptoms arose.

References

1. Rice, R. (1990). Believing, behaving, belonging – Exploring a larger view of faith. *Spectrum, 20*(3), 22–31.
2. Field, C. D. (2015). *Britain's last religious revival? Quantifying belonging, behaving, and believing in the long 1950s*. New York: Palgrave MacMillan.
3. Olson, L. R., & Warber, A. L. (2008). Belonging, behaving, and believing: Assessing the role of religion on presidential approval. *Political Research Quarterly, 61*(2), 192–204.
4. Kosmin, B. A., & Keysar, A. (2008). *American religious identification survey: Summary report*. Hartford: Trinity College.
5. Levin, J. S., & Schiller, P. L. (1987). Is there a religious factor in health? *Journal of Religion and Health, 26*(1), 9–36.
6. Levin, J. S., & Vanderpool, H. Y. (1987). Is frequent religious attendance really conducive to better health? Toward an epidemiology or religion. *Social Science & Medicine, 24*(7), 589–600.
7. Hall, D. E., Meador, K. G., & Koenig, H. G. (2008). Measuring religiousness in health research: Review and critique. *Journal of Religion and Health, 47*(2), 134–163.
8. Koenig, H. G., McCullough, M. E., & Larson, D. B. (2001). *Handbook of religion and health*. New York: Oxford University Press.
9. Galek, K., & Porter, M. (2009). A brief review of religious beliefs in research on mental health and ETAS theory. *Journal of Health Care Chaplaincy, 16*(1–2), 58–64.
10. Krause, N. (2010). God-mediated control and change in self-rated health. *The International Journal for the Psychology of Religion, 20*(4), 267–287.
11. Park, C. L. (2012). Attending to the construct of beliefs in research on religion/spirituality and health: Commentary on 'Beyond belief'. *Journal of Health Psychology, 17*(7), 969–973.
12. Flannelly, K. J., Koenig, H. G., Ellison, C. G., Galek, K., & Krause, N. (2006). Belief in life after death and mental health: Findings from a national survey. *Journal of Nervous and Mental Disease, 194*(7), 524–529.
13. Freud, S. (1914). *Psychopathology of everyday life* (A. A. Brill, Trans.). London: T. Fisher Unwin.
14. Flannelly, K. J., Koenig, H. G., Galek, K., & Ellison, C. G. (2007). Beliefs, mental health, and evolutionary threat assessment systems in the brain. *Journal of Nervous and Mental Disease, 195*(12), 996–1003.
15. Beck, A. T. (1996). Beyond belief: A theory of modes, personality, and psychopathology In P. M. Salkovskis (Ed.), *Frontiers of cognitive therapy* (pp. 1–25). New York: Guilford Press.
16. Beck, A. T., Emery, G., & Greenberg, R. L. (1985). *Anxiety disorders and phobias: A cognitive perspective*. New York: Basic Books.
17. Pargament, K. I., Murray-Swank, N. A., Magyar, G. M., & Ano, G. G. (2005). Spiritual struggle: A phenomenon of interest to psychology and religion. In W. R. Miller, & H. D. Delaney (Eds.), *Judeo-Christian perspectives on psychology: Human nature, motivation, and change*. (pp. 245–268): Washington, DC: American Psychological Association.
18. Ellison, C. G., Roalson, L. A., Guillory, J. M., Flannelly, K. J., & Marcum, J. P. (2010). Religious resources, spiritual struggles, and mental health in a nationwide sample of PCUSA clergy. *Pastoral Psychology, 59*(3), 287–304.
19. Ellison, C. G., Fang, Q., Flannelly, K. J., & Steckler, R. A. (2013). Spiritual struggles and mental health: Exploring the moderating effects of religious identity. *The International Journal for the Psychology of Religion, 23*, 214–229.

Part I
The Origin of Evolutionary Ideas in Historical and Religious Context

Chapter 2
Greek Philosophy, Early Christian Theology, Purpose, and Change

Abstract This chapter examines the main philosophical and religious beliefs of the Western world, from the 5th Century (BCE) through the 13th Century (AD), that posed obstacles to the development of the concept of organic evolution. These include Plato's and Aristotle's belief in teleology (that everything in nature has a purpose), Plato's concept of immutable forms, Aristotle's *Scala Naturae*, and the later Christian belief that the Hebrew Bible's *Book of Genesis* (which describes how God created the world in six days) is literally true. The chapter also describes Thomas Aquinas' integration of Aristotle's philosophical ideas into Christian theology to achieve the goal of 13th Century Scholasticism to reconcile reason and religious faith. Collectively, these philosophical and religious beliefs portrayed the world and all the creatures in it as being immutable (i.e., unchanging), which precluded the possibility of organic evolution. The chapter also introduces Aristotle's four causes, which are the forerunners of the modern concepts of proximate and ultimate causes.

Keywords Aquinas • Aristotle • Augustine • Bible • Book of Genesis • Immutability of species • Natural History • Plato • *Scala Naturae* • Teleology

2.1 Greek Philosophers

Historians frequently trace the origin of scientific ideas back to the philosophers of ancient Greece [1–5]. Hence, it is not surprising that some historians trace the roots of the modern theory of organic evolution to the 5th Century (BCE) Greek philosopher, Empedocles of Agrigentum [6–10].[1] The surviving philosophical writings of Empedocles consist of two poems, one of which appears to be related to evolutionary theory because it proposed that animals arose through a series of episodes in which individual animals were spontaneously created with a random combination of body parts. These random assemblages of body parts mostly produced monstrosities that were unable to survive and thrive. Over time, a series of such creatures

[1] Agrigentum was a Greek city in Sicily.

K.J. Flannelly, *Religious Beliefs, Evolutionary Psychiatry, and Mental Health in America*, Religion, Spirituality and Health: A Social Scientific Approach 1,
DOI 10.1007/978-3-319-52488-7_2

spontaneously appeared, died off, and disappeared from the earth until new animals eventually appeared that were able to thrive and reproduce [10–13].

Modern evolutionary theory is, to some extent, similar to Empedocles' theory in that it claims that new types of animals have arisen over time by random variations in physical characteristics that help them to survive and reproduce. However, Empedocles' ideas do not seem to me to foresee the development of the evolutionary theories of the 18th and 19th Centuries (AD) or anticipate the questions that those theories attempted to address. Rather, it seems to me that Empedocles was trying to explain why the fantastic creatures described in Greek mythology no longer existed in his time. His explanation was that these creatures, which consisted of odd combinations of body parts, existed for awhile and then disappeared. Such creatures in Greek mythology included Centaurs, which had the head and torso of a human and the hindquarters of a horse, the Minotaur, which had the head of a bull and the body of a man, and the Griffin, which had the body of a lion and the head and wings of an eagle – not to mention the winged flying-horse Pegasus [14, 15]. All these creatures and many more mythological creatures were supposed to have existed at some point in time, according to the ancient Greeks, yet they no longer existed in Empedocles' time. Hence, it makes sense that he tried to explain their appearance and disappearance. However, Empedocles' theory was not embraced by other Greek philosophers and there is no reason to believe it ever influenced future evolutionary theorists.

The Greek philosopher who can rightly be said to have had a substantial influence on the history of evolutionary theories is Anaxagoras, a contemporary of Empedocles. Anaxagoras had his own theory of the origin of life, but this theory does not appear to have had any more of an effect than Empedocles' theory did on the development of theories of organic evolution, i.e., the origin and transformation of life on earth. What had a profound effect on the development of future evolutionary theories, however, was Anaxagoras' belief that all natural processes serve a purpose and that they reflect the product of a divine intelligence [12, 16, 17]. The effect of Anaxagoras' belief was to impede the acceptance of theories of organic evolution and, possibly, to delay the development of such theories.

Although Anaxagoras' writings, like those of Empedocles, are fragmentary, the later Greek philosophers Plato and Aristotle accepted Anaxagoras' concept that all natural phenomena serve a purpose – a concept which is called teleology. This teleological interpretation of nature has been common throughout history, even among people who are not familiar with the philosophy of Anaxagoras, Aristotle, or Plato. The American paleontologist Henry Fairfield Osborn identified Anaxagoras as the first known historical figure explicitly to express a belief in "Intelligent Design" [10]. Intelligent Design – the apparent purposefulness of the "design" of animals and plants – is used by some people today as an argument against the modern theory of organic evolution.

The 5th Century (BCE) Greek philosopher Plato, who is one of the most influential philosophers of the Western world [18, 19], presented his own ideas about the creation of the universe in *Timaeus* [20]. The *Timaeus* describes a divinely created universe that is both rationale and purposeful. In it, Plato also expands on an idea he introduced in his earlier *Phaedo* [21],[2] that all things that exist in the world are reflections of intangible, unchanging forms. In a word, Plato's immutable forms are the permanent essence of things, whereas the material objects that reflect them are only transitory, imperfect shadows of these forms [20, 22]. One might think of Plato's forms as the prototypes of material objects, or perhaps, even the causes of material objects [22].

2.2 Aristotle

Aristotle, a student of Plato, was a naturalist as well as a philosopher, and one of the world's first scientists [5, 10]. Aristotle proposed two general principles that influenced the study of nature or Natural History, as it is often called,[3] for over 2000 years [10]. The first, which embraces the teleological stance of Anaxagoras, is that everything in nature exists for a purpose [23–25]. Or, as he said in *De Anima* (*On the Soul*), "nature does nothing in vain" [26]. Based on this principle, Aristotle explicitly rejected Empedocles' idea that animals were created by, or could ever be created by, random processes [27].

Aristotle's second principle was that nature forms a continuous progression from lifeless things (e.g., rocks) to plants, to different types of animals, and ultimately to humans. This conception of nature has been called the *Scala Naturae*, which literally means the "Ladder of Nature" in Latin. The concept also has been called the "Chain of Being" [5, 28]. While Aristotle's *History of Animals* describes the anatomy and behavior of different kinds of animals that are associated with their relative positions on the *Scala Naturae*, the underlying dimension of the *Scala Naturae* is best described by Aristotle in *On the Soul*, because the scale is actually based on his theory of the faculties or the powers of the soul [23, 26]. To Aristotle, the soul is the essence of life, and it governs the behavior and abilities of different types of things. Inanimate objects lack a soul, so they form the lowest rung of the ladder of life. The souls of plants and animals differ with respect to four faculties or functions (nutrition, sensation, locomotion, and intellect) [26], and these differences partly determine their place on Aristotle's continuum of perfection. Though some historians doubt that Aristotle believed his classification of animals in his *History of Animals* should be viewed as a true hierarchy of nature, the *Scala Naturae* influenced scientific thought well into the 19th Century (AD) [29]. The American historian Charles Singer [5] illustrated the *Scala Naturae* in his *A History of Biology*, based on Aristotle's descriptions [5]. Singers' illustration has been reconstructed in Fig. 2.1.

---

[2] The brief discussion of forms in *Phaedo* introduces its main topic, which is the question of whether the human soul is immortal.

[3] A naturalist is someone who studies nature, or Natural History; Natural History is generally defined as the observation of plants and animals in their wild state.

Aristotle's Classification	Modern Classification
Man	Humans
Vivip arous Quadrupeds	Mammals
Cete	Cetaceans (e.g., dolphins, porpoises, whales)
Ovipara	Amphibians, Reptiles, Birds
Malacia	Fish, Cephalapods (e.g., cuttlefish, octopus, squid)
Malacostroca	Crustacea (e.g., crabs, lobsters, shrimp)
Entoma	Arthopods (terrestrial) (e.g., insects, spiders)
Ostracoderma	Mollusks (e.g., clams, oysters, snails)
Zoophyta	(e.g., sea anenomes, sponges)
Plants	Plants
Inanimate Matter	Rocks, Minerals

Fig. 2.1 Reconstruction of Charles Singer's illustration of Aristotle's *Scala Naturae* and the equivalent modern terms

As you see in the figure, rocks and minerals lie at the bottom of the ladder, with plants being the next step up on the ladder. Sponges and related sea animals are just above them because Aristotle recognized they were animals, but they did not have the power of locomotion. Cetaceans are higher on the ladder than amphibians, reptiles, and birds because cetaceans give birth to live offspring (vivipary), whereas amphibians, reptiles, and birds lay eggs (ovipary). Aristotle considered vivipary to be a more perfect form of producing offspring than ovipary. Humans are at the top of the ladder because of their intelligence, and mammals are lower than humans because they are less intelligent than humans.

Another aspect of Aristotle's writings has had long-term consequences for philosophical, religious, and scientific thinking. That is, his ideas about the causes of things. Aristotle described four meanings of the term cause in his books on *Physics* and *Metaphysics* [27, 30]. The first is a thing's material cause: What is it made of? Aristotle's examples of the material causes of things are the bronze used to make a statue and the silver used to make a cup. His second cause, which is called the formal cause of things, is its form or pattern: What is it? or What is its essence? Aristotle offers the example that the essence of an octave in music is its 2:1 ratio. More complex examples would by the formula of a chemical compound, the blueprint of a house, and the human genome. The third cause is a thing's efficient cause; that which has caused something to happen, such as the father of a child, the sculptor of a stature, or the builder of a house. Who made it? Aristotle's fourth cause is the "final cause" of things. Why was it made? or What is its purpose? Aristotle's final cause embodies the concept of teleology. The first three of Aristotle's causes are similar to what are now called "proximate causes," whereas Aristotle's fourth cause is now called the "ultimate cause" of something – its purpose.

Greek became the second language of educated Romans by the 1st Century (BCE) [31], so the major works of some Greek philosophers, notably Aristotle, were not translated into Latin. As few people read Greek after the fall of Rome in the 4th and 5th Centuries (AD) and few of Aristotle's writings were in Latin, Aristotle's ideas were lost for centuries to European philosophers and theologians, who mainly read Latin [31, 32]. However, Aristotle's works had been translated into Arabic and they were highly regarded by Arab scholars [10, 31]. The body of Aristotle's writings began to be translated from Arabic into Latin in Europe at the beginning of the 13th Century (AD) [31].

2.3 Christian Theology and Creation

Early Christian theologians cast Natural History in a Biblical context [10]. Hence, as Christianity began to spread through Europe in the 5th Century (AD), theological and philosophical thought about the origin of life was dominated by the description of creation given in the first Book of Moses in the Hebrew Bible – or Old Testament [33]. Called the *Book of Genesis*, the first book of the Bible describes how God created the world in six days. For centuries, most Christians believed the *Book of Genesis* was a literal account of creation, and many Christians still believe this is true.

Yet, even as Christianity began to spread, the 5th Century theologian *Aurelius Augustinus*, the Bishop of Hippo,[4] wrote several commentaries on *Genesis* that rejected the idea that it gives a factual account of creation [34]. Augustine challenged the belief that God created the world and all its creatures in six days as described in the *Book of Genesis* [35, 36]. Instead, he suggested that creation might have continued through natural processes that God had created [31]. His rejection of a literal interpretation of the account of creation told in the *Book of Genesis* and his suggestion that creation might continue through natural processes had important implications centuries later regarding the development of evolutionary theories [10]. Augustine raised another issue that had implications for evolutionary theory. Even though Augustine believed that God was immutable (i.e., unchanging), he felt that nothing in the *Book of Genesis* implied that God's creations were immutable [36]. In fact, he explicitly stated, that unlike God himself, all of God's creations were subject to change, in particular, a gradual change from the imperfect to the perfect [10, 35].

Although few of Augustine's contemporaries seem to have accepted his notion about the mutability of plants and animals, his critique of the *Book of Genesis* [35, 36] undermined the belief that the *Holy Scriptures* (especially, the Old Testament of

---

[4] Hippo was a Roman city in what is now Algeria, Africa. Augustine is also referred to as Saint Augustine and Augustine of Hippo.

the Bible) are the literal word of God, and opened the door to the idea that the events described in the Old Testament are subject to interpretation. Augustine's other writings reinforced the Platonic conceptions of God, humans, and the world at large, which had seeped into Christian theology, including beliefs about the body and soul, goodness, and unchanging "Platonic Forms" [37]. Thus, various aspects of Plato's philosophy came to have a major influence on later Christian theologians [38, 39].

With the re-discovery of Aristotle's writings in the 13th Century, his ideas began to permeate European philosophy [38]. Despite the many differences between Aristotle's beliefs and Christian beliefs [38], the 13th Century (AD) theologian Thomas Aquinas attempted to find common ground in these sets of beliefs and to integrate Aristotelian philosophy into Christian theology [40]. In the process, Aristotle's conception of the soul as a vital force was replaced with the Christian concept of an immortal soul [29], which Plato himself had endorsed in *Phaedo* [21]. Aquinas' ultimate goal was to demonstrate that faith was compatible with reason and, in fact, that reason supported Christian beliefs. Aquinas' opus, *Summa Theologica*, relies heavily on Aristotle's ideas, including his four causes and his *Scala Naturae* [40, 41].

2.4 Christian Theology and Evolution

Aquinas was one of the most prominent leaders of the Medieval philosophical movement called Scholastic Philosophy or Scholasticism [31]. Scholasticism arose in the 11th Century to become a dominant force in the major Catholic universities of Europe during the 13th Century. Before the translations of Aristotle in the 13th Century, Scholasticism was primarily based on early Christian theologians, especially Augustine, and Latin translations of the works of Plato [31, 42]. The goal of Scholasticism was to reconcile faith and reason or, more prosaically, to establish Christian dogma on a logical basis [31]. To do so, the scholastics relied on the authority of Greek philosophers, particularly Plato and Aristotle. Because it relied exclusively on ancient authority, Scholasticism was a philosophy of argument rather than of observation [31]. Hence, while Aquinas may have reconciled science and faith, Scholasticism did nothing to advance science [29].

Two aspects of Christian dogma undermined the concept of organic evolution. The first was the teleological beliefs of Plato and Aristotle that everything in nature exists for a purpose, which implies that all things exist in harmony with nature. The second was that Aristotle's *Scala Naturae* was accepted by Christian scholars as an expression of the belief that God's creations reflect God's perfection. The *Scala Naturae*, which represented a static unchanging system of nature that did not allow for the possibility of change, was widely accepted until the 19th Century [43]. Augustine held a minority view that creation continued beyond the description given in the *Book of Genesis* and that creatures might change over time [35]. Even though Aquinas' theological analysis in his *Summa Theologica* led him to conclude that the multiplicity of the creatures of the world must be the direct result of God's creation, he discussed Augustine's beliefs that God's creations are subject to change and, thus, that God's creatures have the potential to change [38, 40].

Hence, the position of Aquinas favored the traditional view of an unchanging world created by God, but it could accommodate the contrarian view of Augustine. Nevertheless, Scholasticism itself was a barrier to scientific progress, and, therefore, a barrier to evolutionary thought. By adopting ancient authority as the ultimate source of scientific knowledge, it essentially closed the door on contemporary science. As the historians Sedgwick, Tyler and Bigelow [31] note, although the "thirteenth Century saw a great revival of natural history, [it was] chiefly in the form of huge encyclopedic compilations, rarely containing original observations" [p. 217]. Thus, while Aquinas' theology was open to the study of nature, Scholasticism stifled it as scientific enterprise [29]. More barriers to the concept of evolution arose when the influence of Scholasticism declined in the Catholic Church and the Protestant Reformation promoted the belief that the *Book of Genesis* was literally true [10].

2.5 Chapter Highlights and Comments

In this first chapter, I have tried to provide the reader with an overview of key philosophical and religious ideas from the ancient Greeks up to the 13th Century, which by and large, exerted the greatest influence, directly or indirectly, on the later development of evolutionary theory. Aristotle not only influenced science, especially Natural History, but also Christianity, through the writings of Thomas Aquinas. By the end of 13th Century, both religion and science in Europe accepted two basic beliefs that would be barriers to the development of evolutionary theory: (1) that the world and the plants and animals that inhabit it were created by God as described in the *Book of Genesis,* and (2) that plants and animals have not changed since they were created by God – the belief than plant and animal species are immutable.

References

1. Hall, A. R., & Hall, M. B. (1964). *A brief history of science*. New York: New American Library.
2. Beck, W. S. (1961). *Modern science and the nature of life*. Garden City: Anchor Books.
3. Fidell, O. H. (1966). *Ideas in science*. New York: Washington Square Press.
4. Milne, C. (2011). *The invention of science*. Rotterdam: Sense Publishers.
5. Singer, C. (1950). *A history of biology* (Revised ed.). New York: Henry Schuman.
6. Simpson, G. G. (1949). *The meaning of evolution*. New Haven: Yale University Press.
7. Clodd, E. (1904). *Pioneers of evolution, from Thales to Huxley*. London: Watts & Company.
8. Depew, D. J. (2011). Accident, adaptaton and teleology in Aristotle, Empedocles, and Darwin In G. Auletta, M. L. Leclerc, & R. A. Martínez (Eds.), *Biological evolution: Facts and*

theories – A critical appraisal 150 years after "The Origin of Species". Rome: Gregorian & Biblical Press.
9. Nardo, D. (2009). *The theory of evolution: A history of life on Earth*. Mankato: Capstone.
10. Osborn, H. F. (1894). *From the Greeks to Darwin*. New York: MacMillan.
11. Burt, B. C. (1889). *A brief history of Greek philosophy*. Boston: Ginn & Company.
12. Zeller, E. (1886). *Outlines of the history of Greek philosophy*. London: Longmans, Green & Co.
13. Adamson, R. (1908). *The development of Greek philosophy*. London: William Blackwood & Sons.
14. Hamilton, E. (1942). *Mythology*. New York: Mentor Books.
15. Bulfinch, T. (1959). *Mythology*. New York: Dell Publishing.
16. Mitchell, E. M. (1891). *A study of Greek philosophy*. Chicago: S.C. Griggs & Company.
17. Stace, W. T. (1920). *A critical history of Greek philosophy*. London: Macmillan.
18. Heller, M. (2011). *Philosophy in science: An historical introduction*. New York: Springer.
19. Taylor, A. E. (1953). *Plato: the man and his work*. London: Methuen & Co.
20. Plato. (2009). *Plato's Timaeus* (B. Jowett, Trans.). Rockville: Serenity Publishers.
21. Plato. (1919). *Plato: Euthyphro. Apology. Crito. Phaedo. Phaedrus* (H. N. Fowler, Trans.). London: William Heinemann.
22. Prior, W. J. (2012). *Unity and development in Plato's metaphysics*. New York: Routledge.
23. Aristotle (1951). *Aristotle's De Anima with the commentary of St. Thomas Aquinas* (K. Foster & S. Humphries, Trans.). New Haven: Yale University Press.
24. Grant, M. (1994). *The ancient historians*. New York: Barnes & Noble Books.
25. Aristotle. (1902). *Aristotle's psychology* (W. A. Hammond, Trans.). New York: MacMillan.
26. Aristotle. (1907). *Aristole De Anima* (R. D. Hick, Trans.). Cambridge: Cambridge Univeristy Press.
27. Aristotle. (1961). *Aristotle's Physics* (R. Hope, Trans.). Lincoln: University of Nebraska Press.
28. Lovejoy, A. O. (1936/2001). *The great chain of being: A study of the history of an idea*. Cambridge: Harvard University Press.
29. Mayr, E. (1982). *The growth of biological thought*. London: Belknap Press.
30. Aristotle (1991). *The Metaphysics* (J. H. McMahon, Trans.). Buffalo: Prometheus Books.
31. Sedgwick, W. T., Tyler, H. W., & Bigelow, R. P. (1939). *A short history of science* (Revised ed.). New York: MacMillan.
32. Miall, L. C. (1912). *The early naturalists, their lives and work (1530–1789)*. New York: Macmillan.
33. King James Holy Bible. (1611/1999). Dayton: Greyden Press.
34. Neil, B. (2006). Exploring the limits of literal exegesis: Augustine's reading of Gen 1:26. *Pacifica, 19*(June), 144-155.
35. Augustine. (415/1982). *The literal meaning of Genesis*. Mahwah: Paulist Press.
36. Augustine. (389/2002). *On Genesis: A refutation of the Manichees*. Hype Park: New City Press.
37. Rist, J. M. (1996). *Augustine: Ancient thought baptized*. Cambridge: Cambridge University Press.
38. Weinberg, J. R. (1974). *A short history of Medieval philosophy*. Princeton: Princeton University Press.
39. van Nieuwenhove, T. (2012). *An introduction to Medieval theology*. Cambridge: Cambridge University Press
40. Aquinas, T. (1981). *Summa theologica*. Westminister: Christian Classics.
41. Webb, C. C. J. (1915/2013). *Studies in the history of natural theology*. London: FB &cc Ltd.
42. Rickaby, J. (1908). *Scholasticism*. London: Archibald Constable & Co.
43. Eisely, L. (1970). The dawn of evolutionary theory. In L. B. Young (Ed.), *Evolution on man*. New York: Oxford Univeristy Press.

Chapter 3
The Reformation and The Enlightenment

Abstract This chapter examines key scholars' ideas related to organic evolution during the historical periods known as The Reformation and The Enlightenment. The Protestant Reformation, which began in the early 16th Century, ended the Roman Catholic Church's control over learning and Christian theology. The Reformation's rejection of Scholasticism revitalized interest in science, but its emphasis on the Bible as the core of Christian theology turned the study of Natural History into Natural Theology, which saw the hand of God in every aspect of nature. While significant advances were made in biology and zoology during the 16th and 17th Centuries, as demonstrated by the research of John Ray and the systemization of these fields by *Carolus Linnaeus*, the chapter explains how belief in Biblical literalism and belief in the immutability of plant and animal forms, hampered the development of ideas about organic evolution. Much of the chapter is devoted to explaining how the writings of The Enlightenment thinkers Georges-Louis Leclerc Buffon and Erasmus Darwin during the 18th Century set the stage for the theory of organic evolution proposed by Charles Darwin in the 19th Century.

Keywords Buffon • Biblical literalism • Common ancestor • Darwin • Immutability of species • Natural History • Natural Theology • Protestant Reformation

3.1 The Reformation

At the beginning of the 16th Century, virtually all learning in Europe depended upon the Catholic Church and its universities. However, the Protestant Reformation, which began early in the 16th Century, ended the Roman Catholic Church's control over learning, as well as its control over Christian theology [1]. Martin Luther, the Catholic priest and theologian who started the Reformation, stressed the supremacy of scripture in Christian theology and rejected Scholasticism's goal to found Christianity on reason, saying that he learned little from Scholasticism, and what he did learn he had to unlearn [2]. Instead, Luther emphasized that Christians should find their faith in the Bible, which was believed to be the literal word of God.

K.J. Flannelly, *Religious Beliefs, Evolutionary Psychiatry, and Mental Health in America*, Religion, Spirituality and Health: A Social Scientific Approach 1,
DOI 10.1007/978-3-319-52488-7_3

The Reformation coincided with an increased interest in Natural History [3], and its rejection of Scholasticism [4] seems to have revitalized the biological sciences [5]. Many of the naturalists of the period were Protestant clergy [3] who turned Natural History into Natural Theology, as a way to understand God through his creations [4], and religious beliefs were expressed in the writings of many 16th Century Naturalists [6, 7], the most prominent of which was John Ray.

An ordained Anglican priest [8], John Ray saw the hand of God at work in the design of every creature, and his book *The Wisdom of God Manifested in the Works of Creation* epitomized the blending of science and religion that was traditional in Natural Theology [9, 10]. He was particularly struck by the way God had fashioned each kind of animal so that it is ideally suited or adapted to the environment in which it lives [9, 11, 12]. This perspective was the hallmark of Natural Theology, in which every plant and animal provided proof of the purposiveness of creation [4]. Ray believed each species was created by God and that each species was the same at it was on the day of its creation; that is, that species were immutable [8]. Ernst Mayr, a renowned evolutionary biologist has called *The Wisdom of God*, "not only a powerful argument [for] design but also very sound natural history" (p. 104) [4]. Mayr thought that, in its time "design was really the only possible explanation for adaptation in a static 'created' world" (p. 104) [4].

The Reformation's acceptance of scriptural supremacy made the Bible the centerpiece of Natural History [12], and this was reflected in a wide range of popular beliefs about the world. An often cited example is the 17th Century belief that the earth is only several thousand years old [13]. The origin of this belief is attributed to a 1650 book published by Archbishop Ussher of Ireland [14]. Based on his literal reading of the events in the Old Testament, Archbishop Ussher claimed that the earth was created in 4004 BC [15]. The belief that the earth is only several thousand years old was widely held until the later part of the 19th Century, and some people still believe this is true [16].

3.2 Carl von Linnė (*Carolus Linnaeus*)

The Swiss naturalist Carl von Linnė, better known by his Latinized name Linnaeus, developed a systematic method for classifying plants and animals, which was built, in part, upon Rays' work [17]. Linnaeus' father, who was a minister, had a large garden where he introduced his son Carl to botany. So, despite his family's expectations that he would go into the ministry, the interest in botany that he developed as a child prevailed in Linnaeus' choice of careers [6, 18].

Linnaeus became prominent in science because he developed a taxonomic system of classifying plants and animals, which he introduced his 1735 book *Systemae Naturae*. Linnaeus used a binomial wording system (or nomenclature) in which different kinds of plants and animals are given a two-part name: one for their *species* and one for the next broader category or group of organisms (i.e., plants or animals) to which they belonged – their *genus*. Linnaeus' binomial nomenclature, which

Table 3.1 Comparison of the taxonomic classification of the horse and the ass

	Horse	Ass (Donkey)
Kingdom	Animalia	Animalia
Phyla	Vertebrata	Vertebrata
Class	Mammalia	Mammalia
Order	Perisodacytyla	Perisodacytyla
Family	Equidae	Equidae
Genus	*Equus*	*Equus*
Species	*cabbalus*	*asinus*

uniquely identifies each species by its *genus* and *species* names, is still used today. The genus name of the "big cats" of Africa, for example, is *Panthera*, with the lion being named *Panthera leo*, the leopard being named *Panthera pardus*, and the jaguar being *Panthera onca*.

Linnaeus' original system consisted of four levels, or taxa, which were expanded by later taxonomists to create the seven levels that are used today (see Table 3.1). The table shows the taxonomic relationship between horses and asses (donkeys), using this expanded taxonomic system of classification [8, 19].

While the horse and the ass easily can be distinguished from one another and are classified as separate species, they are sufficiently similar to one another that they are classified as belonging to the same genus, *Equus*, as shown in Table 3.1. As such, they also fall into the same Family (Equidae) and the same Order (Perisodacytyla: which means they have an odd number of toes). They both are mammals because they are warm-blooded (as are birds) and they are viviparous (whereas birds are oviparous). It goes without saying, that they are both vertebrates (or chordates) because they have a spinal cord, and of course, they are animals.

Linnaeus believed for most of his life that God created all the species of plants and animals and that they had not changed since their creation [6, 20, 21]. Because of his scientific prominence, this belief came to be accepted as part of scientific thinking [17, 22], and the immutability of species became the central argument against the concept of organic evolution [17, 22]. Indeed, the evolutionary biologist Ernst Mayr has said that Linnaeus' belief in the immutability of species made the origin of species (i.e., how species evolved) a scientific problem which it would not have been otherwise [4].

3.3 The Enlightenment

The last decade of the 17th Century is generally recognized as the beginning of the intellectual movement called the Age of Enlightenment [23–25], in which people tried to understand the reasons behind everything and questioned accepted beliefs about the world and traditional institutions, including governments and religions [4, 13, 23, 24]. However, this was not an "Age" in which people relied on the reasoning of ancient philosophers; it was an era of empiricism that grew out of the empiricism that followed the rejection of Scholasticism by the Protestant Reformation. Nevertheless, "To the extent that Christianity was based on divine revelation rather than human reason, it lost its credibility among enlightened thinkers" (p. 13) [13].

In the field of Natural History, enlightened thinkers questioned accepted religious beliefs about nature of the world [13, 23, 24]. Three such men challenged the concept of the immutability of species that had become ingrained in Christian theology and science, laying the philosophical and scientific groundwork for the modern theory of organic evolution. The men were Georges-Louis Leclerc Buffon, Erasmus Darwin, and Jean-Baptiste de Monet Lamarck [21, 26]. I discuss Lamarck's contribution to evolutionary theory in Chap. 4.

3.3.1 Georges-Louis Leclerc Buffon

The French mathematician and naturalist Georges-Louis Leclerc Buffon (also known as the Comte de Buffon) was born in the same year as Linnaeus [6]. He was raised in a Catholic family, he attended a Jesuit school, his two brothers were Catholic monks, and his sister was a Catholic nun [27]. Yet, it is not clear whether Buffon himself was religious. Like other Enlightenment thinkers, Buffon acknowledged the existence of God [4, 13, 27], but he firmly believed that science should be founded on physical principles, and he rejected Christian theology as an explanation of the creation of the world [4, 13].

While Linnaeus systematized Natural History, Buffon popularized it [4, 6, 21], publishing three dozen volumes of his encyclopedic *Historie Naturelle* during this lifetime [6, 13, 21]. When the first three volumes were published in 1749, *Historie Naturelle* was the talk of the Paris salons and Buffon became an instant celebrity [27]. The first three volumes covered Buffon's ideas about the history of the earth, the formation of the planets, and human development, and he continued throughout his career to combine the traditional descriptive approach of Natural History with his own sweeping interpretations of the available evidence in all areas of Natural History.

Though some historians have questioned Buffon's contributions to the development of evolutionary theory [28], others have noted that his extensive writings discuss every major topic that Charles Darwin discussed in his 1859 book on evolution [21, 29], and that Buffon's writings set the stage for Charles Darwin and other 19th Century evolutionary theorists, including his protégé, Jean-Baptiste de Monet Lamarck [4]. One of his major contributions to evolutionary theory was his idea that variations in physical form within a species could result in the development of different species through gradual steps, similar to the way in which domestication has produced numerous variants of the same species, such as breeds of dogs. He also noticed the tendency of animals to multiply faster than their food supply, which promotes competition among animals [21]. Moreover, he recognized that the earth was much older than Archbishop Ussher had proposed [15, 21, 29], and that the great age of the earth would have made it possible for wild animals to change in form over time [21, 29].

Buffon presented some of his evolutionary speculations in 1766 (*Historie Naturelle,* volume 14), proposing that the more than 200 species of mammals that were known in his time may have descended from less than 40 original mammalian species [11, 13] through a process he called "degeneration" [13, 21, 30]. He suggested, for example, that all known cats (e.g., leopards, lions, tigers, and even domestic cats) had descended from a common ancestor through physical changes in response to differences in the climate and different aspects of the environments in which they lived [13]. Some of his other writings implied, at least, that climatic differences throughout the world could lead to the degeneration of many different species from a common ancestor.

The initial publication of *Historie Naturelle* in 1749 not only caught the attention of the public, it caught the attention of the Catholic Church, and Buffon received a letter from the Faculty of Theology at the Sorbonne complaining that his ideas about the origin of the earth and planets contradicted the *Book of Genesis* [27, 31]. He published a retraction in Volume 4 of *Historie Naturelle* [27, 32] to avoid further trouble with the Catholic Church.

Historians have said that Buffon's often cryptic and ironic writing style and his occasional refutations of his own arguments when interpreting evidence also were intended to avoid having further trouble with the Catholic Church [21, 27, 32, 33]. The modern historian Loren Eiseley described the sometimes frustrating experience of reading Buffon's theoretical ideas, complaining: "He brought forward an impressive array of facts suggesting evolutionary changes and then arbitrarily denied what he had just been at such pains to propose" (p. 39) [21] (see below[1]). A 19th Century historian, who wrote about Buffon just 20 years after Darwin published his *Origin of Species* in 1859, was more sympathetic than Eiseley was to Buffon's situation during the 18th Century, saying: "Whenever he has shown us clearly what we ought to think, he stopped short on religious grounds" (p. 115) [30].

3.3.2 Erasmus Darwin

There are historians who say Erasmus Darwin would not have a place in history were it not for the fact that he was Charles Darwin's grandfather [4, 21]. However, Erasmus Darwin was quite famous in his own time as a leading figure of The Enlightenment [34–37], and he helped to advance and expand upon Buffon's ideas

[1] Buffon's description of the Ass provides a classic example of Eisely's complaint about Buffon's writing. Buffon begins by saying: "If we consider this animal with some degree of attention, he appears only to be a horse degenerated" after which he devotes over 200 words to support his hypothesis. Then, he devotes another 250 words to rebutting his own hypothesis, finally concluding: "The Ass is then an Ass, and not a horse degenerated".

that species changed over time in response to the environments in which they live [21, 30, 34, 35].

Erasmus Darwin first gained fame in 1753 for a poem he wrote about the death of the Prince of Wales [34]. His poetry brought him even greater acclaim in later life, especially *The Botanic Garden*, which made him the most renown poet of the time in Britain [34–37]. The two-part poem popularized science through poetry. Part I, *The Loves of Plants* (1789) described sexual reproduction in plants. Part II, *The Economy of Vegetation* (1791) emphasized the self-regulating economy of the natural world, and covered a wide of range topics in natural history, including some of his evolutionary ideas [37].

A practicing physician, when Erasmus Darwin published his book *Zoonomia* in 1794 he became Britain's leading medical writer [34]. *Zoonomia* described the circulatory, digestive, and motor systems, physiological functions, and a number of diseases and other ailments [34, 35, 38]. In addition, the book, which was published six years after the death of the Comte de Buffon, laid out Dr. Darwin's ideas about evolution in a chapter titled "Of Generation" [38].

Erasmus Darwin thought that all living things shared a common ancestor, and that new types of plants and animals had developed over "millions of ages" [37]. Changes in form occurred as species of plants and animals improved their ability to meet the demands of the environments in which they lived, with the improvements of each generation being passed along to the next generation [34, 37, 38]. Dr. Darwin thought that animals had three primary "wants" – security, hunger, and lust – and that animals were changed by their efforts to gratify these wants. Certain kinds of animals, for example, developed colored skin (e.g., many insects and lizards) or feathers (e.g., owls) as camouflage that conceal them, turtles developed armored shells that protect them from attack, and birds developed wings that enable them to escape from predators [30, 35, 38]. Other animal species have diversified in form, which enhances their ability to satisfy hunger, according to Dr. Darwin. For instance, elephants developed an elongated nose that makes it possible for them to pull tree branches down so they can eat the leaves. Whole orders of other animals have changed in some way to gratify the "want" of hunger. Carnivores, for instance, developed strong jaws and claws over many generations that make it easy for them capture and kill prey; some birds developed short, hard beaks that make it possible for them to crack seeds, and other birds developed long beaks that make it possible for them to pick insects out of the soil. All this diversification occurred very gradually over a vast number of generations, according to Dr. Darwin [30, 38].

Dr. Darwin thought the gratification of lust has unique effects because it reflects competition for mates rather than for resources (e.g., food). This has led to distinctive male physical characteristics that can aid males in monopolizing access to females, such as weapons (e.g., horns or tusks) that enable males to fight one another for access to females [30, 38]. His grandson Charles Darwin later called the process of behavioral and morphological changes associated with reproductive competition "sexual selection" [37, 39, 40].

Dr. Darwin described several lines of support for his evolutionary ideas. First, the breeding of domestic animals demonstrates that the behavioral and structural characteristics of animals can be transformed from one generation to the next. For example, different breeds of horses have been created over generations for different purposes, such as strength (e.g., Clydesdale and Jutland) and speed (e.g., Thoroughbred), and different breeds of dogs have been created for their speed (e.g., Dalmatian and Greyhound), strength (e.g., Husky and German Shepherd), and sense of smell (e.g., Beagle and Bloodhound). Second, as Linnaeus himself recognized, new species could be created by hybridization, the mating of two different but similar species [18, 38]. Third, the individuals of some species transform themselves during their lives, such as tadpoles, which change into frogs, and caterpillars, which change into butterflies [38]. Finally, Darwin believed that the structural similarities across the vertebrate species, including man, suggested they had a common ancestor [38].

Erasmus Darwin was not religious, and some have called him anti-Christian [35]. Although Dr. Darwin had more freedom to express his unorthodox ideas than Buffon did [30], Darwin was publically criticized for his "transformist view of biodiversity" [41] and his "blasphemous evolutionary ideas" [37]. His evolutionary ideas, which he sketched out in Zoonomia, were expanded upon in yet another poem that was published in 1803, a year after his death: *Temple of Nature; or, The Origin of Society* [34, 37].

3.4 Chapter Highlights and Comments

While the Protestant Reformation probably encouraged scientific progress in some fields, it also imposed constraints on science by making the Bible the centerpiece of Natural History in the form of Natural Theology. Nevertheless, naturalists like John Ray and systematists like Linnaeus helped to advance Natural History, although their belief in the immutability of species probably impeded recognition of the fact that animals and plants have evolved over time. Moreover, Ernst Mayr has argued that Linnaeus' belief in immutability posed a barrier to evolutionary ideas that they would not have faced otherwise. The thinkers of the Age of Enlightenment undermined the influence of religious dogma on science to some extent, just as the Protestant Reformation had undermined the influence of Scholasticism on science. Both the Comte de Buffon and Dr. Erasmus Darwin made important contributions to the development of evolutionary theory, and they publicly presented their evolutionary ideas even though they were counter to the prevailing cultural norms and religious beliefs of their times.

References

1. Sedgwick, W. T., Tyler, H. W., & Bigelow, R. P. (1939). *A short history of science* (Revised ed.). New York: MacMillan.

2. Selden, J. (1984). Aquinas, Luther, Melanchton, and biblical apologetics. *Grace Theological Journal, 5*(2), 181–195.
3. Miall, L. C. (1912). *The early naturalists, their lives and work (1530–1789)*. New York: Macmillan.
4. Mayr, E. (1982). *The growth of biological thought*. London: Belknap Press.
5. Harrison, P. (1998). *The Bible, Protestantism, and the rise of natural science*. Cambridge: Cambridge University Press.
6. Ley, W. (1968). *Dawn of zoology*. Englewood Cliffs: Prentice-Hall.
7. Ogilvie, B. W. (2008). Nature's Bible: Insects in seventeenth-century art and science. *Tidsskrift for Kulturforskning, 7*(3), 5–21.
8. Singer, C. (1950). *A history of biology* (Revised ed.). New York: Henry Schuman.
9. Huxley, R. (2007). John Ray: The English Aristotle. In R. Huxley (Ed.), *The great naturalists* (pp. 92–97). London: Thames & Hudson.
10. MacGillavray, W. (1834). *Lives of eminent zoologists: From Aristotle to Linnaeus*. Edinburgh: Oliver & Boyd.
11. Bowler, P. J. (2003). *Evolution: The history of an idea*. Berkeley/Los Angeles: University of California Press.
12. Bowler, P. J., & Morus, I. R. (2005). *Making modern science: A historical survey*. Chicago: University of Chicago Press.
13. Larson, E. J. (2004). *Evolution: The remarkable history of a scientific theory*. New York: The Modern Library.
14. Ussher, J., Pierce, L., & Pierce, M. (2003). *The annals of the world*. Green Forest: Master Books.
15. Sapp, J. (2003). *Genesis: The evolution of biology*. New York: Oxford University Press.
16. Roberts, M. (2002). The genesis of John Ray and his successors. *Evangelical Quarterly, 74*(2), 143.
17. Eisely, L. (1970). The dawn of evolutionary theory. In L. B. Young (Ed.), *Evolution on man*. New York: Oxford Univeristy Press.
18. Humphries, C. J., & Huxley, R. (2007). Carl Linnaeus: The man who brought order to nature. In R. Huxley (Ed.), *The great naturalists* (pp. 132–139). London: Thames & Hudson.
19. Hanson, E. D. (1972). *Animal diversity* (3rd ed., Prentice-Hall Foundations of Modern Biology Series). Englewood Cliffs: Prentice-Hall.
20. Canguilhem, G. (2008). *Knowledge of life*. New York: Fordham University press.
21. Eiseley, L. (1961). *Darwin's century: evolution and the men who discovered it*. Garden City: Anchor Books.
22. Hall, A. R. (1962). *The scientific revolution: 1500–1800* (2). Boston: Beacon Press.
23. Reill, P. H., & Wilson, E. J. (2004). *Encyclopedia of the enlightenment* (Revised ed.). New York: Book Builders.
24. Venn, C. (2006). The enlightenment. *Theory, Culture & Society, 23*(2–3), 477–498.
25. Hall, A. R., & Hall, M. B. (1964). *A brief history of science*. New York: New American Library.
26. Dendy, A. (1915). Progressive evolution and the origin of species. *The American Naturalist, 49*(579), 149–182.
27. Roger, J. (1997). *Buffon: A life in natural history* (S. L. Bennefoi, Trans.). Ithaca: Cornell University Press.
28. Eddy, J. H. (1994). Buffon's histoire naturelle: History? A critique of recent interpretations. *Isis, 88*, 644–661.
29. Eiseley, L. (1970). The dawn of evolutionary theory. In L. B. Young (Ed.), *Evolution on man*. New York: Oxford University Press.
30. Butler, S. (1879). *Evolution, old and new; or, The theories of Buffon, Dr. Erasmus Darwin, and Lamarck, as compared with that of Mr. Charles Darwin*. London: Hardwicke and Bogue.
31. Knapp, S. (2007). Comte de Buffon: A grand theorist. In R. Huxley (Ed.), *The great naturalists* (pp. 140–148). London: Thames & Hudson.

32. Curtis, W. C. (1922). *Science and human affairs from the viewpoint of biology*. New York: Harcourt, Brace and Company.
33. Buffon, G. -L. L. (1831). *Buffon's natural history of the globe and of man*. London: Thomas Tegg.
34. Kormondy, E. J. (2011). Erasmus Darwin, 18th-Century Polymath. *The American Biology Teacher, 73*(2), 68–71.
35. Press, R. (2007). Erasmus Darwin: Evolutionary beginnings. In R. Huxley (Ed.), *The great naturalists* (pp. 159–164). London: Thames & Hudson.
36. Page, M. (2005). The Darwin before Darwin: Erasmus Darwin, visionary science, and romantic poetry. *Papers on Language and Literature, 41*(2), 146–169.
37. King-Hele, D. (2003). The furtive evolutionist. *New Scientist, 177* (2390), 48–49.
38. Darwin, E. (1794). *Zoonomia: Or the laws of organic life*. London: J. Johnson.
39. Darwin, C. (1871). *The descent of man and selection in relation to sex* (Vol. 1). London: John Murray.
40. Smith, C. U. M. (2009, May 21). Erasmus Darwin saw sexual selection before his grandson. *Nature, 429*, 321.
41. Friedman, W. E. (2009, September 10). Evolution pioneers: Celebrating Lamarck at 200, Darwin 215. *Nature, 461*, 167.

Chapter 4
19th Century Evolutionary Thought Before Charles Darwin

Abstract The chapter describes ideas that undermined and fostered the concept of organic evolution during the first half of the 19th Century. The prevailing Western view about nature at the beginning of the 19th Century was expressed in Reverend William Paley's popular 1802 book, *Natural Theology*. The book was based on the idea that animals are so well suited to the environment in which they live that they must be the result of a Divine plan, and it presented the often repeated analogy that the parts of the body are like the parts of a watch, which are so complicated and inter-related that they must be the product of an "intelligent and designing Creator." By 1809, however, the French zoologist Jean Baptiste Lamarck, who is recognized as the founder of evolutionary theory, published his *Philosophie Zoologique*, which claimed that forces of nature, not the direct hand of God, had molded plants and animals to adapt them to the worlds in which they live. As the chapter explains, Lamarck offered two theories of what he called, transformism, which changed generations of animals over vast amounts of time from one form of animal into another form. Although Lamarck's theories were never widely accepted, *Philosophie Zoologique* was the best argument at that time for organic evolution, and it even traced the evolution of modern animals from a common ancestor. Despite the rejection of Lamarck's theories, his book seemed to spur others to develop theories of evolution that culminated in Charles Darwin's *Origin of Species*.

Keywords Adaptation • Common ancestor • Evolution • Intelligent Design • Natural Theology • Lamarck

4.1 Geology and the Fossil Record

By the beginning of the 19th Century, two lines of geological evidence were converging that were ultimately crucial for helping to establish the scientific basis of organic evolution. One was that the earth is extremely old, and the other was the recognition that fossils are the remains of extinct animals and plants [1].[1] At the

[1] Fossils are created in sedimentary rock when minerals slowly replace the organic matter that comprise and animal or plant.

K.J. Flannelly, *Religious Beliefs, Evolutionary Psychiatry, and Mental Health in America*, Religion, Spirituality and Health: A Social Scientific Approach 1,
DOI 10.1007/978-3-319-52488-7_4

time, however, fossils were just pieces of a puzzle whose importance was not recognized by most naturalists [2–6].

Late in the 18th Century, some naturalists who were studying the earth's geology came to realize that the massive layers of exposed rock observed throughout Europe must have taken vast amounts of time to accumulate [2, 4]. This conclusion was primarily predicated on geological evidence that suggested that the topographical features of the earth were the products of uniform, continuous processes, like those that occur today, such as erosion, deposition, and volcanism. As these processes are very slow, they concluded that the earth must be very old [4, 5, 7].

Many of these rock formations in Europe contained stone impressions of the bodies of plants and animals, which came to be called fossils. Fossils had been recognized as the remnants or traces of plants and animals by several philosophers of ancient Greece, [1, 8, 9] but some later naturalists dismissed them as flukes of nature that were not actually what they appeared to be [10]. As most of the fossils discovered in Europe up until the 19th Century were the petrified remains of shellfish and many of these were found in rock beds that were far away from the sea, their existence implied that the land was once submerged [8, 10]. The increasing numbers of fossils found during the 17th and 18th Centuries were taken by Christian scholars and theologians as proof of the Biblical Flood of Noah. Fossils of land animals, which were relatively rare, were assumed to be animals that perished in the flood, and fossils of sea creatures, which were very common, were assumed to be animals that were stranded on land and died when the flood waters receded [1, 8, 10]. During the early part of the 19th Century, it became evident that fossils represented not just individual animals that had died, but entire species of animals that had died off and no longer existed, i.e., that species had become extinct.

4.2 William Paley's *Natural Theology*

In 1802, the prominent Anglican priest and theologian William Paley published a book in England titled, *Natural Theology; or Evidences of the Existence and Attributes of the Deity, Collected from the Appearances of Nature* [11]. *Natural Theology* expanded upon the themes John Ray expressed in *The Wisdom of God* – i.e., that God designed each plant and animal species to fit perfectly into the habitat in which it lives. *Natural Theology* makes the frequently repeated analogy that the parts of the body are like the parts of a watch, which are so complicated and interrelated that they must be the product of "Intelligent Design," or as Paley put it, an "intelligent and designing Creator," (p. 154) and "an intelligent, designing mind" (p. 280) [12].

Paley uses the human eye as an example of a biological contrivance (i.e., something skillfully crafted to serve a particular purpose) that is so complicated that it had to be created by a Divine craftsman. The eyes of every animal are fashioned for its own peculiar way of life, such as the eyes of fish, which are be best suited for life underwater. Paley described hundreds of examples of how the anatomy of different kinds of animals makes them uniquely adapted to their environmental niche, and he explicitly believed that no law of nature could account for such diverse adaptations. The evolutionary biologist Ernst Mayr has praised *Natural Theology* as "an excellent introduction to natural history and the study of adaptation" (p. 397) [9]. Indeed, Mayr said that Natural Theology, as a scientific and theological endeavor, was a necessary development in Natural History because Divine creation offered the only explanation for adaptation until adaptation was recognized to be the product of evolution [9].

The book was popular among the British public and British academic circles, the latter of which opposed even discussing the possibility of organic evolution. European academics were more open to evolutionary ideas. During the last decade of the 18th Century and the first decade of the 19th Century, several philosophers and naturalists in Germany, Italy, and France speculated about the origin of life on earth [8, 13, 14]. Hence, the time was right on the Continent, if not in Britain, for a comprehensive theory of the evolution of life [14].

4.3 Jean Baptiste de Monet Lamarck

Jean Baptiste Lamarck, who was born in 1744, attended a Jesuit college before joining the French army. He subsequently attended medical school and eventually turned to the study of botany in Paris in 1778, where he met the Comte de Buffon. Buffon mentored him and helped him to obtain membership in the French Academy of Science in 1779 and a position at the Royal Garden in Paris in 1781 [15]. In the midst of the French Revolution, the revolutionary government reorganized the Royal Garden into the Museum of Natural History in 1793 and Lamarck became a professor of, essentially, insects and worms [15–18]. Although he knew little about the subject matter at the time, he mastered the field and developed a classification system for what he called invertebrates [18], i.e., animals without vertebral columns [19, 20].

Lamarck is recognized as the founder of evolutionary theory because his 1809 book *Philosophie Zoologique* [21] contains the first thorough formulation of the causes of organic evolution and the first attempt to trace a possible path of descent from a common ancestor across the animal kingdom (Fig. 4.1) [15, 22–24]. Although Lamarck had thought that species were immutable, he changed his mind based on the evidence that fossils were extinct species of animals. Lamarck refused to believe that nature would be so fickle as to allow species to become extinct [23, 25, 26], writing in *Philosophie Zoologique*: "I am still doubtful whether the means adopted by nature to ensure the preservation of species or races have been so inadequate that entire races are now extinct or lost" (p. 44) [27]. So, Lamarck thought there must be a reason, other than extinction, why some animals had disappeared. His explanation was that the species that apparently had become extinct, had instead, evolved to become other species. His *Philosophie Zoologique (Zoological Philosophy* in

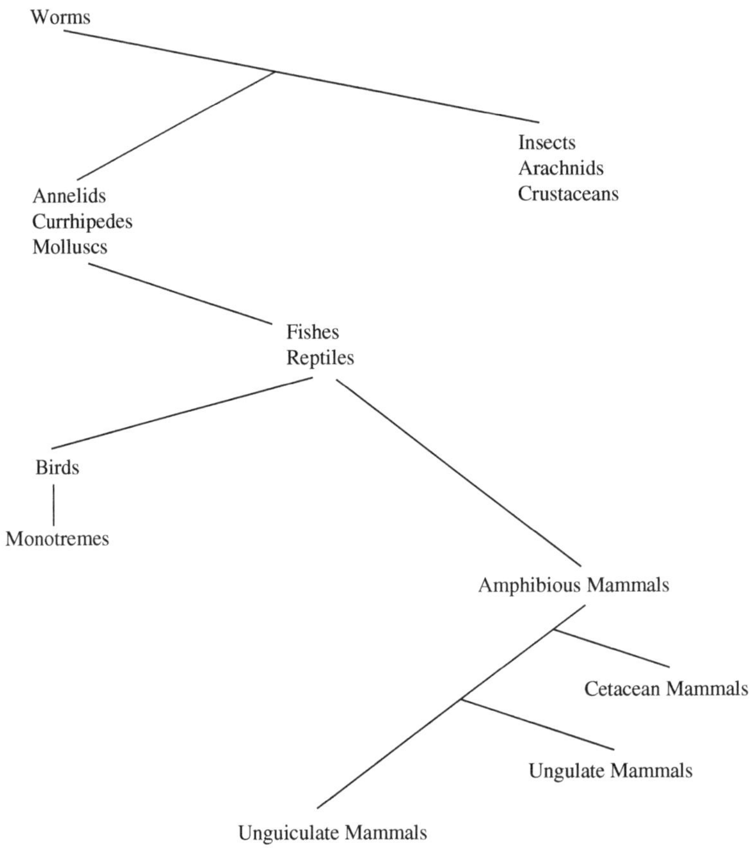

Fig. 4.1 Redrawing of the main features of Lamarck's figure in *Philosophie Zoologique* "showing the origins of various animals"

English) presents two theories of evolution [23, 25, 26], which became known in France as tranformisme and transformism in England [26].

Though some historians have questioned Lamarck's religious commitment [17, 18, 28], he began his book with a statement that is similar to the viewpoint of Saint Augustine: "Assuredly, nothing can exist but by the will of the Supreme Author, but can we venture to assign rules to him in the execution of his will? May not his infinite power have chosen to create an order of things which should evolve in succession all that we know as well as all that we do not know?" (p. 36) [27]. Some historians have concluded that Lamarck's words were sincere, citing related passages from Lamarck's other writings that indicate he was a pious man [29, 30]. Other historians share the view that Lamarck was religious [16], whereas some think he was a deist who [26, 31], like Buffon, sought to separate divine action from material explanations of causation in the natural world [31].

Like the Comte de Buffon and Erasmus Darwin before him, Lamarck believed the earth was very old, and the dramatic changes that humans can produce in domesticated animals through selective breeding provide evidence that wild animals also could change dramatically in behavior, shape, size, and other characteristics over vast amounts of time [27]. Over time, species of animals could transform into entirely new species; species could change so much that they could form new genera, and new genera could change so much they could form new families of animals, and so on. Given enormous amounts of time, families could form new orders and new orders could form new classes of animals.

Lamarck thought that all 13 classes of animals that were recognized in his time were related to one another in some way, and he traced the origin of most of them back to worms, based on a series of anatomical comparisons. I have redrawn his path of common descent from worms to the different Orders of mammals recognized in his day in Fig. 4.1.[2] Lamarck hypothesized that the transformation of worms branched off into two lineages, one of which led to Insects, Arachnids (spiders), and Crustaceans (e.g., crabs, lobsters, and shrimp). The other lineage eventually led to the evolution of fish, reptiles, birds, and various kinds of mammals. This general scheme reflects Lamarck's first theory of transformation, i.e., that lower forms of life progressed into higher forms in terms of complexity and perfection [21, 27]. Like Aristotle, Lamarck thought plants and different kinds of animals formed a hierarchy of life that represented degrees of perfection. Unlike Aristotle, Lamarck did not think this was a static hierarchy. Instead, he thought that there was a natural force in living things that drove them to perfect themselves [23, 25–27].

Lamarck's study of geology also led him to realize that since the earth constantly changes, plants and animals must be able to adapt to these changes in order to survive and thrive [16, 23, 25, 26]. Hence, the basic premise of Lamarck's second theory of transformation is that animals are indirectly affected by changes in their environment, such as climatic changes, and that they are transformed as they attempt to adapt to these changes [23, 25–27]. Like Erasmus Darwin, Lamarck believed that three main needs drove transformation in response to the environment: nourishment, reproduction, and self-self-defense. Unlike Erasmus Darwin, however, Lamarck considered adaptation to the environment to be an anomalous process that interfered with the normal progression of increasing complexity and perfection. Formally,

[2] The reader should keep in mind the figure reflects Lamarck's best guess about descent from a common ancestor, when the true ancestry of Fish was not known. Lamarck was partially correct in thinking that Reptiles evolved from Fish, although Reptiles actually evolved from Amphibians, which had evolved from Fish. He is also correct that Birds evolved act least indirectly from Reptiles. Monotremes, which are primitive mammals, evolved from Reptiles, not from Birds. Lamarck also mistakenly thought that land mammals (the Ungulate Mammals and Unguiculate Mammals) evolved from Cetacean Mammals, which are sea creatures; Cetacean Mammals actually evolved from Ungulate Mammals, which lived on land. The Cetacean Mammals have adapted to spend their entire lives in water, having flipper-like front limbs and broad tails with horizontal flukes: e.g., dolphins, porpoises, and whales. Like other mammals, however, they breath air and are warm-blooded and viviparous. Ungulate Mammals are animals with hooves, such as antelope, buffalo, deer, horses, and pigs. Unguiculate Mammals are animals that have nails or claws rather than hooves; most of the species of Unguiculate Mammals are carnivorous, such as bears, cats, wolves.

Lamarck's second theory consists of a set of three propositions, from which are deduced two general laws. Briefly, Lamarck's second theory states that: (a) animals alter their behavior to adjust to environmental demands; (b) that these behavioral changes modify structures, such as muscles, bones, and other organs; (c) that structures that are used more often in adapting to the environment will be strengthened, whereas those that are used less often will deteriorate; and (d) the modifications of the structures of parents are transmitted to their offspring. This has led the theory to be called "the theory of the inheritance of acquired characteristics" [23, 24], which has been definitively refuted by scientific research [23].[3]

4.4 Between Lamarck and Darwin

Although Lamarck's theories were never fully accepted and even some of his colleagues criticized them, they did influence the thinking of philosophers and other scientists, and Lamarck's theories were a breakthrough in advancing the concept of organic evolution [9, 15]. Lamarck's first theory envisioned the concept of descent from a common ancestor, and his second theory embodied evolutionary change in response to the demands of life. Both these concepts were major themes in Charles Darwin's 1859 *Origins of Species.*

The zoologist Kamales Kumar Misra identified six theories of evolution that were proposed between Lamarck's *Philosophie Zoologique* and Darwin's *Origins of Species*, which addressed, or failed to address, three key elements of evolution: common descent, gradual change, and "speciation" (i.e., the differentiation of new species) [15]. None of these six theories, however, was accepted by the scientific community. At least two other naturalists presented ideas that anticipated the arguments that Charles Darwin published his 1859 *Origins of Species,* but these ideas received little attention at the time [10].

By the 1830's, the assemblages of fossils in different geological strata led to the development of a crude scale of geological time based on sequential layers of rock [1, 2, 32], which suggested that the earth was several hundred million years old

[3] Formally, the theory consists of a set of three propositions, from which are deduced two general laws. The three propositions are: (1) That every considerable and sustained change in the surroundings of any animal involves a real change in its needs. (2) That such change of needs involves the necessity of changed action in order to satisfy these needs, and, in consequence, of new habits. (3) It follows that such parts, formerly less used, are now more frequently employed, and in consequence become more highly developed; new parts also become insensibly evolved in the creature by its own efforts from within.

The two laws are: First. that in every animal which has not passed its limit of development, the more frequent and sustained employment of any organ develops and aggrandizes it, giving it a power proportionate to the duration of its employment, while the same organ in default of constant use becomes insensibly weakened and deteriorated, decreasing imperceptibly in power until it finally disappears. Second, that these gains or losses of organic development, due to use or disuse, are transmitted to offspring, provided they have been common to both sexes, or to the animals from which the offspring have descended.

[32–35]. This time-scale provided more than ample time for the successive changes in animals to create new species, genera, families, orders, and classes of animals, as Lamarck had proposed. These layers of rock also indicated that successively younger rock strata contained progressively more advanced animals, which implied a gradual transformation towards increased complexity [3, 9, 36]. Finally, the fact that many fossil specimens were similar in some ways but different in other ways from existing animals lent support to the notion that many species of ancient animals had become extinct [3, 36].

Although no theory of evolution had yet attained scientific acceptance, the 1844 book *Vestiges of the Natural History of Creation* [37] prompted popular interest in Britain about the possibility of evolution. The book, which was anonymously published by a philosophically inclined author and journalist named Robert Chambers [38], summarized the existing geological evidence of the time to argue that life on earth had gradually evolved as Lamarck had proposed over an extremely long period of time. The *Vestiges* created a furor in intellectual circles in Britain, where it was condemned by British theologians as Godless and heretical, and by British scientists as "foolish fantasies" and "a work of fiction." However, because it received so much attention it became a best seller among the general public who seemed more open to its ideas [9, 10].

4.5 Chapter Highlights and Comments

The present chapter discussed how the conception of the world expressed by Natural Theology was widely accepted in England at the beginning of the 19th Century. By the middle of the century, however, the British public had been exposed to and expressed a strong interest in ideas that contradicted the worldview of Natural Theology. In the meantime, Jean Baptiste Lamarck presented the first systematic theories of the evolution of plants and animals in his 1809 book *Philosophie Zoologique*. Although Lamarck's theories were not well received in the scientific community in Europe, and they received little attention in England, his book presented the first thorough formulation of the causes of organic evolution. Despite the poor reaction to Lamarck's book, philosophers and naturalists began publishing their own ideas about organic evolution, which included some of the elements that were central to Charles Darwin's 1959 treatise on evolution. The notion of organic evolution was "in the air" during the 19th Century, as the American historian Edward J. Larson put it [3]. I think this is a very important point, since some people may think that the theory of evolution can be dismissed as the product of a single individual. In all likelihood, a comprehensive theory of organic evolution, akin to Darwin's, would have been published before the end the 19th Century even if Darwin had never published his *Origin of Species*.

References

1. Berry, E. W. (1922). The geological evidence of evolution. *The Scientific Monthly, 19*(2), 97–118.
2. Gohau, G., Carozz, A. V., & Carozzi, M. (1990). *A history of geology*. New Brunswick: Rutgers University Press.
3. Larson, E. J. (2004). *Evolution: The remarkable history of a scientific theory*. New York: The Modern Library.
4. Dean, D. R. (1992). *James Hutton and history of geology*. Ithaca: Cornell University Press.
5. Hutton, J. (1795). *Theory of the earth*. Edinburgh: W. Creech.
6. Hunt, G. (2010). Evolution in fossil lineages: Paleontology and the origin of species. *The American Naturalist, 176*(S1), S61–S76.
7. Berry, W. B. N. (1968). *Growth of the prehistoric time scale*. San Francisco: W.H. Freemann
8. Osborn, H. F. (1894). *From the Greeks to Darwin*. New York: MacMillan.
9. Mayr, E. (1982). *The growth of biological thought*. London: Belknap Press.
10. Eiseley, L. (1961). *Darwin's century: Evolution and the men who discovered it*. Garden City: Anchor Books.
11. Ferre, F. (2001). William Paley. In P. B. Dematteis, & P. S. Fosi (Eds.), *Dictionary of literary biography: British philosophers, 1500–1799* (Vol. 252, pp. 299–306). Farington Hills: The Gale Group.
12. Paley, W. (1802/1881). *Natural theology*. New York: American Trust Society.
13. Corsi, P. (2005). Before Darwin: Transformist concepts in European natural history. *Journal of the History of Biology, 38*(1), 67–83.
14. Corsi, P. (1988). *The age of Lamarck: Evolutionary theories in France 1790–1830* (J. Mandelbaum, Trans.). Berkeley: University of California Press.
15. Misra, K. K. (2011). Philosophie zoologique – 200: Lamarck in retrospect. *Science and Culture, 77*(5–6), 198–207.
16. Stafleu, F. A. (1971). Lamarck: The birth of biology. *Taxon, 20*(4), 397–442.
17. Gisis, S. (2009). Interactions between social and biological thinking: The case for Lamarck. *Perspectives on Science, 17*(3), 237–306.
18. Sapp, J. (2003). *Genesis: The evolution of biology*. New York: Oxford University Press.
19. Knapp, S. (2007). Jean-Baptiste Lamarck: The inheritance of life characteristics. In R. Huxley (Ed.), *The great naturalists* (pp. 190–196). London: Thames & Hudson.
20. Singer, C. (1950). *A history of biology* (Revised ed.). New York: Henry Schuman.
21. Lamarck, J. B. (1809/1873). *Philosophie zoologique*. Paris: Librairie F. Savy.
22. Curtis, W. C. (1922). *Science and human affairs from the viewpoint of biology*. New York: Harcourt, Brace and Company.
23. Mayr, E. (1972). Lamarck revisited. *Journal of the History of Biology, 5*(1), 55–94.
24. Butler, S. (1879). *Evolution, old and new; or, the theories of Buffon, Dr. Erasmus Darwin, and Lamarck, as compared with that of Mr. Charles Darwin*. London: Hardwicke and Bogue.
25. Burkhardt, R. W. (1972). The inspiration of Lamarck's belief in evolution. *Journal of the History of Biology, 5*(2), 413–438.
26. Gillispie, C. C. (2006). The formation of Lamarck's theory. *Transactions of the American Philosophical Society, 65*(5), 47–62.
27. Lamarck, J. B. (1809/1914). *Zoological philosophy* (H. Elliot, Trans.). London: MacMillan and Company.
28. Corsi, P. (2012). Idola tribus: Lamarck, politics and religion in the early nineteenth century. In A. Fasolo (Ed.), *The theory of evolution and its impact*. Milan: Springer-Verlag Italia.
29. Packard, A. S. (1901). *Lamarck: The founder of evolution*. New York: Longmans, Green & Co.
30. Packard, A. S. (1900). Lamarck's views on the evolution of man, on morals, and the relation of science to religion. *The Monist, 11*(1), 30–49.
31. Grumett, D. (2007). Teilhard de Chardin's evolutionary natural philosophy. *Zygon, 42*(2), 519–534.

32. Dodick, J., & Orion, N. (2003). Geology as an historical science: Its perception within science and the educational system. *Science & Education, 12*, 197–211.
33. Lyell, C. (1830). *Principles of geology* (Vol. 1). London: John Murray.
34. Lyell, C. (1832). *Principles of geology* (Vol. 2). London: John Murray.
35. Lyell, C. (1833). *Principles of geology* (Vol. 3). London: John Murray.
36. Francis, K. A. (2007). *Charles Darwin and the origin of species*. Westport: Greenwood Press.
37. Anonymous (1844). *Vestiges of the natural history of creation*. London: John Churchill.
38. Schwartz, J. S. (1990). Darwin, Wallace, and Huxley, and *Vestiges of the Natural History of Creation*. *Journal of the History of Biology,* 23(1), 127–153.

Part II
Charles Darwin's Theories of Evolution and Reactions to Them

Chapter 5
Charles Darwin's *Origin of Species*

Abstract The chapter traces the development of Charles Darwin's ideas about the concept of organic evolution, discusses the reasons why he delayed publishing his ideas for many years, and describes the major elements of the theories of evolution presented in his 1859 book, *On the Origin of Species by Means of Natural Selection*. The influence of his grandfather's ideas about evolution is also discussed, as well as the common themes found in Charles Darwin's *Origin of Species* and the writings of Erasmus Darwin (his grandfather), the Comte de Buffon, and Jean-Baptiste Lamarck. These similarities include their emphasis on the similarities between the breeding of domesticated plants and animals (which Charles Darwin called Artificial Selection) and the natural processes underlying the evolution of wild plants and animals (which Charles Darwin called Natural Selection). The chapter discusses key elements of Darwin's theories of evolution, including that: (1) animals reproduce at a rate that exceeds their food resources, (2) which creates competition for resources, (3) that members of a species vary in terms of their inherited characteristics, (4) that some inherited characteristics enhance survival and reproduction, (5) that such adaptive characteristics are inherited by offspring, (6) which leads to the spread of these adaptive characteristics within the population, such that (7) successive generations of the descendants of members of the original species may become sufficiently different from their ancestors that they become a different kind of animal over time through the accumulation of adaptive characteristics.

Keywords Adaptation • Common ancestor • Darwin • Evolution • Natural Selection • *Origin of Species*

5.1 Development of Darwin's Ideas

Charles Darwin was born into an affluent English family in 1809 [1, 2], the same year Lamarck published his book about evolution, *Philosophie Zoologique* [3]. In 1825, Charles went to Edinburgh University, where his older brother Robert was studying medicine, to try his hand at medicine too. While there, he did coursework in geology and zoology and became interested in Natural History, especially invertebrate sea animals, which he studied throughout the rest of his life. Abandoning the

K.J. Flannelly, *Religious Beliefs, Evolutionary Psychiatry, and Mental Health in America*, Religion, Spirituality and Health: A Social Scientific Approach 1,
DOI 10.1007/978-3-319-52488-7_5

idea of becoming a physician, Darwin enrolled in Cambridge University in 1827 to study for the clergy, where he continued to pursue his interest in Natural History [2].

The idea of becoming a clergyman was his father's idea, as had been the idea of becoming a physician and, as Darwin wrote in his autobiography, the idea of becoming a clergyman "died a natural death" (p. 40) when he had an opportunity to be a naturalist [4]. However, Darwin said in his autobiography: "I did not then in the least doubt the strict and literal truth of every word in the Bible"(p. 40) [4]. Nevertheless, as his private notebooks indicate, by the time he was developing his ideas about evolution he no longer believed in the major tenets of Christianity [5, 6].

Darwin's opportunity to become a naturalist came shortly after graduating from Cambridge University in 1831, when he joined the crew of the British Navy's *HMS Beagle* [1, 2], which sailed around the world between December of 1931 and October 1836 [2, 7]. Most of the voyage was devoted to exploring the east and west coasts of South America, where Darwin made detailed observations of the geology and collected specimens of terrestrial and aquatic plants and animals. The *Beagle* also stopped at Atlantic and Pacific islands, including the now famous Galapagos Islands off the coast of Chile [8]. The scientific papers Darwin wrote based on the voyage brought him acclaim within the British scientific community, and his popular description of the expedition in his *The Voyage of the Beagle* became a bestseller, making him a prominent scientific figure among the British public [2].

Charles Darwin's observations during the voyage led him to think about the possibility of evolution, which he called "transmutation," and he began a series of "transmutation notebooks" in March of 1837. The first entry in his first notebook was "*Zoonomia*," the name of his grandfather's book [9], under which Charles wrote comments about some of the things his grandfather (Erasmus Darwin) wrote in *Zoonomia*. In particular, he noted that his grandfather said sexual reproduction results in variation among offspring, whereas asexual reproduction does not produce variation [10, 11]. Within a year, Charles Darwin developed his concept of Natural Selection in which he envisioned individual variation as the raw material that made evolution possible [11]. Despite the apparent connection between Charles's idea and his grandfather's ideas about variation, Charles often denied that his grandfather's writings about evolution had influenced his own ideas. Indeed, he said in his autobiography, although he admired *Zoonomia* when he was younger, when he was older he "was much disappointed [at] the proportion of speculation [in the book] being so large [compared] to the facts given [in *Zoonomia*]" (p. 25) [4]. This observation by Charles Darwin about *Zoonomia* appears to have had a great influence on him, even if his grandfather's ideas did not, because Charles spent decades amassing facts to support his own speculations about evolution before he published *On the Origin of Species by Means of Natural Selection, or the Preservation of Favoured Races in the Struggle for Life* in 1859. Presumably, Charles gathered as many facts as he could because he feared his theory of evolution would be attacked, just as his grandfather's theory had been.

Charles Darwin became convinced of the transmutation of species in 1837 [7], but he did not formulate his concept of Natural Selection until 1938, after reading *An Essay on the Principle of Population* by an economist named Thomas Malthus

[1, 2, 4]. Malthus argued that animal and human populations, if unchecked, naturally reproduce at a rate that outstrips their food supply, which creates a "struggle for existence" in which some individuals will win and some will lose [12]. Darwin reasoned that if the individuals comprising a species must compete for their existence, and individuals within a species vary to some degree, some individuals will be better than others at competing for necessary resources (such as food). Since those individuals that are more successful in such competition should be more likely to survive and reproduce, they should pass their helpful or advantageous characteristics on to their offspring [1, 13], a process that the English philosopher and Herbert Spencer later called "survival of the fittest" [14]. Thus, Darwin argued, over successive generations individuals with these advantageous characteristics should become more common than individuals without these advantageous characteristics, as the latter would be less likely to survive and reproduce [13]. He thought that this shift in the characteristics of increasing numbers of individuals over successive generations could lead to the creation of new species.

Charles Darwin, like his grandfather Erasmus Darwin, the Comte de Buffon, and Lamarck, saw the process of evolutionary change as being analogous to the selective breeding of domesticated plants and animals. The practice of selective breeding of animals, or Artificial Selection as Charles called it, over thousands of years had created new and very different varieties of dogs, horses, cattle, etc., by breeding only those individuals that had the particular characteristics which the breeder thought were desirable. Likewise, Charles Darwin thought nature has selected those animals with characteristics that enhance survival and reproduction, and this process over time has yielded, different varieties, species, genera, and families of animals, and so on [1].

5.2 Darwin's Delay in Publishing

Although Charles Darwin initially articulated his theory of evolution in 1938, he did not publish anything about it until 1859 [1, 2], when he published *The Origin of Species* [13]. Authors have offered a number of possible explanations for this long delay. One explanation, which I already mentioned, is that he wanted to collect all the facts he could to support his theory before presenting it [15]; this is consistent with the comment in his notebook that his grandfather's book *Zoonomia* contained more speculation than facts [1, 2]. Another related explanation, which I alluded to earlier, is that Charles was sensitive to the social climate of his time [1, 15], and he was acutely aware that the transmutation of species was a politically and religiously controversial topic in Britain [16].

Darwin finally wrote a long, detailed essay about his theory in 1844 [2], the same year the *Vestiges of the Natural History of Creation* was published [17]. Darwin expressed concern to friends that his book about transmutation would be as fiercely attacked and as readily dismissed as the *Vestiges* had been by the British establishment [2, 18]. Darwin hoped, however, that the *Vestiges* might have made organic evolution a more socially acceptable notion in Britain than it had been previously [18], as suggested by the popular appeal of the *Vestiges* [6, 9].

Darwin finally gave his full attention to writing his book in 1854 [2], around the same time a Welch naturalist named Alfred Russell Wallace was developing his own ideas about the how new species could arise [2]. Darwin received an essay from Wallace in 1858 describing his own ideas about the evolution of species, along with a letter asking Darwin for his opinion about the essay. Darwin was astonished by the similarity of Wallace's theory to his own theory [2], and he had friends make arrangements for Wallace's paper and a portion of his own 1844 paper to be read at a meeting of the Linnean Society in London [2, 15], so that both he and Wallace could share credit for the theory. The incident finally prompted Darwin to publish his *Origin of Species* in 1859 [2].

5.3 Darwin's *Origin of Species*

The Origin of Species begins by describing the nature of individual differences in domestic and wild animals, as well as plants, and how variations in individual characteristics underlie the modification of species over time. Like his grandfather, Buffon, and Lamarck, Charles Darwin used the domestication of plants and animals as evidence that the morphology of plants and animals could change dramatically over time. Like them, he argued, if morphological and behavioral changes could be produced in animals by humans through selective breeding (i.e., Artificial Selection), they certainly could be produced by nature. Unlike his grandfather, Buffon, and Lamarck, however, Charles Darwin was able to offer a mechanism (i.e., Natural Selection) that he claimed could select which individuals of a species would survive and reproduce in a way analogous to Artificial Selection [13].

Darwin said that believed the "diversity of inheritable deviations of structure is endless" (p. 12) [13] in plants and animals and that individual variation in characteristics made it possible to modify plants and animals by Artificial Selection. This is most clearly seen in the breeding of dogs, cattle, and other animals for specific characteristics. Though Buffon, Lamarck, and Erasmus Darwin had all made the analogy between changes in animals produced by selective breeding and changes in wild animals, which they proposed were produced by evolution, Charles Darwin was able to make a more compelling case for this analogy because: (a) he had a mechanism for evolutionary change (Natural Selection); (b) he provided more extensive evidence of the changes produced by selective breeding; and (c) he understood selective breeding better than they did because he talked to many animal breeders and he conducted his own experiments on the selective breeding of pigeons. The use of the analogy between selective breeding (Artificial Selection) and evolution (Natural Selection) in *The Origin of Species* was particularly well-suited for its British audience because many British people were familiar with breeding plants and pigeons and the British gentry were particularly familiar with the breeding of livestock, hounds, and horses [1].

The Origin of Species also discusses how individual differences among wild animals creates great diversity even within the same species, such that some groups of animals that are recognized as varieties of a species could just as easily be classified as sub-species of the species. Charles Darwin thought that these varieties or sub-species were incipient species and could change so much over time that they would be recognized as separate species – a view shared by Lamarck [3, 13]. Charles Darwin stressed, to varying degrees, that the capacity of nature to modify plant and animal characteristics depends on the existence of various natural forces impinging on every organism, including: (a) climatic fluctuations and their effects on food and other resources; (b) competition for resources among members of the same species; and (c) other forces, such as prey-predator and host-parasite relationships. Buffon, Lamarck, and Erasmus Darwin had stressed, to varying degrees, the influence of these same natural forces on evolution, but Charles Darwin embodied these natural forces in the concept of the "struggle for existence." He said, because animals and plants face a struggle to survive, "any variation, however slight … if it be in any degree profitable to an individual of any species, will lend to the preservation of that individual, and will generally be inherited by its offspring" (p. 61) [13]. The offspring, then, will also have a better chance of surviving. This is the essence of Darwin's theory of Natural Selection. In *The Origin of Species*, Darwin often refers to such profitable variations as adaptations [13].

According to Charles Darwin, Natural Selection works solely by preserving structural variations that, by chance, happen to benefit an individual in the struggle for existence; that is, those modifications that help an animal or plant survive and have offspring. As these beneficial modifications are inherited by an individual's offspring, they accumulate over time to make successive generations of offspring better suited (or better adapted) to their environment. However, Natural Selection does not produce the best possible way to adapt to environmental conditions. For example, the wings of bees, birds, and bats reflect different structural mechanisms that have evolved to enable flight, but they may not be the best way for an animal to fly. Natural Selection can only preserve modifications to existing structural components (i.e., bones, muscles, nerves, etc.) that, by chance, enhance survival and reproductive success (which is sometimes referred to as "increased fitness").

As these modifications accumulate over successive generations, individuals tend to diverge from their ancestral forms. This is a central element of Darwin's theory, which he repeatedly called his "theory of descent with modification." He claimed that this divergence accounts for the hierarchical organization of animals observed in the Linnaean and subsequent classification systems [19]. Such taxonomic systems, he thought, were classifications of genealogy that reflect descent from a common ancestor.

Some of the best evidence Darwin presented for descent from a common ancestor was the anatomical evidence that different animals share homologous or corresponding organs and structures. In vertebrates, for example, homology is readily apparent in the structural order of the bones of the limbs [13]. Each forelimb and hindlimb is composed of a series of bones that are arranged in the same serial order across all the vertebrate species. Even though the bones may differ in shape and size, their arrangement is always the same regardless of the vertebrate's species, genus, order, or class. The same homologous bones even exist in the same arrangement in the fins of fish because all vertebrates share a common ancestor with fish. This structural evidence for common descent was apparent, then as it is now, not only in the homologies among existing vertebrates, but also in the homologous structures of extant species and extinct species (i.e., fossils).

In addition to demonstrating the feasibility of evolution and presenting a plausible mechanism of evolution, *The Origin of Species* undermined the central tenants of Natural Theology that each animal is perfectly designed and ideally suited for the world in which it lives [1, 13]. Darwin noted, for example, that there are numerous cases in nature of animals with rudimentary organs that no longer serve a purpose: snakes have the rudimentary bones of a pelvis and hind limbs even though snakes cannot use them to walk; cave-dwelling animals have rudimentary eyes that are incapable of vision; and some island-dwelling birds have rudimentary wings that are no longer capable of flight. Darwin's explanation was similar to Lamarck's explanation that organs would atrophy from disuse over many generations because they no longer served a purpose. Darwin claimed that these and numerous other examples of animals that have useless organs or other structures indicated that animals were not perfectly designed.

A central argument in *The Origin of Species* is that different types of animals came to be the way they are, not by Divine design, but by a very slow process of gradual evolution over vast amounts of time. Darwin presented several lines of evidence to dispute Divine design. One, as just mentioned, was the fact that some animals have useless structures, which undermine the notion that their anatomy reflects the work of a Divine clock-maker. Another was that some animals grow organs during their embryonic development that disappear before they are born, which, to him, was further evidence of an imperfect design rather than a Divine design. Instead of being the result of design, Darwin proposed, animals and plants came to be the way they are by chance: (a) they inherit characteristics that happen by chance to enhance their survival and reproductive success; (b) these adaptive characteristics (adaptations) are passed along to (are inherited by) their offspring; and (c) hence, these adaptive characteristics are spread within the breeding population. Evolution does not produce the best design of a structure for a function or purpose because Natural Selection can only modify already existing structures to perform new functions; it cannot "go back to the drawing board" to create something "from scratch" that would produce the best fit between structure and function [20].

5.4 Chapter Highlights and Comments

Charles Darwin's *Origin of Species* explains how animals and plants could change in form over time by a process he called Natural Selection. Like, Buffon, Erasmus Darwin, and Lamarck, his explanation hinged, in part, on the analogy between evolution and the selective breeding of domestic animals that has been practiced for thousands of years. To summarize Darwin's argument: (1) animals reproduce at a rate that exceeds their food resources; (2) this creates a "struggle for existence" for resources between members of the same species, as well as between different species; (3) members of a species vary in terms of their inheritable, individual characteristics ("diversity of inheritable deviations"); (4) in the struggle for existence, some of these inherited characteristics will enhance survival and reproduction (adaptive characteristics or adaptations); (5) these adaptive characteristics will be inherited by offspring and enhance their likelihood of survival and reproduction; (6) this will lead to the spread of these adaptive characteristics within the breeding population; and (7) successive generations of the descendants of members of the original species may become sufficiently different from their ancestors that they become a different kind of animal over time through the accumulations of adaptive characteristics [13, 21, 22]. This process applies not only to the emergence of different species, but also to the emergence of different genera, families, orders, classes, etc., as adaptations accumulate over time. This process forms the basis for both the concept of evolution, in general, and the concept of descent from a common ancestor, which were both explicitly proposed by Erasmus Darwin and Lamarck, and implied by Buffon.

Although I only alluded to the fact that Alfred Russell Wallace developed a theory of evolution that was similar to Charles Darwin's theory, Henry Fairfield Osborne published the major elements of their theories side by side to show how similar their theories were [23]. These similarities made it inevitable that a theory of evolution closely akin to Darwin's would have been published in the 19th Century even if Darwin had not published his *Origin of Species*. Beyond establishing the feasibility of evolution, *The Origin of Species* severely undermined the central tenets of Natural Theology: (1) that each animal is perfectly suited to its environment by Divine design; and (2) that the match between an animal and its world could not be achieved by natural means.

References

1. Larson, E. J. (2004). *Evolution: The remarkable history of a scientific theory*. New York: The Modern Library.
2. Francis, K. A. (2007). *Charles Darwin and the Origin of Species*. Westport: Greenwood Press.
3. Lamarck, J. B. (1809/1873). *Philosophie zoologique*. Paris: Librairie F. Savy.
4. Barlow, N. (1958). *The autobiography of Charles Darwin*. London: Collins.
5. Dilley, S. (2012). Charles Darwin's use of theology in the Origin of Species. *British Journal for the History of Science, 45*(1), 29–56.
6. Mayr, E. (1982). *The growth of biological thought*. London: Belknap Press.
7. Sulloway, F. J. (1982). Darwin's Conversion: The *Beagle* voyage and its aftermath. *Journal of the History of Biology, 15*(3), 325–396.
8. Darwin, C. (1845). *The voyage of the Beagle*. London: J.M. Dent & Sons.
9. Eiseley, L. (1961). *Darwin's century: Evolution and the men who discovered it*. Garden City: Anchor Books.
10. Darwin, E. (1794). *Zoonomia: Or the laws of organic life* (Vol. I). London: J. Johnson.

11. Colp, R., Jr. (1986). The relationship of Charles Darwin to the ideas of his grandfather, Dr. Erasmus Darwin. *Biography, 9*(1), 1–24.
12. Malthus, T. (1798). *An essay on the principle of population*. London: J. Johnson.
13. Darwin, C. (1859). *On the origin of species by means of natural selection, or the preservation of favoured races in the struggle for life*. London: John Murray.
14. Spencer, H. (1868). *Principles of biology*. New York: D. Appleton and Company.
15. Richards, R. J. (1983). Why Darwin delayed, or interesting problems and models in the history of science. *Journal of the History of the Behavioral Sciences, 19*(1), 43–53.
16. Endersby, J. (2009). Sympathetic science: Charles Darwin, Joseph Hooker, and the passions of Victorian naturalists. *Victorian Studies, 51*(2), 299–320.
17. Vestiges (1844). *Vestiges of the natural history of creation*. London: John Churchill.
18. Schwartz, J. S. (1990). Darwin, Wallace, and Huxley, and Vestiges of the Natural History of Creation. *Journal of the History of Biology, 23*(1), 127–153.
19. Singer, C. (1950). *A history of biology* (Revised ed.). New York: Henry Schuman.
20. Gilbert, P. (2002). Evolutionary approaches to psychopathology and cognitive therapy. *Journal of Cognitive Psychotherapy: An International Quarterly, 16*(3), 263–294.
21. Beck, W. S. (1961). *Modern science and the nature of life*. Garden City: Anchor Books.
22. Campbell, N. A., & Reece, J. B. (2005). *Biology* (7ed.). San Francisco: Pearson Education.
23. Osborn, H. F. (1894). *From the Greeks to Darwin*. New York: MacMillan.

Chapter 6
Reactions to Darwin's *Origin of Species*

Abstract The chapter describes the initial reaction of the British general public to the 1859 publication of Charles Darwin's *Origin of Species*, the immediate and later reactions of the scientific community, and the 20th Century response of Conservative Christians in the U.S. The British public had a generally favorable reaction to *Origin of Species* when it was first published, and it has been said that the British public widely accepted that the theory of evolution was true within a decade of the book's publication. As the chapter explains, Darwin's "theory of descent with modification" was widely accepted among scientists in Britain and the U.S. by the 1870s, but many biologists were not convinced that Darwin's "theory of Natural Selection" was the mechanism of evolution until the early 20th Century, when the field of genetics showed that individual characteristics were expressed through and transmitted by genes and that random mutations in genes could produce significant changes in genetic characteristics upon which Natural Selection could act. The chapter also describes that most Christian denominations came to accept the theory of evolution, but strong objections to the theory arose among Conservative Christians in America in the early 1920s. Their objection to the concept of evolution, which is predicated on their literal interpretation of the description of God's creation of the world in the *Book of Genesis*, has been expressed in educational movements in the U.S. that oppose the teaching of evolution in the public schools, including "Creation Science" and "Intelligent Design."

Keywords Adaptation • Common ancestor • Darwin • Evolution • Intelligent Design • Modern Synthesis • Natural Selection • *Origin of Species*

6.1 Initial Reactions to the *Origin of Species*

When Darwin's *Origin of Species* was published in 1859, it was immediately controversial in religious and scientific circles [1], just as the *Vestiges* had been. However, the logic of Darwin's arguments, the depth and breadth of the evidence from many different fields that he included in *The Origin of Species*, and his synthesis of that evidence made a compelling case for the reality, not just the theory of evolution. Moreover, the *Vestiges* had, it seemed, made the British public more

K.J. Flannelly, *Religious Beliefs, Evolutionary Psychiatry, and Mental Health in America*, Religion, Spirituality and Health: A Social Scientific Approach 1,
DOI 10.1007/978-3-319-52488-7_6

receptive to the concept of organic evolution [2], and the public's primary reaction to *The Origin of Species* was, according to some scholars, more one of fascination than anything else [3]. *The Times of London* published a very favorable review of the book's central premise, leaving it to scientists to decide its ultimate fate [2]. Within a decade of its publication, the British public generally accepted the theory as being true [4]. The concept of organic evolution also was readily embraced in Germany, although it was rejected in France [5].

By the 1870s, Darwin's "theory of descent with modification"(i.e., descent from a common ancestor) was widely accepted among scientists in Britain and the United States [2, 6], and some historians say that it was accepted as a scientific fact by then [7]. Whether they considered evolution to be a plausible theory or a fact, scientists overwhelmingly rejected the idea that plants and animals were created by God as a valid explanation of the origin of species [2, 4]. Nevertheless, many biologists were not convinced that Darwin's "theory of Natural Selection" was the mechanism of evolution until the 20th Century [2, 8].

6.2 Creation Science and Intelligent Design

As the scientific community came to endorse evolution, the Roman Catholic Church and most Protestant denominations also came to accept or, at least, tolerate it, claiming that God used evolution as a means to create the diversity of life on earth [9, 10]. However, Conservative Christians in America, who believed in the literal truth of the Old Testament, including the *Book of Genesis*, sought to ban the teaching of evolution in American public schools [2, 10]. The movement had some success in the 1920s, convincing the legislatures of several states, including Arkansas and Tennessee, to prohibit the teaching of evolution in public schools [9, 10]. In 1968, however, the U.S. Supreme Court said it was unconstitutional to ban the teaching of evolution [9, 10], based on the "Establishment Clause" of the First Amendment of the U.S. Constitution, which is generally described as the "separation of Church and State."[1]

"Creation Science," which was created in the 1920s to promote the belief that the *Book of Genesis* was literally true, included the beliefs that the earth was created several thousand years ago, as Bishop Ussher had proclaimed, and that fossils are the result of the great flood described in the Bible [9, 11]. Creation Science was used in a second wave of Conservative Christian efforts in the 1970s and 1980s to attack

[1] The first amendment to the U.S. Constitution begins with the following clause, which has come to be known as the "Establishment Clause": "Congress shall make no law respecting an establishment of religion, or prohibiting the free exercise thereof." The U.S. Supreme Court has interpreted this clause to mean than no government entity in the U.S. should promote or hinder the practice of religion, and that allowing the expression of religious beliefs and practices in public schools constitutes the promotion of religion by the government. Banning the teaching of evolution in public schools because it is contrary to the story of creation in the "Book of Genesis" thereby constitutes the promotion of religion by the government. The first ten amendments to the U.S. Constitution are called, collectively, the "Bill of Rights."

the teaching of evolution in response to the Supreme Court decision that prohibited the ban on teaching evolution in American public schools. The political goal of proponents of Creation Science was to have Creation Science taught in public schools whenever evolution was taught. One of the rationales for doing so was to assure that students were given a balanced perspective about the creation of plants and animals, including humans. This movement had some success, in that Arkansas and Louisiana passed laws in the early 1980s mandating that Creation Science be taught along with evolution in public schools [9, 10, 12]. However, these laws were struck down by the U.S. Supreme Court in 1987, when the Court ruled that Creation Science was not science but religion, and that the purpose of the Arkansas and Louisiana laws was to advance the religious belief that humans were created by a supernatural being [9–12].

Yet, a dissenting Supreme Court opinion argued that the people of a state had the right to present secular evidence against evolution in the public schools [9]. Hence, Creation Science was recast as "Intelligent Design" in the early 1990s [9, 11], as a way to get religion into the classroom [10]. The advocates of Intelligent Design claimed that some forms of life, notably humans, are too complex to have been created by the chance processes of evolution, and that they must have been created by design [9, 11, 13, 14]. Moreover, they argued, since evolution is only a theory, teaching Intelligent Design in conjunction with evolution is a way to promote students' critical thinking [9]. Although a federal judge stopped the teaching of Intelligent Design in a Pennsylvania school district because it is fundamentally the same thing as Creation Science, the Supreme Court has not addressed the issue [12].

The U.S. appears to remain unique in the Western World with respect to its rejection of the reality of organic evolution [15, 16], and efforts have continued to undermine the teaching of evolution in public schools. A 2009 study by The Pew Research Center reported that State laws in Louisiana, South Carolina, Tennessee, and Wisconsin allow local school districts to decide if Intelligent Design should be taught in science classes. As of 2009, the school board of Cobb County, Georgia, placed stickers on school biology books that said "evolution is a theory, not a fact." Although the state school board of Kansas no longer warns students that evolution is just a theory, it cautions them that it is controversial, and the state of Alabama continues to place stickers on biology books that evolution is a "controversial theory" [17].

6.3 The Modern Synthesis

As mentioned above, although scientists accepted Darwin's "theory of descent with modification," many scientists remained skeptical that Darwin's "theory of Natural Selection" was the mechanism of evolution. The problem was twofold: the source of variation upon which Natural Selection supposedly worked was not known and the mechanism of inheritance was unknown. Answers to these questions did not begin to emerge until the science of genetics was developed in the early 1900s, when the botanical experiments of a Moravian monk named Gregor Mendel were rediscovered [5, 18, 19]. Mendel had published a little noticed scientific paper in 1866 that summarized the findings of his decade of research on the inherited characteristics of pea plants (e.g., stem length, flower position, shape and color of seeds) and described the basic rules or laws of inheritance in plants that he had derived from his research [19, 20]. By 1918, mathematicians began to develop models of genetic variation based on Mendel's laws, which showed that the inheritance of adaptive characteristics in plants and animals spread within a population, as predicted by Charles Darwin's theory of Natural Selection [2, 4].

Yet, a complete understanding of evolutionary processes was not achieved until the mechanism of inheritance (i.e., the gene) and the major cause of variations in individual characteristics (random mutations in genes) were discovered [21]. These discoveries allowed Theodosius Dobzhansky to put the mathematic models of evolution into concrete terms in his 1937 book, *Genetics and the Origin of Species*, which explains how genetic variations drive the evolutionary process [2, 4, 21].

In the meantime, evolutionary biologists clarified concepts that had been ill-defined or loosely used when describing Darwin's theory of Natural Selection, particularly the concepts of adaptation and fitness. The modern concept of fitness is defined as the degree to which a trait or characteristic of an organism contributes to the ability to survive and reproduce [22]. Therefore, a trait is considered to be adaptive, "if it contributes to the fitness … of an organism" [22]. Ernst Mayr provides a more formal definition of adaptation: "an adaptation is a property of an organism, whether a structure, physiological trait, behavior, or any other attribute, the possession of which favors the individual in the struggle for existence" (p. 179) [22]. Adaptations are believed to arise by chance and to be maintained within a species by Natural Selection. That is, an adaption does not arise to serve a purpose in the teleological sense. Instead, the fact that some change in a characteristic turns out to serve a useful purpose that promotes fitness, leads to its selection and spread (or diffusion) in a population [22]. Contrary to Lamarck's theory that evolution was an active process in which organisms strove to perfect themselves, Charles Darwin thought adaptation was a passive process that was not driven by a striving for perfection and was not under the control of the individual organism [22].

Although I have only alluded to different components of the theory of evolution Darwin presented in *The Origin of Species*, Mayr [23] identified five distinct theories about evolution in Darwin's *Origin of Species*. The first is the theory of evolution, per se, that species change into a new form over time, and the second theory is that the process of evolution is gradual, as opposed to occurring in bursts, as some recent theories have proposed [24, 25]. Mayr further distinguished these two theories from the theory of common descent (i.e., that all animals and plants have a single common ancestor), and he explained that all three of these theoretical concepts are independent from the theory (which I have not until now mentioned) that the evolution of species causes an increase in the number of species, which increases organic diversity. Finally, Mayr made the distinction, between the theory that evolution occurs and the theory of how evolution occurs, which Darwin claimed was Natural Selection [23]. The gradual nature of evolution was, of course, specifically proposed by both Darwin's grandfather and Lamarck.

6.4 Chapter Highlights and Comments

Although the part of Darwin's theory that is called "the theory of descent with modification" was accepted relatively quickly by scientists and the public, it took many years and the discovery of genes and gene mutations for the process of evolution to be fully understood. While most people have come to accept that organic evolution is a fact, some American Christians continue to be opposed to the concept of evolution because it is contrary to their religious beliefs, especially their belief that the *Book of Genesis* is literally true

It should also be kept in mind that Darwin's theories of evolution are not static and that evolutionary theory continues to evolve. For instance, whereas Charles Darwin proposed that evolution is a very gradual process, more recent theories have proposed that evolution is a sporadic process in which very little change in species may occur over long periods of time, until some dramatic environmental change provides the opportunity for new species to proliferate [24, 25].

References

1. Colp, R., Jr. (1986). The relationship of Charles Darwin to the ideas of his grandfather, Dr. Erasmus Darwin. *Biography, 9*(1), 1–24.
2. Larson, E. J. (2004). *Evolution: The remarkable history of a scientific theory*. New York: The Modern Library.
3. Fleming, C., & Goodall, J. (2002). Dangerous Darwinism. *Public Understanding of Science, 11*, 259–271.
4. Francis, K. A. (2007). *Charles Darwin and the origin of species*. Westport: Greenwood Press.
5. Singer, C. (1950). *A history of biology* (Revised ed..). New York: Henry Schuman.
6. Bowler, P. J. (2004). The specter of Darwinism: The popular image of Darwinism in early twentieth century Britain. In A. Lustig, R. J. Richards, & M. Ruse (Eds.), *Darwinian heresies*. Cambridge: Cambridge University Press.
7. Huxley, T. H. (1880). The coming of age of "The origin of species." *Science, 1*(2), 15–17., 20.
8. Waller, J. (2005). Evolution's inside man: Other people could have had Darwin's insights, but no one else could have gotten them accepted by the establishment. *New Scientist, 187*(2513), 42–44.
9. Pennock, R. T. (2003). Creationism and intelligent design. *Annual Review of Genomics and Human Genetics, 4*(1), 143–163.
10. Dixon, T. (2009). America's difficulty with Darwin. *History Today, 59*(2), 22–28.
11. Bailey, D. H. (2010). Creationism and intelligent design: Scientific and theological difficulties. *Dialogue: A Journal of Mormon Thought, 43*(3), 62–87.
12. Brown, S. (2014). The evolution of creationism. *Church and State, 67*(3), 9–12.
13. Wald, D. (2000). Special section on intelligent design: The new creationism. *Skeptic, 8*(2), 12.
14. Melott, A. L. (2002). Intelligent design is creationism in a cheap tuxedo. *Physics Today, 55*(6), 48.
15. Blancke, S., Hjermitslev, H. H., Braeckman, J., & Kjaergaard, P. C. (2013). Creationism in Europe: Facts, gaps, and prospects. *Journal of the American Academy of Religion, 81*(4), 996–1028.
16. Coyne, J. A. (2012). Science, religion, and society: The problem of evolution in America. *Evolution, 66*(8), 2654–2663.

17. Masci, D., & Lipka, M. (2009). *Fighting of Darwin, state by state*. Washington, DC.: Pew Research Center.
18. Winchester, A. M. (1966). *Genetics: A survey of the principles of heredity* (3rd ed.). New York: Houghton Mifflin.
19. Olby, R. C. (1966). *Origins of Medelsim*. New York: Schocken Books.
20. Mendel, G. (1866/1996). *Experiments on plant hybridization* (W. Bateson, Trans.). Electronic scholarly publishing project. In Mendel Retrieved from http://www.esp.org/foundations/genetics/classical/gm-65.pdf
21. Dobzhansky, T. (1937). *Genetics and the origin of species*. New York: Columbia Univsersity Press.
22. Mayr, E. (2002). *What is evolution*. London: Phoenix.
23. Mayr, E. (1991). *One long argument: Charles Darwin and the genius of modern evolutionary thought*. Cambridge, MA: Hazen University Press.
24. Gould, S. J., & Eldredge, N. (1977). Punctuated equilibria: The tempo and mode of evolution reconsidered. *Paleobiology, 3*(2), 115–151.
25. Simpson, G. G. (1944/1984). *Tempo and mode in evolution*. New York Columbia University Press.

Chapter 7
Darwin's *Descent of Man* and *The Expression of Emotions*

Abstract The chapter discusses the major topics presented in Charles Darwin's books *The Descent of Man* and *The Expression of Emotions*. As the chapter explains, the primary scientific importance of *The Descent of Man* is that it extends the evolutionary concept of descent from an ancient common ancestor, which was proposed by Charles Darwin, Erasmus Darwin, the Comte de Buffon, Jean-Baptise Lamarck and others, to humans. However, by the time *The Descent of Man* was published, two other books had already made the claim that humans had evolved from lower types of animals. The other major contribution of the book, from a psychological perspective, was its claim that the mental abilities of animals and humans differ only in degree, not in kind, a concept that has come to be called the theory of the "continuity of mind." As the chapter explains, the major contribution of *The Expression of Emotions*, which has been called the first book on Evolutionary Psychiatry, is that it explicitly extends the concept of the continuity of mental abilities in humans and other animals to the experience and expression of emotions. The chapter describes the parallels Darwin saw between the human and animal expression of anger, fear, and other emotions.

Keywords Common ancestor • Continuity of mind • Darwin • *Descent of Man* • *Expression of Emotions* • Evolutionary Psychiatry

7.1 Darwin's *Descent of Man*

Darwin wrote two more books about evolution after *The Origin of Species*. One was *The Descent of Man, and Selection in Relation to Sex* [1] and the other book was *The Expression of Emotions in Man and Animals* [2]. Volume 1 of *The Descent of Man* formally extends the theory of common descent to humans, which Darwin avoided doing in *The Origin of Species*, and Volume 2 presents his theory of sexual selection, which greatly expands upon his grandfather's idea that competition for mates has led to unique adaptations among the males of many species that enhance their reproductive success.

The critical evidence that Darwin presents in *The Descent of Man* to demonstrate the common descent of humans from lower animals is the same kind of morphologi-

K.J. Flannelly, *Religious Beliefs, Evolutionary Psychiatry, and Mental Health in America*, Religion, Spirituality and Health: A Social Scientific Approach 1,
DOI 10.1007/978-3-319-52488-7_7

cal evidence he presented in *The Origin of Species* to demonstrate the descent of other animals from a common ancestor. This evidence included, for example, the fact that the functions and structures of the skeletal, muscular, circulatory, digestive, and respiratory system are all fundamentally the same across all classes, orders and families of vertebrate species, including humans [1, 3, 4]. These similarities are particularly strikingly when one compares the skeletal systems of humans and other vertebrate animals.

After describing the anatomical similarities between humans and other animals in *The Descent of Man*, Darwin turns his attention to similarities in their "mental faculties," arguing that humans and animals share basic instincts, including self-preservation, sexual love, and a mother's love for her child, and that other animals experience many of the same emotions that we do. Darwin even claimed that humans and animals shared "more intellectual faculties," such as curiosity, imitation, attention, memory, reason, and language. Although "articulate language," as Darwin called it, was obviously unique to humans, he recognized that other animals communicated through vocalizations, gestures, and other means. To the extent that humans and animals differed in mental faculties, Darwin believed the differences were a matter "of degree and not of kind" (p. 105) [1]. This expression encapsulates what is now called the theory of the "continuity of mind" [5, 6].

The publication of *The Descent of Man* in 1871 was not as controversial as *The Origin of Species* was in 1859, partly because other books had already been published in Britain, which proposed that humans had evolved the way as other animals had evolved and, therefore, that humans had a common ancestor with other animals.[1] In fact, two such books about human evolution were published in 1863 by Darwin's scientific colleagues and long-time supporters: Thomas Huxley's *The Evidence as to Man's Place in Nature*, and Charles Lyell's *The Geological Evidence of the Antiquity of Man* [7, 8].

7.2 Darwin's *Expression of Emotions*

Darwin's third book about evolution, *The Expression of Emotions* [2], has been called the first book on "evolutionary psychiatry" [9], and it seems to have prompted some early psychiatrists, most notably Sigmund Freud, to speculate about the evolutionary origins of mental disorders [10, 11]. *The Expression of Emotions* expands on the concept, which was mentioned several times in *The Descent of Man* [1], that animals and humans have similar mental faculties, particularly with respect emotions. Since it is considered by some to be the first book on evolutionary psychiatry (e.g., [9]), I will devote more time to it than I did to *The Descent of Man*.

[1] Darwin proposed in *The Descent of Man* than humans descended from the "Old World" monkeys in Africa before the apes diverged from the monkeys. We now know that humans evolved from apes long after the apes evolved from "Old World" monkeys.

The Expression of Emotions has been called a "Milestone in Natural History" (p. 6) [12], because it extensively describes the actions of animals and humans that Darwin believed conveyed emotional states, or "states of mind," as he usually referred to them. The book covers a wide range of emotions in animals and humans, with several chapters concentrating on anger and fear, and other chapters discussing joy, love, and pain. The book attempts to demonstrate the similarity of emotional expressions across animal groups (i.e., species, genera, and classes of animals) and humans.

Although Darwin included a variety of species of animals in his analysis, his examples were primarily drawn from domestic animals and wild animals that were held in captivity. Many of the latter observations were anecdotes from zoo keepers. To obtain information about the expression of emotions by native peoples throughout the world, Darwin mailed surveys to missionaries and other Europeans in foreign countries. He also showed people pictures and paintings that were intended to depict different emotions, and asked them to identify what each depicted emotion was.

7.2.1 Expressions of Fear and Anger

Darwin described two nearly universal behavioral expressions of fear. The first is trembling of the muscles, and the second is standing motionless (or "freezing") for a time "in order" for an animal "to collect it senses and to ascertain the source of danger, and sometimes for the sake of escaping detection" (pp. 77–78) [2]. Much like frightened animals, Darwin says, "The frightened man at first stands like a statue motionless and breathless ... The heart beats quickly and violently, ... The skin instantly becomes pale, ... [and] the hairs ... on the skin stand erect; and the superficial muscles shiver" (p. 290) [2].

Darwin used the words anger and rage almost interchangeably, considering rage to be a more intense state of mind than anger. In humans, he said, "Rage exhibits itself in the most diversified manner. The heart and circulation are always affected; the face reddens or becomes purple, with the veins on the forehead and neck distend" (p. 240) [2]. Darwin gave examples of rage in various animals, and described how the human expression of rage is much like that of apes.

7.2.2 Expression of Other Emotions

Darwin emphasized the importance of facial expressions in human emotions, which he sometimes compared to the facial expressions of other primates. His descriptions included the positioning of the eyebrows, eyelids, and lips, the degree to which the mouth is open, and the muscles that control them. Darwin noted that the facial expressions exhibited in surprise and astonishment were very similar to the facial expressions exhibited for fear.

The Expression of Emotions also contains descriptions of joy in animals, which Darwin thought was expressed through laughter in other primates, in addition to humans, and he mentioned that chimpanzees and orangutans were observed to grin or smile when laughing. Although other mammals may not laugh, Darwin described how some make seemingly joyful sounds during meetings between parents and offspring, as well as other members of their own social group. Darwin recognized that laughter does not always express joy in humans, and he comments on the fact that humans frequently employ a forced laugh to conceal their actual state of mind, including shame or shyness. The book also devotes a great deal of space to the description and discussion of disgust in animals and humans.

7.2.3 Common Descent of Emotions

Darwin believed "that the chief expressive actions, exhibited by man and by the lower animals, are … innate or inherited – that is, [they] have not been learnt by the individual" (p. 351) [2]. Being innate, they "cannot be said to depend on the will of the individual" (p. 353) [2]. Although Darwin thought the similarities in the expressions of emotions by different animals demonstrated common descent, it was not as easy to demonstrate the common descent of behaviors as it was to demonstrate the common descent of structures as he had done in *The Origin of Species* and *The Descent of Man*. Thus, *The Expression of Emotions* provided extensive descriptions of the similarities in the expression of emotions and the muscles used in their expression, as well as numerous pictures of emotional expressions. However, muscles and bones can only tell us so much about emotions [13, 14] because emotions are seated in the brain [15, 16], and though the gross anatomy of the brain was known when *The Expression of Emotions* was published, the relationship between brain structure and function was not [17].

7.3 Chapter Highlights and Comments

Darwin's second book about evolution, *The Descent of Man*, extends the theory of common descent to humans and expands upon his grandfather's notion that competition for mates has lead to unique adaptations among males of a species that enhance their reproductive success. Darwin introduced the ideas that human and animals have similar mental faculties (now called the theory of the "continuity of mind") [5, 6] in *The Descent of Man*, and expanded upon this with regard to emotions in *The Expression of Emotions*. However, knowledge about the overt expression of emotions provides only a limited understanding of emotions, which are products of the brain.

References

1. Darwin, C. (1871). *The descent of man and selection in relation to sex* (Vol. 1). London: John Murray.
2. Darwin, C. (1872). *The expression of emotions in man and animals*. London: John Murray.
3. Romer, A. S. (1970). *The vertebrate body* (4th ed.). Philadelphia: W.B. Saunders.
4. Romer, A. S. (1959). *The vertebrate story* (4th ed.). Chicago: University of Chicago Press.
5. Bolhuis, J. J., & Wynne, C. D. L. (2009). Can evolution explain how minds work? *Nature, 548*, 832–833.
6. Hauser, M. (2009, September). The mind. *Scientific American*, pp. 44–51.
7. Moore, J. (1991). The politics of evolution in the 1860s. *Journal of the History of Biology 24*(3), 353–408.
8. Francis, K. A. (2007). *Charles Darwin and The Origin of Species*. Westport: Greenwood Press.
9. O'Connell, H. P. (2008). 150 years of evolutionary theory. *British Journal of Psychiatry, 193*, 258–259.
10. Adriaens, P. R., & de Block, A. (2010). The evolutionary turn in psychiatry: A historical overview. *History of Psychiatry, 21*(2), 131–143.
11. Cuzzillo, S. L. W. (1991). Historical contingencies in the evolution of human behavior and psychopathology. *Psychiatry, 54*(2), 187–207.
12. Thorpe, W. H. (1973). Ethology as a new branch of biology. In M. W. Fox (Ed.), *Readings in ethology and comparative psychology* (pp. 5–23). Monterey: Books/Cole.
13. Hinde, R. H., & Tinbergen, N. H. (1973). The comparative study of species-specific behavior. In M. W. Fox (Ed.), *Readings in ethology and comparative psychology* (pp. 30–48). Monterey: Books/Cole.
14. Atz, J. W. (1970). The application of the idea of homology to behavior. In L. R. Aronson, E. Tobach, D. S. Lehrman, & J. S. Rosenblatt (Eds.), *Development and evolution of behavior* (pp. 53–74). San Francisco: W. H. Freeman and Company.
15. Panksepp, J. (2005). Affective consciousness: Core emotional feelings in animals and humans. *Consciousness and Cognition, 14*(1), 30–80.
16. Panksepp, J. (1998). *Affective neuroscience: The foundations of human and animal emotions*. New York: Oxford University Press.
17. Finger, S. (2004). *Minds behind the brain: A history of the pioneers and their discoveries*. Oxford: Oxford University Press.

Chapter 8
Reactions to *The Expression of Emotions*

Abstract The chapter describes how psychologists and biologists reacted to Charles Darwin's *The Expression of Emotions*, which has been called the first book on Evolutionary Psychiatry. The reactions of psychologists have been mixed over the years. Evolution became an element of the Functionalist school of American psychology in the early 20th Century, but evolution was ignored by the Behaviorist school of American psychology for the rest of the century. As the chapter explains, it was not until the end of the century that a group of U.S. researchers began the field of Evolutionary Psychology to apply evolutionary principles to understand the cognitive processes underlying human culture and social relationships, including gender roles, mate selection, and parental investment. *The Expression of Emotions* and evolutionary theory, in general, had a more profound and sustained effect on the field of ethology, which originated in Europe as a branch of biology that studies the evolutionary adaptiveness of instinctive behavior in animals. The chapter introduces the ethological concept of fixed-action patterns in animals, which has implications for understanding certain human psychiatric symptoms, as discussed in later chapters. The chapter also explains the relationship between Aristotle's four causes and the modern scientific concepts of the proximate causes (or proximate mechanisms) and the ultimate causes of behavior (and anatomy), and gives examples of the proximate causes and ultimate causes of territorial aggression in animals and eating in humans.

Keywords Continuity of mind • Ethology • Evolutionary psychology • *Expression of Emotions* • Fixed-action patterns • Proximate cause • Ultimate cause

The publication of *The Expression of Emotion* led, directly or indirectly, to the development of several schools of thought and scientific fields. The first field that can be directly linked to the book is comparative psychology [1], which was founded by a young colleague of Charles Darwin, George J. Romanes. Romanes wrote a series of books, not about animal emotions, but about animal intelligence, which primarily consisted of compilations of anecdotes about animal behavior [2–4]. Romanes completely accepted the "theory of continuity of mind" at face value. Hence, he seems to have seen intelligence in every creature and everything they did

K.J. Flannelly, *Religious Beliefs, Evolutionary Psychiatry, and Mental Health in America*, Religion, Spirituality and Health: A Social Scientific Approach 1,
DOI 10.1007/978-3-319-52488-7_8

[2], saying of microscopic animals: "No one can watch the movements of [protozoa] without feeling it difficult to believe that these little animals are not actuated by some amount of intelligence" (p. 18) [5]. The British psychologist William McDougall [3] appears to have taken the opposite message from *The Expression of Emotions*, as he believed that human behavior was mainly the product of innate or native abilities [6].

8.1 American Psychology

American psychology has been inconsistent in its reaction to Darwin's *Expression of Emotions* and his theory of evolution, in general. Several prominent American psychologists endorsed Darwin's theory of evolution around the turn of the century [7]. These like-minded psychologists and the philosopher and psychologist John Dewy created the Functional school of psychology, or Functionalism, in the 1890s to apply Darwin's approach to the study of the mind and mental processes [3, 7]. However, the brief ascendance of Functionalism in American psychology was undercut by John B Watson, who founded Behaviorism in 1913 [8]. Watson sought to change American psychology from a science of consciousness, or mind, to a science of behavior [9]. He not only dismissed the notion of studying consciousness in animals, he dismissed the notion of studying it in humans, saying that consciousness should be abolished from psychology [9]. Later Behaviorists claimed that all behaviors were learned and they denied the existence of innate or instinctive behavior except for simple reflexes [10, 11]. B.F. Skinner, who came to personify Behaviorism [12, 13] and its emphasis on learned behavior, claimed to accept that evolution had shaped animals over time, but he ignored its influence on animal behavior and doubted its influence on human behavior [14–16].

Behaviorism was the major force in American psychology until the 1970s [3, 17] when renewed interest emerged in the study of the mind [17], and by the 1980s cognitive psychology dominated psychological research in the U.S. [17]. A small group of these researchers began the field of "evolutionary psychology" to apply evolutionary principles to the cognitive processes underlying human culture and social relationships [18–22], including gender roles, mate selection, and parental investment, which are phenomena that are closely tied to Darwin's theory of sexual selection [19, 23].

Although evolutionary psychologists are obviously interested in the degree to which evolution has influenced human psychology, their interest to date has been relatively narrow, and most of their research does not directly address mental health, per se. However, one research topic in evolutionary psychology is particularly pertinent to mental health – i.e., the human ability to detect cheating in social relations [21]. Since humans are highly social animals, reciprocity in social exchanges is extremely important; thus, cheating (i.e., non-reciprocity) can be advantageous.[21] Leda Cosmides and John Tooby, two of the founders of evolutionary psychology, have suggested that both cheating and the ability to detect cheating have evolved relatively recently in humans [21]. Their analysis of cheating and its detection is quite interesting although they ignore paranoia, which appears to be a very old mechanism to detect cheating that probably antedates the evolution of humans. Their later analysis of fear is also superficial, [24, 25] in that it seems to imply that fear evolved as an adaptation in humans, when fear actually evolved in our ancient animal ancestors as a warning signal of potential danger.

There are several basic assumptions of evolutionary psychology that have been the subject of criticism. One assumption is that the period of earth history called the Pleistocene [20, 26], which extended from roughly 1.8 million years ago to 11,000 years ago [26], is a critical period for human adaption. Evolutionary psychologists call this period the "Environment of Evolutionary Adaptedness" because they believe this is the timeframe in which current humans evolved adaptations that led to their unique reproductive success and allowed them to populate the world. This may be a reasonable assumption with respect to the evolution of certain aspects of human cognition; however, it minimizes the importance of the adaptations of our animal ancestors that occurred during the vast periods of geological time before the Pleistocene [27]. Another assumption is that Natural Selection would have favored the evolution of specific cognitive systems, or "modules," to solve specific types of problems, rather than a general problem-solving system, as psychologists long have presumed [19, 28]. While neuroscience research has identified numerous special-purpose neural circuits in sub-cortical areas of the brain, which evolved long before the Pleistocene, there is no evidence of special-purpose neural circuits in the cortical areas that are involved in cognition [27, 29] Finally, the presumption of evolutionary psychology that human adaptations for addressing social relationships are primarily cognitive excludes the interplay between emotional and cognitive brain systems, as I will discuss later [27].

8.2 European Ethology

The modern field of ethology began to take form in the 1920s and 1930s, with the research of the European naturalists Karl von Frisch [30], Konrad Lorenz [31, 32], and Nikolaas Tinbergen [33, 34] who jointly won the 1973 Nobel Prize in "Medicine or Physiology" for their naturalistic research on animal behavior. While American Behaviorists studied learning in college students and domesticated (i.e., laboratory) rats [35, 36], European ethologists studied innate behavior patterns in insects, fish, birds, and other wild animals [30, 31, 33, 34, 37]. Like students of Natural History before them, ethologists devote a great deal of time to observing animals in their natural environments to make detailed descriptions of the animal in its world [38–40]. It is only after extensive observation that ethologists conduct "naturalistic" experiments to examine how the instinctive behaviors of different species of animals are adaptive [40].

Konrad Lorenz realized the key to understanding instinctive behaviors (i.e., inherited behaviors) was to identify discrete sets or units of behavior that were rigidity performed in specific sequences by individuals of the same species, which he called fixed-action patterns [1, 32, 40, 41]. Fixed-action patterns are used for many types of functions, including nest-building, grooming, courtship and mating, and agonistic behaviors (e.g., attack, threat, defense, and submission). Agonistic behaviors are used in establishing and maintaining social hierarchies and territory. Fixed-actions patterns are not only highly ritualized, they often are very repetitive.

Fixed-action patterns are also called "species-specific" behaviors because they are performed in nearly the exact same way by all members of the same species [40, 42]. However, many so-called "species-specific" behaviors actually are quite similar across related species and the commonalties among the fixed-action patterns of different species have been used to provide evidence of their common evolutionary heritage, similar to the way in which common anatomical features are used to demonstrate common descent [1, 42–45]. This is possible because the ritualistic (or stereotypical) nature of fixed-action patterns provides a kind of structure to behavior that permits units of behavior and combinations of units to be compared across species, genera, families, and orders of animals [45, 46].

As the behavioral branch of biology [40], a key question in ethology is: What is a given behavior for? [32, 40] which corresponds to Aristotle's final cause. In modern terminology, Aristotle's final cause [47, 48] is called the ultimate cause or distal cause of something. Within biology, including ethology, another way of expressing this question is: How is this characteristic (a structure or behavior) adaptive for an animal? Another type of question one may ask about a behavior or other characteristic is: How does it work? This type of question refers to what is called a proximate cause of something. Just as Aristotle proposed different ways of considering the cause of something, so do modern biologists. The proximate causes of modern science (also called proximate mechanisms) are grossly similar to Aristotle's first three causes in that they define how the ultimate cause is achieved.

The ethologist Robert Hinde illustrated different perspectives one might take in trying to answer questions of causation, using the thumb as an example: "Why does your thumb move in a different way than the other fingers?" Hinde's first response to this question illustrated an answer from the perspective of proximate causes or proximate mechanisms: The thumb moves in a different way than the other fingers because of "differences in the skeletal structure and muscle attachments between the thumb and the other fingers." Another of his examples illustrated an answer from the perspective of ultimate cause: The thumb moves in a different way than the other fingers because "an opposable thumb makes it easier for us to pick things up, climb trees, and so on" (p. 21) [46]. One might ask a similar question about animal behavior: Why do male animals of the same species fight each other? Based on Darwin's theory of sexual selection, the ultimate cause is to secure access to females in order to reproduce. However, the proximate causes, at different levels of explanation, may be: (a) to defend their territory; (b) because they respond aggressively to the sight or odor of nearby males; (c) increased testosterone levels at certain times of the year make them aggressive; (d) the presence of another male activates the part of the brain that elicits aggression; or (e) part of their brain is genetically programmed to attack another male. A question more in keeping with our everyday experience, might be, Why do we eat? The ultimate cause is to obtain the nourishment we need to live. However, the proximate causes, may be: (a) the sight and smell of food; (b) our blood sugar is low; (c) we feel a sense of hunger; (d) a part of the brain that monitors blood sugar triggers hunger; or (e) part of the brain is genetically programmed to trigger hunger when our blood sugar is low.

Finally, Hinde makes a very important point concerning evolution when he discusses that Natural Selection does not act on specific traits or characteristics, but on individuals. As such, selection reflects a balance between different adaptations, some of which may have potentially adverse as well as beneficial effects on an individual, and some of which may conflict with one another, but collectively enhance survival and/or reproductive success [46].

8.3 Chapter Highlights and Comments

Darwin's book, *The Expression of Emotions*, initially caught the attention of psychologists, but interest in evolution among American psychologists has fluctuated over the years. The current field of evolutionary psychology reflects the post-Behaviorist surge in interest in the mind among American psychologists, and it has re-introduced evolutionary principles to psychology. However, it has focused on putative human adaptations that are assumed to have evolved very recently in geological time. Ethology, a branch of biology, has made significant contributions to our understanding of the evolution of innate behavior in animals, which as we will see, have important implications for understanding the relationship between the brain and behavior, including psychiatric symptoms. The concept of proximate mechanisms is particularly important for understanding the evolutionary basis of psychiatric symptoms.

References

1. Thorpe, W. H. (1973). Ethology as a new branch of biology. In M. W. Fox (Ed.), *Readings in ethology and comparative psychology* (pp. 5–23). Monterey: Books/Cole.
2. Breed, M. D., & Moore, J. (2011). *Animal behavior*. Waltham: Academic Press.
3. Boring, E. G. (1950). *A history of experimental psychology* (2 ed.). New York: Appleton Century Crofts which will.
4. Greeberg, G. (2013). Historical review of the use of captive animals and comparative psychology. In E. Tobach (Ed.), *Historical perspectives and the international status of comparative psychology*. East Sussex: Psychology Press.
5. Romanes, G. J. (1882). *Animal intelligence*. London: Kegan Paul, Trench & Co.
6. McDougall, W. (1933). *The energies of men*. New York: Charles Scribner's Sons.
7. Green, C. D. (2009). Darwinian theory, functionalism, and the first American psychological revolution. *American Psychologist, 64*(2), 75–83.
8. Heidbreder, E. (1933). *Seven psychologies*. New York: Appleton-Century-Crofts.

9. Watson, J. B. (1913). Psychology as a behaviorist views it. *Psychological Review, 20*(2), 158–177.
10. Beach, F. A. (1955). The descent of instinct. *Psychological Review, 62*(6), 401–100.
11. Herrnstein, R. J. (1972). Nature as nurture: Behaviorsm and the instinct doctrine. *Behaviorism, 1*(1), 23–32.
12. Herrnstein, R. J. (1977). The evolution of behaviorism. *American Psychologist, 32*(8), 593–603.
13. Skinner, B. F. (1938). *The behavior of organisms: An experimental analysis*. New York: Appleton-Century-Crofts.
14. Skinner, B. F. (1990). Can psychology be a science of the mind? *American Psychologist, 45*(11), 1206–1210.
15. Skinner, B. F. (1968). The phylogeny and ontogeny of behavior. *Science, 153*(3741), 1205–1213.
16. Skinner, B. F. (1976). *About Behaviorism*. New York: Vintage Books.
17. Robins, R. W., Gosling, S. D., & Craik, K. H. (1999). An empirical analysis of trends in psychology. *American Psychologist, 54*(2), 117–128.
18. Barkow, J., Cosmides, L., & Tooby, J. (Eds.). (1992). *The adapted mind: Evolutionary psychology and the generation of culture*. New York: Oxford University Press.
19. Buss, D. M. (1990). Evolutionary social psychology: Prospects and pitfalls. *Motivation and Emotion, 14*(4), 265–286.
20. Tooby, J., & Cosmides, L. (1989). Evolutionary psychology and the generation of culture, Part I: Theoretical considerations. *Ethology and Sociobiology, 10*(1), 29–49.
21. Cosmides, L., & Tooby, J. (1992). Cognitive adaptations for social exchange. In J. Barkow, L. Cosmides, & J. Tooby (Eds.), *The adapted mind: Evolutionary psychology and the generation of culture*. New York: Oxford University Press.
22. Buss, D. M. (1994). *The evolution of desire*. New York: Basic Books.
23. Nisbett, R. E. (1990). Evolutionary psychology, biology, and cultural evolution. *Motivation and Emotion, 14*(4), 255–263.
24. Cosmides, L., & Tooby, J. (2000). Evolutionary psychology and the emotions. In M. Lewis, & J. M. Haviland-Jones (Eds.), *Handbook of emotions* (pp. 91–115). New York: Guilford Press.
25. Cosmides, L., & Tooby, J. (2008). Evolutionary psychology and the emotions and their relationship to internal regulatory variables. In M. Lewis, J. M. Haviland-Jones, & L. F. Barrett (Eds.), *Handbook of emotions* (3rd ed., pp. 114–137). New York: Guilford Press.
26. Eastwick, P. W. (2009). Beyond the Pleistocene: Using phylogeny and constraint to inform the evolutionary psychology of human mating. *Psychological Bulletin, 135*(5), 794–281.
27. Panksepp, J., & Panksepp, J. B. (2000). The seven sins of evolutionary psychology. *Evolution and Cognition, 6*(2), 108–131.
28. Tooby, J., & Cosmides, L. (1992). The psychological foundations of culture. In J. Barkow, L. Cosmides, & J. Tooby (Eds.), *The adapted mind: Evolutionary psychology and the generation of culture*. New York: Oxford University Press.
29. Panksepp, J. (1998). *Affective neuroscience: The foundations of human and animal emotions*. New York: Oxford University Press.
30. von Frisch, K. (1966). *The dancing bees: An account of the life and senses of the honey bee*. London: Methuen.
31. Lorenz, K. A. (1961). *King Solomon's ring* (M. K. Wilson, Trans.). London: Methuen.
32. Lorenz, K. (1981). *The foundations of ethology*. New York: Spinger-Verlag.
33. Tinbergen, N. (1972). *The animal in its world: Explorations of an ethologist* (Vol. 1). Cambridge, MA: Harvard University Press.
34. Tinbergen, N. (1968). *Curious naturalists*. Garden City: Anchor Books.
35. Hall, J. F. (1966). *The psychology of learning*. Philadelphia: J.B. Lippincott.
36. Deese, J., & Hulse, S. H. (1967). *The psychology of learning* (3rd ed.). New York: McGraw-Hill.

37. Schiller, C. H. (Ed.). (1975). *Instinctive behavior: The development of the modern concept*. New York: International Universities Press.
38. von Uexkull, J. (1975). A stroll through the world of animals and men. In C. H. Schiller (Ed.), *Instinctive behavior: The development of the modern concept* (pp. 5–80). New York: International Universities Press.
39. Tinbergen, N. (1975). Preface. In C. H. Schiller (Ed.), *Instinctive behavior: The development of the modern concept* (pp. 15–19). New York: International Universities Press.
40. Tinbergen, N. (1963). On the aims and methods of ethology. *Zeitschrift furTierpsychologie, 26*, 410–433.
41. Moltz, H. (1965). Contemporary instinct theory and the fixed action pattern. *Psychological Review, 72*(1), 27–47.
42. Hinde, R. H., & Tinbergen, N. H. (1973). The comparative study of species-specific behavior. In M. W. Fox (Ed.), *Readings in ethology and comparative psychology* (pp. 30–48). Monterey: Books/Cole.
43. Atz, J. W. (1970). The application of the idea of homology to behavior. In L. R. Aronson, E. Tobach, D. S. Lehrman, & J. S. Rosenblatt (Eds.), *Development and evolution of behavior* (pp. 53–74). San Francisco: W. H. Freeman and Company.
44. Mayr, E. (1958). Behavior and systematics. In A. Roe (Ed.), *Behavior and evolution* (pp. 341–362). New Haven: Yale University Press.
45. Lorenz, K. (1975). Comparative study of behavior. In C. H. Schiller (Ed.), *Instinctive behavior: The development of the modern concept* (pp. 239–263). New York: International Universities Press.
46. Hinde, R. H. (1982). *Ethology: Its nature and relations with other sciences*. Oxford: Oxford University Press.
47. Aristotle (1961). *Aristotle's physics* (R. Hope, Trans.). Lincoln: University of Nebraska Press.
48. Aristotle (1991). *The metaphysics* (J. H. McMahon, Trans.). Buffalo: Prometheus Books.

Part III
Evolutionary Psychiatry

Chapter 9
Brain Evolution and Emotions

Abstract The chapter explains the American neuroscientist Paul MacLean's concept of the "Triune Brain," illustrates its basic structure, and discusses the evolution and functions of the major brain structures involved in instinctual and emotional behavior in animals and humans. These include the brain stem and basal ganglia, which form the most primitive parts of the brain, and are involved in self-protection and other basic functions needed to survive. The basal ganglia, for instance, is known to control species-specific, fixed-action patterns related to eating, drinking, courtship, and territorial behaviors in lizards. The limbic system, which MacLean thought evolved in early mammals and incorporated many of the functions of the brain stem and the basal ganglia in animals, has been implicated in at least six basic emotions in mammals: anger/aggression, fear, grief, lust/mating, maternal love, and joy. As the chapter explains, emotions, which probably did not exist until the evolution of the limbic system, provided mammals with superior flexibility to respond to life challenges and other circumstances. The chapter further explains that the evolution of the neocortex added even greater flexibility to respond to a variety of life situations by inhibiting the more or less automatic reactions of the brain stem, basal ganglia, and the limbic system. Finally, the chapter introduces the idea that the expansion of the neocortex reflects the evolution of causal beliefs about the nature of the world in our primitive human ancestors.

Keywords Basal ganglia • Brain • Brain stem • Causal beliefs • Emotions • Evolution • Evolutionary psychiatry • Limbic system • MacLean • Neocortex • Triune Brain

9.1 The Triune Brain and Behavior

The American physician and neuroscientist Paul D. MacLean coined the term "evolutionary psychiatry" and established its neuro-anatomical foundations [1–3]. MacLean started publishing his ideas about the association between evolution and psychiatric problems in the late 1940s and early 1950s [4, 5]. Over the years, MacLean developed and elaborated the premise that the human brain is composed of three distinctive "brains" that evolved at different points in time [1, 2, 6, 7].

K.J. Flannelly, *Religious Beliefs, Evolutionary Psychiatry, and Mental Health in America*, Religion, Spirituality and Health: A Social Scientific Approach 1,
DOI 10.1007/978-3-319-52488-7_9

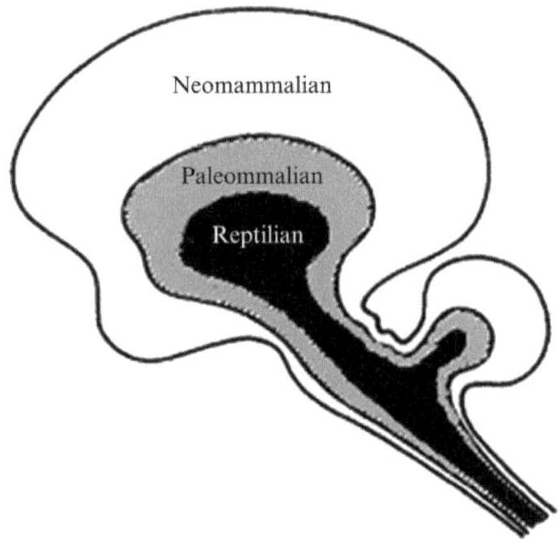

Fig. 9.1 Adapted drawing of Paul MacLean's "Triune Brain" (Maclean, 1967) [8]

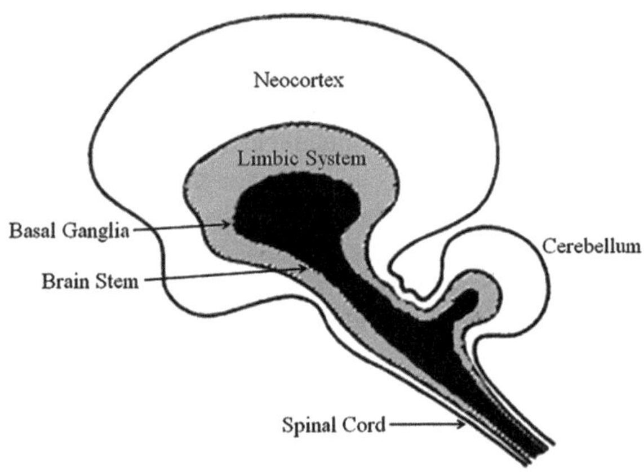

Fig. 9.2 Adapted drawing of Paul MacLean's "Triune Brain" (Maclean, 1967) [8], replacing his terminology with commonly accepted terminology. Additional brain areas have been labeled

MacLean's concept of the "Triune Brain" is depicted in Fig. 9.1 [2, 6–8], which shows the left half of the human brain. Although MacLean's model is a gross simplification of the anatomy of the brain, it is generally accurate and it is useful for our purposes in that it illustrates that newer parts of the brain evolved by developing outside of already existing brain systems [9]. MacLean called the oldest part of the brain of modern mammals the reptilian brain (shown in black) because it is structurally and functionally similar to the brain of reptiles. He thought the paleomammalian brain evolved in early mammals and the neomammalian brain evolved in modern mammals. The size of the neomammalian brain depicted in his model reflects its expansion during the evolution of primates and humans. Figure 9.2 shows the common technical terms used in reference to the brain regions illustrated in MacLean's model [9]. Many species of animals do not even have a brain [10] and the brains of vertebrate species vary greatly in terms of their complexity [11, 12]. The brain stem, which is part of MacLean's reptilian brain, extends roughly from the arrow marked "Spinal Cord" to the arrow marked "Brain Stem" in Fig. 9.2. It probably evolved in primitive early fish [13] to regulate vital reflexes, such as heart rate, respiration, sleeping, and eating, and to coordinate reflexive muscle activity, which it still controls in humans and other vertebrates. The cerebellum, which also is involved in muscle movements, is not a central feature of MacLean's model.

The other portion of MacLean's reptilian brain (the black bulge above the brain stem) contains the basal ganglia, whose main structures are the striatum and the pallidum. The basal ganglia evolved in later fish [14, 15] and they are the capstone of brain development in early amphibians and some reptiles [15]. Although their structure is similar in amphibians, reptiles, and mammals [14–18], their structural elaboration from amphibians to reptiles probably contributed to the increased behavioral repertoire of reptiles [15]. The basal ganglia are known to control species-specific, fixed-action patterns related to eating, drinking, courtship, and territorial behaviors in lizards [2, 19]. They also are known to control the highly repetitive, fixed-action patterns used for digging and grooming in mammals [20–24].

9.2 The Triune Brain and Emotions

MacLean, who coined the terms "limbic system" [25] and "paleomammalian brain," referred to the limbic system as the paleomammalian brain because of its prominent role in the evolution of mammalian behavior, even though limbic structures existed in a rudimentary form in reptiles, amphibians, and some fish [2, 9, 13, 26]. MacLean's research indicated that the limbic system is associated with maternal behavior in mammals and he expanded our knowledge about its role in emotions, which had been established by the classic work of James W. Papez in 1937 [27]. The limbic system is closely connected to the brain stem [28] and the basal ganglia in animals, and as the limbic system evolved it incorporated some of their functions [29, 30], especially the regulation of species-specific behaviors related to mating, territoriality, and self-defense, which were and still are, to some extent, controlled by the basal ganglia [31]. Further animal research has confirmed MacLean's findings [32] that the limbic system is involved in maternal behavior in mammals [31, 33]. It also receives extensive internal (e.g., visceral) and external (e.g., visual, auditory and, and olfactory) sensory input [2, 9].

Although many neuroscientists dismiss the idea that the limbic system is, itself, a neural circuit or system, the structures that the term encompasses are involved in a number of emotional systems. Indeed, Jaak Panksepp, an American psychologist and neuroscientist, has indentified six basic emotional systems in mammals that involve limbic structures: (1) anger and aggression, (2) fear (3), grief, (4) courtship and mating, (5) maternal care, and (6) play and joy [9, 33–35]. One of the major evolutionary adaptations of the limbic system is that it provided mammals with superior flexibility to recognize and respond to immediate threats of harm and other life challenges compared to the primitive brain of reptiles [9].

9.3 The Neocortex

Early mammals, which evolved 280 million years ago or so, were about the size of a mouse or rat, and they had disproportionately small brains for their size [36]. Their neocortex was also small and thin [36, 37]. As mammals evolved, the neocortex became larger due to an increase in its number of layers and the development of specialized areas of the cortex [9, 36, 37].

The size of the neocortex increased tremendously in the primates [38, 39], which first appeared in the fossil record around 60 million years ago [40]. There are two major hypotheses about the increase in the size of the neocortex [38, 41–43]. One hypothesis is that the enlargement of the neocortex reflects the increased cognitive ability of primates to adapt to environments with different ecologies. The other hypothesis is that the enlargement of the neocortex reflects the increased cognitive ability of primates to deal with more complex social relationships [38, 41]. There is support for both hypotheses and it is likely that both factors influenced cortical evolution to some extent [41–43].

In any case, the neocortex, like the limbic system before it, added greater flexibility to the functioning of lower brain systems [9]. This greater flexibility is partly due to the capacity of cortical structures to inhibit the activity of subcortical structures [9, 44]. Although the neocortex is involved in the regulation of emotions [33, 45, 46], the generation of emotions is thought to be the product of subcortical structures in the limbic system, basal ganglia, and brain stem [2, 9, 33]. An area of the neocortex called the prefrontal cortex (PFC), which has reciprocal connections with the brain stem [45], the basal ganglia [47–49], the and limbic system [47–51], is thought to be involved in the regulation of emotions in non-human primates and other mammals.

The size of the human brain has continued to increase since the human lineage separated from the other primates 3.5 million years ago [52]. The neocortex, in particular, has grown much larger in humans, and it is even larger than the neocortex of the "great apes," who are our nearest living relatives [53]. Specific areas of the cortex also have enlarged in humans, especially the PFC [54–56]. One reason for the larger size of the PFC in humans is the fact that it is involved in language [57], but another reason is that the human PFC has extensive interconnections with other brain areas [54]. These neural interconnections include connections with the brain stem, basal ganglia, and the limbic system [50, 51, 58–60], which may have allowed the PFC to extend its control over the subcortical structures that generate innate defensive reactions and fear.

A 2007 book by the British evolutionary biologist Dr. Lewis Wolpert [61, 62] proposed that much of the increase in the size of the human neocortex is attributable to the manufacture and use of tools by early members of our own species (*Homo sapiens*) and our immediate human predecessor (*Homo erectus*) [63–65]. *Homo habilis,* which evolved before and overlapped in time with *Homo erectus* [63–65], was given its Latin name (the English equivalent of "handy man") by its discovers (archeologist Mary Leakey and paleontologist Louis Leaky) because of the large quantity of stone tools uncovered in association with its fossilized remains [64, 65]. Wolpert argued that tool use and tool making led to the development of causal beliefs about why things happen and how things work, which, along with the later evolution of language, greatly contributed to the expansion of the human neocortex [61, 62]. I will talk more about Wolpert's ideas in Chap. 13.

9.4 Chapter Highlights and Comments

The gross structure of the modern mammalian brain roughly reflects the evolutionary development of the brains of later mammals and the early mammals and reptiles that preceded them. Here, I have attempted to explain how the different regions of Paul MacLean's "Triune Brain" are involved in the processing of emotions. The brain stem is the most primitive portion of the brain, and the basal ganglia, which evolved later, are both involved in innate defensive behaviors, which are so primitive that they probably evolved before emotions, per se, existed. The primary emotional area of the brain, the limbic system, is involved in several distinct emotional systems, including aggression, fear, and grief.

The evolution of the limbic system created a more flexible response to environmental challenges to survival. The evolution of the neocortex provided even greater flexibility, partially through its capacity to inhibit the activity of subcortical structures. The area of the neocortex called the prefrontal cortex is the principal area of the cortex regulating emotions, especially fear.

The increased size of the neocortex in humans and other primates appears to be the result of several factors, including the social complexity or primate social groups and the need to adapt to environments with different ecologies. However, the even greater expansion of the human neocortex has been attributed to the evolution of causal beliefs about the nature of the world and the subsequent evolution of language.

References

1. MacLean, P. D. (1985). Evolutionary psychiatry and the triune brain. *Psychological Medicine, 15*(2), 219–221.
2. MacLean, P. D. (1990). *The triune brain in evolution: Role in paleocerebral functions*. New York: Plenum Press.
3. Newman, J. D., & Harris, J. C. (2009). The scientific contributions of Paul D. MacLean (1913–2007). *Journal of Nervous and Mental Disease, 197*(1), 3–5.
4. Ploog, D. W. (2003). The place of the Triune Brain in psychiatry. *Physiology and Behavior, 79*(3), 487–493.
5. MacLean, P. D. (1952). Some psychiatric implications of physiological studies on frontotemporal portion of limbic system (visceral brain). *Electroencephalography and Clinical Neurophysiology, 4*(4), 407–418.

6. MacLean, P. D. (1977). The Triune Brain in conflict. *Psychotherapy and Psychosomatics, 28*, 207–220.
7. MacLean, P. D. (1972). Cerebral evolution and emotional processes: New findings on the striatal complex. *Annals of the New York Academy of Sciences, 193*, 137–149.
8. MacLean, P. D. (1967). The brain in relation to empathy and medical education. *Journal of Nervous and Mental Disease, 144*(5), 374–382.
9. Panksepp, J. (1998). *Affective neuroscience: The foundations of human and animal emotions*. New York: Oxford University Press.
10. Farries, M. A. (2013). How 'basal' are the basal ganglia? *Brain, Behavior and Evolution, 82*(4), 211–214.
11. Romer, A. S. (1970). *The vertebrate body* (4th ed.). Philadelphia: W.B. Saunders.
12. Kent, G. C. (1973). *Comparative anatomy of the vertebrates*. Saint Louis: C.V. Mosby.
13. Aboitiz, F., & Montiel, J. (2007). *Origin and evolution of the vertebrate telencephalon, with special reference to the mammalian neocortex*. New York: Springer.
14. Medina, L., Abellan, A., Vicario, A., & Desfilis, E. (2014). Evolutionary and developmental contributions for understanding the organization of the basal ganglia. *Brain, Behavior and Evolution, 83*(2), 112–125.
15. Reiner, A., Medina, L., & Veenman, C. L. (1998). Structural and functional evolution of the basal ganglia in vertebrates. *Brain Research Reviews, 28*(3), 235–285.
16. Marín, O., Smeets, W. J., & González, A. (1998). Evolution of the basal ganglia in tetrapods: A new perspective based on recent studies in amphibians. *Trends in Neurosciences, 11*(1), 487–494.
17. Medina, L., & Reiner, A. (1995). Neurotransmitter organization and connectivity of the basal ganglia in vertebrates: Implications for the evolution of basal ganglia. *Brain, Behavior and Evolution, 46*(4–5), 235–246.
18. Smeets, W. J., Marin, O., & Gonzalez, A. (2000). Evolution of the basal ganglia: New perspectives through a comparative approach. *Journal of Anatomy, 196*(4), 501–517.
19. Tarr, R. S. (1982). Species typical display behavior following stimulation of the reptilian striatum. *Physiology & Behavior, 29*(4), 615–620.
20. Liu, C., & Cerny, V. (1976). Release of grooming responses in basal ganglia and thalamic cats. *Anatomical Record, 184*(3), 464.
21. Strazielle, C., Lefevre, A., Jacquelin, C., & Lalonde, R. (2012). Abnormal grooming activity in Dab1 scm (scrambler) mutant mice. *Behavioural Brain Research, 233*(1), 24–28.
22. Cromwell, H. C., & Berridge, K. C. (1996). Implementation of action sequences by a neostriatal site: A lesion mapping study of grooming syntax. *Journal of Neuroscience, 16*(10), 3444–3458.
23. Thompson, R., Huestis, P. W., Shea, C. N., Crinella, F. M., & Yu, Y. (1990). Brain structures important for solving a sawdust-digging problem in the rat. *Physiology & Behavior, 48*(1), 107–111.
24. Aldridge, J. W., Berridge, K. C., & Rosen, A. R. (2004). Basal ganglia neural mechanisms of natural movement sequences. *Canadian Journal of Physiology and Pharmacology, 82*, 732–739.
25. Holden, C. (1979). Paul MacLean and the triune brain. *Science, 204*(4397), 1066–1068.
26. Cory, G. A., & Gardner, R. (Eds.). (2002). *The evolutionary neuroethology of Paul MacLean: Convergences and frontiers*. Westport: Greenwood Publishing Group.
27. Papez, J. W. (1937). A proposed mechanism of emotion. *Archives of Neurology and Psychiatry, 38*, 725–745.
28. Price, J. L. (2003). Comparative aspects of amygdala connectivity. *Annals of the New York Academy of Sciences, 985*, 50–58.
29. Laberge, F., Muhlenbrock-Lenter, S., Grunwald, W., & Roth, G. (2006). Evolution of the amygdala: New insights from studies in amphibians. *Brain, Behavior and Evolution, 67*, 177–187.

30. Gray, T. S. (1999). Functional and anatomical relationships among the amygdala, basal forebrain, ventral striatum, and cortex. An integrative discussion. *Annals of the New York Academy of Sciences, 29*, 439–444.
31. Sokolowski, K., & Corbin, J. G. (2012). Wired for behaviors: From development to function of innate limbic system circuitry. *Frontiers in Molecular Neuroscience, 5*(55), 1–15.
32. MacLean, P. D. (1985). Brain evolution relating to family, play, and the separation call. *Archives of General Psychiatry, 42*(4), 405–417.
33. Panksepp, J. (2011). The basic emotional circuits of mammalian brains: Do animals have affective lives? *Neuroscience & Biobehavioral Reviews, 35*(9), 1791–1804.
34. Panksepp, J. (2005). Affective consciousness: Core emotional feelings in animals and humans. *Consciousness and Cognition, 14*(1), 30–80.
35. Panksepp, J. (2010). Affective neuroscience of the emotional Brain Mind: Evolutionary perspectives and implications for understanding depression. *Dialogues in Clinical Neuroscience, 12*(4), 533–544.
36. Kaas, J. H. (2011). Reconstructing the areal organization of the neocortex of the first mammals. *Brain, Behavior and Evolution, 78*(1), 7–21.
37. Kaas, J. H. (2011). Neocortex in early mammals and its subsequent variations. *Annals of the New York Academy of Sciences, 1225*, 28–36.
38. Dunbar, R. I. M. (1992). Neocortex size as a constraint on group size in primates. *Journal of Human Evolution, 20*(469–493).
39. Finlay, B. L., & Darlington, R. B. (1995). Linked regularities in the development and evolution of mammalian brains. *Science, 268*, 1578–1584.
40. Seiffert, E. R. (2012). Early primate evolution in Afro-Arabia. *Evolutionary Anthropology, 21*(6), 239–253.
41. Boesch, C. (2012). The ecology and evolution of social behavior and cognition in primates. In J. Vonk, & T. K. Shackelford (Eds.), *The Oxford handbook of comparative evolutionary psychology* (pp. 489–503). Oxford: Oxford University Press.
42. Reader, S. M., & Laland, K. N. (2002). Social Intelligence, innovation, and enhanced brain size in primates. *Proceedings of the National Academy of Sciences, 99*(7), 4436–4441.
43. Reader, S. M., Hager, Y., & Laland, K. N. (2011). The evolution of primate general and cultural intelligence. *Philosophical Transactions of the the Royal Society, B, 366*(1567), 1017–1027.
44. Burgdorf, J., & Panksepp, J. (2006). The neurobiology of positive emotions. *Neuroscience and Biobehavioral Reviews, 30*(2), 173–187.
45. Groenewegen, H. J., & Uylings, H. B. M. (2000). The prefrontal cortex and the integration of sensory, limbic and autonomic information. *Progress in Brain Research, 126*, 3–28.
46. Panksepp, J., Fuchs, T., & Iacobucci, P. (2011). The basic neuroscience of emotional experiences in mammals: The case of subcortical FEAR circuitry and implications for clinical anxiety. *Applied Animal Behaviour Science, 129*(1), 1–17.
47. Groenewegen, H. J., Wright, C. I., & Uylings, H. B. M. (1997). The anatomical relationships of the prefrontal cortex with limbic structures and the basal ganglia. *Journal of Psychopharmacology, 11*(2), 99–106.
48. Groenewegen, H. J., Berendse, H. W., & Wolters, J. G. (1990). The anatomical relationship of the prefrontal cortex with the striatopallidal system, the thalamus and the amygdala: Evidence for parallel organization. *Progress in Brain Research, 85*, 95–116.
49. Masterman, D. L., & Cummings, J. L. (1997). Frontal-subcortical circuits: The anatomic basis of executive, social and motivated behaviors. *Journal of Psychopharmacology, 11*(2), 107–114.
50. Gee, D. G., Humphreys, K. L., Flannery, J., Goff, B., Telzer, E. H., Shapiro, M., et al. (2013). A developmental shift from positive to negative connectivity in human amygdala-prefrontal circuitry. *Journal of Neuroscience, 33*(10), 4584–4593.
51. Petrides, M., & Pandya, D. N. (2002). Comparative cytoarchitectonic analysis of the human and the macaque ventrolateral prefrontal cortex and corticocortical connection patterns in the monkey. *European Journal of Neuroscience, 16*(2), 291–310.

52. Roth, G., & Dicke, U. (2005). Evolution of the brain and intelligence. *Trends in Cognitive Sciences, 9*, 250–257.
53. Franks, D. D. (2010). *Neurosociology*. New York: Springer.
54. Schoenemann, P. T., Sheehan, M. J., & Glotzer, L. D. (2005). Prefrontal white matter volume is disproportionately larger in humans than in other primates. *Nature Neuroscience, 8*(2), 242–252.
55. Seyfarth, R. M., & Cheney, D. L. (2002). What are big brains for? *Proceedings of the National Academy of Sciences, 99*(7), 4141–4142.
56. Semendeferi, K., Armstrong, E., Schleicher, A., Zilles, K., & Van Hoesen, G. W. (2001). Prefrontal cortex in humans and apes: A comparative study of area 10. *American Journal of Physical Anthropology, 114*, 224–241.
57. Gabrieli, J. D. E., Poldrack, R. A., & Desmond, J. E. (1998). The role of left prefrontal cortex in language and memory. *Proceedings of the National Academy of Sciences, 95*(3), 906–913.
58. Middleton, F. A., & Strick, P. L. (2000). Basal ganglia output and cognition: Evidence from anatomical, behavioral, and clinical studies. *Brain and Cognition, 42*(2), 183–200.
59. Middleton, F. A., & Strick, P. L. (2000). Basal ganglia and cerebellar loops: Motor and cognitive circuits. *Brain Research Reviews, 31*(2–3), 236–250.
60. Jarbo, K., & Verstynen, T. D. (2015). Converging structural and functional connectivity of orbitofrontal, dorsolateral prefrontal, and posterior parietal cortex in the human striatum. *Journal of Neuroscience, 35*(9), 3865–3878.
61. Wolpert, L. (2007). *Six impossible things before breakfast: The evolutionary origins of beliefs*. New York: W.W. Norton & Co.
62. Flannelly, K. J. (2008). Review of the book *Six impossible things before breakfast: The evolutionary origins of beliefs* by L. Wolpert. *Journal of Nervous and Mental Disease*, *196*(7), 581–582.
63. Lewin, R. (2009). *Human evolution: An illustrated introduction* (5th ed.). Malden: Blackwell Publishing.
64. Tuttle, R.H. (2014). *Apes and human evolution*. Cambridge, MA: Harvard University Press.
65. Wood, B. (2014). Human evolution: Fifty years after *Homo habilis*. *Nature*, *508*(7494), 31–33.

Chapter 10
Fear in the Animal and Human Brain

Abstract The chapter summarizes current knowledge about the brain structures involved in fear in animals and humans. The periaqueductal gray of the brain stem is the most primitive structure known to be involved in defensive and fear-related behavior in animals and fear in humans. The basal ganglia are also involved in defensive and fear-related behavior in animals, but their role in human fear is not clear. As the chapter explains, the amygdala, which is a part of the limbic system, is the neural nexus of fear in the brain, and it appears to be the primary source of fear in mammals, including humans. Fear as we know it may not have existed before the evolution of the amygdala. The amygdala generates fear as part of its function to assess potential threats of physical harm and to warn us about them. The chapter explains how the amygdala, which is said to operate under the "better safe than sorry principle," tends to over-react to ambiguous stimuli as if they are threats, and therefore, produces fear even when something may not actually pose a threat of harm. This over-reaction can be countered by the prefrontal cortex, which makes it own threat assessments and can suppress the fear generated by the amygdala if it decides the fear is not justified.

Keywords Amygdala • Basal ganglia • Brain • Brain stem • Defense • Fear • Limbic system • Prefrontal cortex • Self-defense • Uncertainty

10.1 Fear in the Animal Brain

Figure 10.1 shows the major structures of the brain that are known to be involved in emotional behaviors in animals: the brain stem, the basal ganglia, the limbic system, and the prefrontal cortex (PFC). The PFC is set off from the rest of the neocortex by two grays lines in the figure. The arrow labeled "Brain Stem" points to the top of the brain stem, as in Fig. 9.2 [1].

The general location of three structures that play important roles in fear have been added to the figure. The round gray circle in the PFC is the ventromedial prefrontal cortex (vmPFC). The white oval in the limbic system is the amygdala, and the white line in the brain stem is the periaqueductal gray (PAG).

K.J. Flannelly, *Religious Beliefs, Evolutionary Psychiatry, and Mental Health in America*, Religion, Spirituality and Health: A Social Scientific Approach 1,
DOI 10.1007/978-3-319-52488-7_10

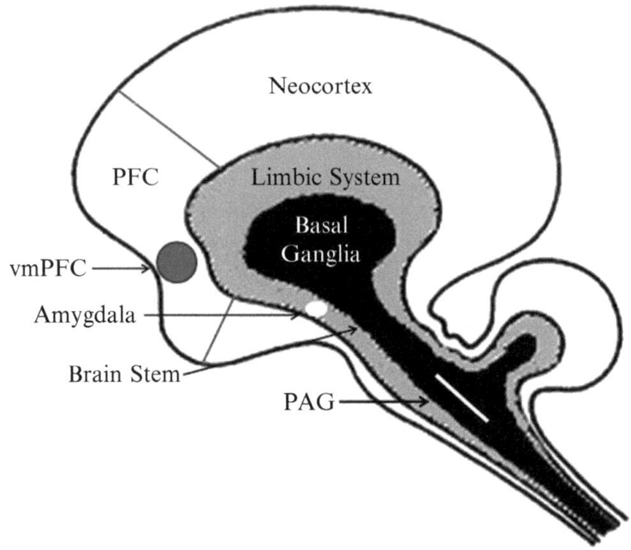

Fig. 10.1 Adapted drawing of Paul MacLean's "Triune Brain" showing key brain areas involved in fear and self-defense

10.1.1 Brain Stem

Early vertebrates were aquatic and they relied mainly on olfaction or other chemical senses to detect potential threats [2, 3]. Their simple brains, which were comparable to the brain stem, probably detected general threats posed by noxious chemicals using the concentration of a chemical to determine the proximity of danger. They may have assessed the presence of predators, which posed a specific threat to them, in a similar way.

As vertebrates evolved, vision began to play a larger role in threat detection. Fixed-action patterns, which already existed in primitive vertebrates, appear to have taken on a special role in intra-specific (with-in species) communication in fish, since they typically perform certain fixed-action patterns in response to specific visual signals or displays related to reproduction and aggression [4]. For example, extensive ethological research has demonstrated that specific signals (called sign stimuli) that denote threat automatically elicit specific defensive fixed-action-patterns in fish and other vertebrates.

Although I know of no research that directly connects brain stem activity to self-defense in fish, amphibians, or reptiles, limited research on mammals indicates that the brain stem clearly is involved in self-defense. The specific brain-stem structure involved in self-defense is the PAG, which activates innate, reflexive reactions to threats, including freezing and flight [5–11]. Animal research also shows that the reaction of the periaqueductal gray to threats is independent of input from higher brain structures [12, 13], which is not surprising since it evolved long before them.

10.1.2 Basal Ganglia

As mentioned previously, the basal ganglia are known to be involved in the territorial behaviors of lizards. The most extensively studied behaviors are fixed-action patterns related to social threats in agonistic encounters, including dominance/subordinance relationships in lizards [14–18]. The basal ganglia also have been found to be involved in defensive behaviors in fish [19].

10.1.3 Limbic System

Emotions, as we know them, probably did not exist before the existence of the limbic system. The evolution of emotions allowed animals to respond to the physical and social environment with greater flexibility because a given stimulus can elicit an emotion rather than a specific response and emotions prepare an animal to make a range of possible responses. Fear, is a case in point. The perception of a predator elicits fear in an animal, and fear prepares the animal to flee from the predator, prepare to fight it or try to scare it away, freeze in place to avoid detection, or hide from in it in some other way [20]. The specific reactions depend on the proximity of the predator [20].

The amygdala, which is a part of the limbic system, is the neural nexus of fear in the brain [21], probably evolved from the bed nucleus (another limbic structure) that is found in amphibians, reptiles, and birds [22], and is involved in fear in humans, particularly anxiety [23]. However, the amygdala appears to be the primary source of fear in mammals, including humans [24–26]. The amygdala generates fear as part of its function to assess potential threats of physical harm and to warn us about them. One should keep in mind, of course, that we cannot be sure that other mammals experience fear as we do, but they certainly appear to experience fear, based on their behavior.

The amygdala interacts with the other subcortical structures, especially the PAG of the brainstem [27, 28] and the bed nucleus of the limbic system [22, 23, 29]. The amygdala also interacts with other limbic structures, such as the anterior cingulate cortex (ACC) and the insula [26, 30, 31], which are also involved in fear [26, 31]. Many studies have reported that an area of the limbic system called the hippocampus is involved in fear, but most of these studies have investigated "fear conditioning" (i.e., learned fear), and the hippocampus plays a critical role in learning. Hence, the hippocampus does not seem to be essential to the experience of fear. Similarly, many studies have reported that a brain area called the thalamus, which is near the limbic system, is involved in fear. However, this is due to the fact that the amygdala processes visual and auditory input from the thalamus [32, 33], which is a preliminary processing center of visual and auditory stimuli, and the function of the thalamus is not unique to emotional or fear-related stimuli.

10.1.4 Prefrontal Cortex

The PFC is divided into several regions (dorsolateral, dorsomedial, orbitofrontal, and ventromedial PFC), all of which have been implicated in emotional processing [34–38]. Research shows that the PFC alters the expression of species-specific defensive behaviors controlled by the periaqueductal gray [39], and that it modulates fear by moderating the activity of the amygdala in rodents [39–42], monkeys, and other primates [43–45]. A 2006 article by Quirk and Beer reviewed animal and human research that suggests the ventromedial PFC (vmPFC) is the specific PFC structure that regulates the amygdala, and that increased activity in the PFC reduces the activity of the amygdala, thereby reducing fear [46, 47].

10.2 Fear in the Human Brain

10.2.1 Brain Stem

Patients with a problem called propopanosia, or blindsight, cannot recognize faces because of damage to their visual cortex. Yet, a 1999 study found that a patient with blindsight was able to recognize the emotions expressed in pictures of faces, despite the fact the patient did not recognize the facial expressions themselves, and he was not consciously aware of the facial expressions [48]. Subsequent neuroimaging research indicated that this is possible because the brain stem has its own visual input (that does not depend on the neocortex) through which it is able to detect emotional facial expressions, such as fear. This makes sense since the brain stem of animals had to interpret and respond to visual input from the eyes long before the visual cortex evolved. Other neuroimaging research has found that the periaqueductal gray of the brain stem in humans reacts to fear-related visual stimuli [13] and the threat of imminent physical harm [49]. This assessment of sensory information is passed along to the amygdala.

10.2.2 Basal Ganglia

Even though the basal ganglia are involved in the defensive behavior of animals, the evidence of their involvement is human fear is limited. Experimental research has shown that the area of the basal ganglia called the striatum is involved in learned or conditioned fear in humans [50–52], and that it is active during the anticipation and avoidance of physical harm [53–56]. Other research indicates that the striatum and another part of the basal ganglia called the globus pallidus react to pictures of angry and fearful faces [57, 58]. Overall, then, the research suggests that the basal ganglia have a limited role in human fear. This is not unexpected, since they antedate the evolution of the amygdala, which is the primary source of fear in humans and other mammals. Nevertheless, future research may find that the basal ganglia play a larger role in human fear than current research suggests.

10.2.3 Limbic System

The amygdala has long been suspected to be the major source of fear and anxiety in humans, based on the results of animal research and some clinical evidence [32, 59]. A growing body of research, especially neuroimaging studies, has confirmed this suspicion [60]. The human amygdala, which looks somewhat like an almond and is about the size of an almond, consists of a dozen or more regions that have connections to various parts of the brain [33]. One of these regions, the central nucleus, is known to be connected to the bed nucleus, which appears to play a role in human anxiety [23, 29].

The human amygdala is thought to assess or evaluate stimuli for different kinds of emotional content [61], including positive and negative emotions. Experimental studies have shown that positive emotional (or pleasant) stimuli tend to decrease the activity of the amygdala, whereas negative emotional stimuli tend to increase its activity [61], especially fear-related (i.e., threat-related) stimuli [62, 63]. Although human research has primarily used visual stimuli to study the amygdala, the amygdala of humans and other mammals assesses and responds to visual, auditory, gustatory, and olfactory stimuli [34, 61].

The most commonly used visual stimuli in human research on the brain's reactions to emotions are pictures of facial expressions, including faces expressing anger, disgust, fear, happiness, and sadness [64, 65]. There is some evidence that the amygdala responds differentially to the emotional expressions of happiness and sadness [65, 66], but it clearly reacts more strongly to anger and fear [61, 66–68]. The amygdala's reaction to an angry face probably reflects its assessment that the person in the picture poses an immediate threat of harm, whereas its reaction to a fearful face probably reflects its assessment that the facial expression indicates a potential threat of harm is nearby [66, 68, 69]. Related research indicates that the human amgydala also reacts to bodily expressions of fear and anger exhibited by other people [67].

The amygdala's reaction to certain kinds of threatening or fear-eliciting stimuli, such as snakes and spiders, is unconscious and occurs without cortical or cognitive input [61, 62, 70, 71]. The amygdala's response to such stimuli is essentially automatic [70], and its assessment of danger appears to be based, in part, on information from other subcortical structures [71]. This information includes sensory input that travels along neural circuits that go directly to the amygdala [32, 33, 60], and information from the brain stem [70, 72]. The amygdala also reacts to the facial expression of fear in the absence of conscious awareness [65, 73], based on input from subcortical structures, including the brain stem [71, 74]. The amygdala's conscious response to fear activates two other areas of the limbic system: the ACC and the insula [63, 68, 70].

It must be kept in mind that the amygdala operates under the "better safe than sorry principle"; therefore, it responds to ambiguous stimuli that may or may not pose a threat of harm as if they are dangerous [75, 76]. Since the amygdala has its own memory, it also may generalize what constitutes a threat from specific stimuli or situations that have posed a threat in the past [33, 60]. Moreover, the amygdala treats unpredictability, the inability to control current events, and uncertainty about future events as forms of threat [75, 77–82].

10.2.4 Prefrontal Cortex

The PFC of humans is best known for its role in awareness [37, 83], language [37, 84], reasoning [37, 85], and its "executive" control over cognitive processing, including decision making [37, 86, 87]. However, it also has a central role in the regulation of emotions [37, 87], especially fear [41].

The PFC attends to threat-related stimuli [88] and it is involved in the conscious assessment of threats of harm [89]. Like the amygdala, it reacts to pictures of threatening faces and to auditory stimuli that are fear-related or signal a threat of harm [90]. Although animal research implicates both the vmPFC and the orbitofrontal PFC (OFC) in the processing of fear in primates [91, 92], the vmPFC is particularly important in processing and regulating fear in humans [93, 94].

Research has demonstrated that the vmPFC modulates amygdala activity, and therefore, fear [46, 95]. Although there is evidence that all the regions of the PFC modulate amygdala activity to some degree [70, 96],[1] recent research indicates that the vmPFC is essential for controlling the amygdala and, consequently, human fear [94]. Specifically, the vmPFC directly inhibits the activity of the amygdala [94, 97]. Some researchers have suggested that the vmPFC assigns emotional values or valences to stimuli, and that stimuli with positive emotional valences increase its activity [93]. This increased activity, in turn, decreases the activity of the amygdala, suppressing fear when the vmPFC does not concur with the assessment of the amygdala that a stimulus poses a threat of harm. The mechanisms by which the vmPFC makes decisions about potential threats will be discussed further in Chap. 14.

10.3 Chapter Highlights and Comments

Emotions probably did not exist before the existence of the limbic system, and defensive behaviors in lower animals were elicited automatically before the evolution of emotions. The periaqueductal gray of the brain-stem, which is involved in self-defense in animals, also is involved in the human recognition of threatening

[1] The dorsomedial PFC, which has been implicated in fear and anxiety in a handful of human studies, will be discussed in Chap. 14 with respect to threat assessment and anxiety.

stimuli. Similarly, the basal ganglia, which are known to be involved in territorial defense in lower animals, are activated during the anticipation and avoidance of physical harm; however, they do not appear to be involved directly in human fear. Fear, itself, may not have existed before the evolution of the amygdala (which is part of the limbic system), although something similar to fear may have existed. In any case, numerous animal and human studies have demonstrated that the amygdala is the primary source of fear.

As the amygdala operates under the "better safe than sorry principle" it overreacts to ambiguous stimuli, in that it tends to identify stimuli as potential threats, and therefore, produces fear even when they may not actually pose a threat of harm. There is good evidence that the amygdala even reacts with fear to the perceived inability to control current events and to the perceived uncertainty or unpredictability of future events.

Different areas of the prefrontal cortex have been implicated in defensive behavior and fear in animals and humans. One particular area of the prefrontal cortex (the vmPFC) makes its own threat assessments, which can override the threat assessments of the amygdala and other subcortical structures. Thus, the vmPFC can suppress fear generated by the amygdala if the vmPFC decides the fear is not justified.

References

1. MacLean, P.D. (1967). The brain in relation to empathy and medical education. *Journal of Nervous and Mental Disease, 144*(5), 374–382.
2. Aronson, L.R. (1970). Functional evolution of the forebrain in lower vertebrates. In L. R. Aronson, E. Tobach, D. S. Lehrman, & J. S. Rosenblatt (Eds.), *Development and evolution of behavior* (pp. 75–107). San Francisco: W. H. Freeman.
3. Derby, C.D., & Sorensen, P.W. (2008). Neural processing, perception, and behavioral responses to natural chemical stimuli by fish and crustaceans. *Journal of Chemical Ecology, 34*(7), 898–914.
4. McLennan, D.A., & Ward, J.L. (2008). Conservation and variation in the agonistic repertoire of the brook stickleback, *Culaea inconstans* (Kirtland). *Environmental Biology of Fishes, 82*(4), 377–384.
5. McNaughton, N., & Corr, P.J. (2044). A two-dimensional neuropsychology of defense: Fear/anxiety and defensive distance. *Neuroscience & Biobehavioral Reviews, 28*(3), 285–305.
6. Morgan, M.M., & Clayton, C.C. (2005). Defensive behaviors evoked from the ventrolateral periaqueductal gray of the rat: Comparison of opioid and GABA disinhibition. *Behavioural Brain Research, 64*, 61–66.
7. Vianna, D.M.L., Graeff, F.G., Brandao, M.L., & Landeira-Fernandez, J. (2001). Defensive freezing evoked by electrical stimulation of the periaqueductal gray: Comparison between dorsolateral and ventrolateral regions. *Neuroreport, 12*(18), 4109–4112.
8. Misslin, R. (2003). The defense system of fear: Behavior and neurocircuitry. *Neurophysiologie Clinique/Clinical Neurophysiology, 33*(2), 55–66.
9. Carrive, P. (1993). The periaqueductal gray and defensive behavior: Functional representation and neuronal organization. *Behavioural Brain Research, 58*(1–2), 27–47.
10. Harris, J.A. (1996). Descending antinociceptive mechanisms in the brainstem: Their role in the animal's defensive system. *Journal of Physiology, 90*(1), 15–25.

11. Behbehani, M.M. (1995). Functional characteristics of the midbrain periaqueductal gray. *Progress in Neurobiology, 46*(6), 575–605.
12. Prather, M.D., Lavenex, P., Mauldin-Jourdain, M.L., Mason, W.A., Capitanio, J.P., Mendoza, S.P., et al. (2001). Increased social fear and decreased fear of objects in monkeys with neonatal amygdala lesions. *Neuroscience & Biobehavioral Reviews, 106*(4), 653–658.
13. Pichon, S., Grezes, J., & De Gelder, B. (2011). Threat prompts defensive brain responses independently of attentional control. *Cerebral Cortex, 22*(2), 274–285.
14. Tarr, R.S. (1982). Species typical display behavior following stimulation of the reptilian striatum. *Physiology & Behavior, 29*(4), 615–620.
15. Baxter, L.R. (2003). Basal ganglia systems in ritualistic social displays: Reptiles and humans; function and illness. *Physiology & Behavior, 79*, 451–460.
16. MacLean, P.D. (1990). *The triune brain in evolution: Role in paleocerebral functions.* New York: Plenum Press.
17. Baxter, L.R., Jr., Ackermann, R.F., Clark, E.C., & Baxter, J.E. (2001). Brain mediation of Anolis social dominance displays. I. Differential basal ganglia activation. *Brain Behavior and Evolution, 57*(4), 169–183.
18. Greenberg, N., MacLean, P.D., & Ferguson, J.L. (1979). Role of the paleostriatum in species-typical display behavior of the lizard (*Anolis carolinensis*). *Brain Research, 172*(2), 229–241.
19. Demski, L.S. (2013). The pallium and mind/behavior relationships in teleost fishes. *Brain Behavior and Evolution, 82*(1), 31–44.
20. Blanchard, R.J., Flannelly, K.J., & Blanchard, D.C. (1986). Defensive behaviors of laboratory and wild *Rattus norvegicus*. *Journal of Comparative Psychology, 100*(2), 101–107.
21. Panksepp, J. (1998). *Affective neuroscience: The foundations of human and animal emotions.* New York: Oxford University Press.
22. Goodson, J.L. (2005). The vertebrate social behavior network: Evolutionary themes and variations. *Hormones and Behavior, 48*(1), 11–22.
23. Walker, D.L., Toufexis, D.J., & Davis, M. (2003). Role of the bed nucleus of the stria terminalis versus the amygdala in fear, stress, and anxiety. *European Journal of Pharmacology, 463*(1), 199–216.
24. Panksepp, J. (2011). The basic emotional circuits of mammalian brains: Do animals have affective lives? *Neuroscience & Biobehavioral Reviews, 35*(9), 1791–1804.
25. Panksepp, J., Fuchs, T., & Iacobucci, P. (2011). The basic neuroscience of emotional experiences in mammals: The case of subcortical FEAR circuitry and implications for clinical anxiety. *Applied Animal Behaviour Science, 129*(1), 1–17.
26. Toyoda, H., Xiang-Yao, L., Long-Jun, W., Ming-Gao, Z., Descalzi, G., Tao, C., et al. (2011). Interplay of amygdala and cingulate plasticity in emotional fear. *Neural Plasticity, 2011*, 1–9.
27. Martinez-Garcia, F., Novejarque, A., & Lanuza, E. (2008). Two interconnected functional systems in the amygdala of amniote vertebrates. *Brain Research Bulletin, 75*(2), 206–213.
28. Price, J.L. (2003). Comparative aspects of amygdala connectivity. *Annals of the New York Academy of Sciences, 985*, 50–58.
29. Grillon, C. (2008). Models and mechanisms of anxiety: Evidence from startle studies. *Psychopharmacology, 199*(3), 421–437.
30. Torta, D.M., & Cauda, F. (2011). Different functions in the cingulate cortex, a meta-analytic connectivity modeling study. *NeuroImage, 56*, 2157–2172.
31. Fiddick, L. (2011). There is more than the amygdala: Potential threat assessment in the cingulate cortex. *Neuroscience and Biobehavioral Reviews, 35*(4), 1007–1018.
32. LeDoux, J.E. (1995). Emotion: Clues from the brain *Annual Review of Psychology, 46*, 209–235.
33. LeDoux, J.E. (2000). Emotion circuits in the brain. *Annual Review of Neuroscience, 23*(1), 155–184.
34. Davidson, R.J. (2002). Anxiety and affective style: Role of prefrontal cortex and amygdala. *Biological Psychiatry, 51*, 68–80.

35. Zelikowsky, M., Hersman, S., Chawla, M.K., Barnes, C.A., & Fanselow, M.S. (2014). Neuronal ensembles in amygdala, hippocampus, and prefrontal cortex track differential components of contextual fear. *Journal of Neuroscience Methods, 34*(25), 8462–8466.
36. Golkar, A., Lonsdorf, T.B., Olsson, A., Lindstrom, K.M., Berrebi, J., Fransson, P., et al. (2012). Distinct contributions of the dorsolateral prefrontal and orbitofrontal cortex during emotion regulation. *PLoS ONE, 7*(11), e48107.
37. Fuster, J. (2008). *The prefrontal cortex*. London: Academic Press.
38. Radley, J.J., Williams, B., & Sawchenko, P.E. (2008). Noradrenergic innervation of the dorsal medial prefrontal cortex modulates hypothalamo-pituitary-adrenal responses to acute emotional stress. *The Journal of Neuroscience, 28*(22), 5806–5816.
39. Chan, T., Kyere, K., Davis, B.R., Shemyakin, A., Kabitzke, P.A., Shair, H.N., et al. (2011). The role of the medial prefrontal cortex in innate fear regulation in infants, juveniles, and adolescents. *Journal of Neuroscience Methods, 31*(13), 4991–4999.
40. Maroun, M. (2013). Medial prefrontal cortex: Multiple roles in fear and extinction. *The Neuroscientist,* 19(4), 370–383.
41. Sotres-Bayon, F., Sierra-Mercado, D., Pardilla-Delgado, E., & Quirk, G.J. (2012). Gating of fear in prelimbic cortex by hippocampal and amygdala inputs. *Neuron, 76*(4), 804–812.
42. Charney, D.S. (2003). Neuroanatomical circuits modulating fear and anxiety behaviors Neuroanatomical circuits modulating fear and anxiety behaviors. *Acta Psychiatrica Scandinavica, 108*, 38.
43. Agustin-Pavon, C., Braesicke, K., Shiba, Y., Santangelo, A.M., Mikheenko, Y., Cockroft, G., et al. (2012). Lesions of ventrolateral prefrontal or anterior orbitofrontal cortex in primates heighten negative emotion. *Biological Psychiatry, 72*(4), 266–272.
44. Kalin, N.H. (2002). The neurobiology of fear. *Scientific American,* 12(1), 72–81.
45. Chudasama, Y., Kralik, J.D., & Murray, E.A. (2007). Rhesus monkeys with orbital prefrontal cortex lesions can learn to inhibit prepotent responses in the reversed reward contingency task. *Cerebral Cortex, 17*, 1154–1159.
46. Quirk, G.J., & Beer, J.S. (2006). Prefrontal involvement in the regulation of emotion: Convergence of rat and human studies. *Current Opinion in Neurobiology, 16*, 723–727.
47. Stern, C.A.J., Do-Monte, F.H., Gazarini, L., Carobrez, A.P., & Bertoglio, L.J. (2010). Anxiety disorders and anxiolytics – Anxiety disorders (basic): Ventromedial prefrontal cortex activity is required for anxiety expression: Distinct neurochemical mechanisms evidence *European Neuropsychopharmacology*, *20*(Suppl. 3), S538–S539.
48. de Gelder, B., Vroomen, J., Pourtois, G., & Weiskrantz, L. (1999). Non-conscious recognition of affect in the absence of striate cortex. *Neuroreport, 10*(18), 3759–3763.
49. Mobbs, D., Petrovic, P., Marchant, J.L., Hassabis, D., Weiskopf, N., Seymour, B., et al. (2007). When fear is near: Threat imminence elicits prefrontal-periaqueductal gray shifts in humans. *Science, 317*(5841), 1079–1083.
50. Linnman, C., Rougemont-Bucking, A., Beucke, J.C., Zeffiro, T.A., & Milad, M.R. (2011). Unconditioned responses and functional fear networks in human classical conditioning. *Behavioural Brain Research, 221*(1), 237–245.
51. Feng, T.Y., Feng, P., & Chen, Z.C. (2013). Altered resting-state brain activity at functional MRI during automatic memory consolidation of fear conditioning. *Brain Research, 1523*, 59–67.
52. Klucken, T., Tabbert, K., Schweckendiek, J., Merz, C.J., Kagerer, S., Vaitl, D., et al. (2009). Contingency learning in human fear conditioning involves the ventral striatum. *Human Brain Mapping, 30*(11), 3636–3644.
53. Schlund, M.W., Siegle, G.J., Ladouceur, C.D., Silk, J.S., Cataldo, M.F., Forbes, E.E., et al. (2010). Nothing to fear? Neural systems supporting avoidance behavior in healthy youths. *NeuroImage, 52*, 710–719.
54. Schlund, M.W., Hudgins, C.D., Magee, S., & Dymond, S. (2013). Neuroimaging the temporal dynamics of human avoidance to sustained threat. *Behavioural Brain Research, 257*, 148–155.

55. Collins, K.A., Mendelsohn, A., Cain, C.K., & Schiller, D. (2014). Taking action in the face of threat: Neural synchronization predicts adaptive coping. *Journal of Neuroscience, 34*(44), 14733–14738.
56. Drabant, E.M., Kuo, J.R., Ramel, W., Blechert, J., Edgc, M.D., Cooper, J.R., et al. (2010). Experiential, autonomic, and neural responses during threat anticipation vary as a function of threat intensity and neuroticism. *NeuroImage, 55*, 401–410.
57. Mühlberger, A., Wieser, M.J., Gerdes, A.B., Frey, M.C., Weyers, P., & Pauli, P. (2011). Stop looking angry and smile, please: Start and stop of the very same facial expression differentially activate threat- and reward-related brain networks. *Social Cognitive and Affective Neuroscience, 6*(3), 321–329.
58. Preibisch, C., Lanfermann, H., Wallenhorst, T., Walter, H., & Erk, S. (2009). Neuroanatomical correlates of visual field bias: A sensitive system for detecting potential threats? *Brain Research, 1263*, 69–77.
59. Davis, M. (1992). The role of the amygdala in fear and anxiety. *Annual Review of Neuroscience, 15*(1), 353–375.
60. Phelps, E.A., & LeDoux, J.E. (2005). Contributions of the amygdala to emotion processing: From animal models to human behavior. *Neuron, 48*, 175–187.
61. Zald, D.H. (2003). The human amygdala and the emotional evaluation of sensory stimuli. *Brain Research Reviews, 41*(1), 88–123.
62. Lipka, J., Miltner, W.H.R., & Straube, T. (2011). Vigilance for threat interacts with amygdala responses to subliminal threat cues in specific phobia. *Biological Psychiatry, 70*(5), 472–478.
63. Bishop, S.J., Duncan, J., & Lawrence, A.D. (2004). State anxiety modulation of the amygdala response to unattended threat-related stimuli. *Journal of Neuroscience, 24*(46), 10364–10368.
64. Fitzgerald, D.A., Angstadt, M., Jelsone, L.M., Nathan, P.J., & Phan, K.L. (2006). Beyond threat: Amygdala reactivity across multiple expressions of facial affect. *NeuroImage, 30*, 1441–1448.
65. Calder, A.J., Lawrence, A.D., & Young, A.W. (2001). Neuropsychology of fear and loathing. *Nature Reviews Neuroscience, 2*(5), 352–363.
66. Mattavelli, G., Sormaz, M., Flack, T., Asghar, A.U.R., Siyan, F., Frey, J., et al. (2014). Neural responses to facial expressions support the role of the amygdala in processing threat. *Social Cognitive and Affective Neuroscience, 9*(11), 1684.
67. Kret, M.E., Pichon, S., Grezes, J., & de Gelder, B. (2011). Similarities and differences in perceiving threat from dynamic faces and bodies. An fMRI study. *NeuroImage, 54*(2), 1755–1762.
68. Klumpp, H., Angstadt, M., Phan, K.L., & Nathan, P.J. (2010). Amygdala reactivity to faces at varying intensities of threat in generalized social phobia: An event-related functional MRI study. *Psychiatry Research: Neuroimaging, 183*(2), 167–169.
69. Anderson, A.K., Christoff, K., Panitz, D., De Rosa, E., & Gabrieli, J.D.E. (2003). Neural correlates of the automatic processing of threat facial signals. *The Journal of Neuroscience, 23*(13), 5627–5633.
70. Öhman, A. (2005). The role of the amygdala in human fear: Automatic detection of threat. *Psychoneuroendocrinology, 30*(10), 953–958.
71. Ohman, A., Carlsson, K., Lundqvist, D., & Ingvar, M. (2007). On the unconscious subcortical origin of human fear. *Physiology & Behavior, 92*, 180–185.
72. Williams, L.M., Das, P., Liddell, B.J., Kemp, A.H., Rennie, C.J., & Gordon, E. (2006). Mode of functional connectivity in amygdala pathways dissociates level of awareness for signals of fear. *Journal of Neuroscience, 26*(36), 9264–9271.
73. Adolphs, R. (2008). Fear, faces, and the human amygdala. *Current Opinion in Neurobiology,* 18, 166–172.
74. Morris, J.S., Öhman, A., & Dolan, R.J. (1999). A subcortical pathway to the right amygdala mediating "unseen" fear. *Proceedings of the National Academy of Sciences, 96*(4), 1680–1685.

75. Rosen, J.B., & Donley, M.P. (2006). Animal studies of amygdala function in fear and uncertainty: Relevance to human research. *Biological Psychology, 73*(1), 49–60.
76. Zaretsky, M., Mendelsohn, A., Mintz, M., & Hendler, T. (2010). In the eye of the beholder: Internally driven uncertainty of danger recruits the amygdala and dorsomedial prefrontal cortex. *Journal of Cognitive Neuroscience, 22*(10), 2263–2275.
77. Sarinopoulos, I., Grupe, D.W., Mackiewicz, K.L., Herrington, J.D., Lor, M., Steege, E.E., et al. (2010). Uncertainty during anticipation modulates neural responses to aversion in human insula and amygdala. *Cerebral Cortex, 20*(4), 929–940.
78. Grupe, D.W., & Nitschke, J.B. (2013). Uncertainty and anticipation in anxiety: An integrated neurobiological and psychological perspective. *Nature Reviews Neuroscience, 14*(7), 488–501.
79. Thompson, S.C. (1981). Will it hurt less if I can control it? A complex answer to a simple question. *Psychological Bulletin, 90*(1), 89–101.
80. Williams, L.E., Oler, J.A., Fox, A.S., McFarlin, D.R., Rogers, G.M., Jesson, M.A.L., et al. (2015). Fear of the unknown: Uncertain anticipation reveals amygdala alterations in childhood anxiety disorders. *Neuropsychopharmacology, 40*(6), 1428–1435.
81. Morriss, J., Christakou, A., & van Reekum, C.M. (2015). Intolerance of uncertainty predicts fear extinction in amygdala-ventromedial prefrontal cortical circuitry. *Biology of Mood & Anxiety Disorders, 5*(1), 1–13.
82. Hsu, M., Bhatt, M., Adolphs, R., Tranel, D., & Camerer, C.F. (2005). Neural systems responding to degrees of uncertainty in human decision-making. *Science, 310*(5754), 1680–1683.
83. Badgaiyan, R.D. (2005). Conscious awareness of retrieval: An exploration of the cortical connectivity. *International Journal of Psychophysiology, 55*(2), 257–262.
84. Hagoort, P., Hald, L., Bastiaansen, M., & Petersson, K.M. (2004). Integration of word meaning and world knowledge in language comprehension. *Science, 304*(5669), 438–441.
85. Bunge, S.A., Wendelken, C., Badre, D., & Wagner, A.D. (2005). Analogical reasoning and prefrontal cortex: Evidence for separable retrieval and integration mechanisms. *Cerebral Cortex, 15*(3), 239–249.
86. Miller, E.K., & Cohen, J.D. (2001). An integrative theory of prefrontal cortex function. *Annual Review of Neuroscience, 24*, 167–202.
87. Domenech, P., & Koechlin, E. (2015). Executive control and decision-making in the prefrontal cortex. *Current Opinion in Behavioral Sciences, 1*, 101–106.
88. Bishop, S., Duncan, J., Brett, M., & Lawrence, A.D. (2004). Prefrontal cortical function and anxiety: Controlling attention to threat-related stimuli. *Nature Neuroscience, 7*(2), 184–188.
89. Mechias, M.-L., Etkin, A., & Kalisch, R. (2010). A meta-analysis of instructed fear studies: Implications for conscious appraisal of threat. *NeuroImage, 49*, 1760–1768.
90. Klumpp, H., Fitzgerald, D. A., & Phan, K.L. (2013). Neural predictors and mechanisms of cognitive behavioral therapy on threat processing in social anxiety disorder. *Progress in Neuropsychopharmacology and Biological Psychiatry, 45*, 83–91.
91. Timbie, C., & Barbas, H. (2014). Specialized pathways from the primate amygdala to posterior orbitofrontal cortex. *The Journal of Neuroscience, 34*(24), 8106–8118.
92. Shiba, Y., Kim, C., Santangelo, A.M., & Roberts, A.C. (2015). Lesions of either anterior orbitofrontal cortex or ventrolateral prefrontal cortex in marmoset monkeys heighten innate fear and attenuate active coping behaviors to predator threat. *Frontiers in Systems Neuroscience, 21*, 250.. Retrieved from http://journal.frontiersin.org/article/10.3389/fnsys.2014.00250/full
93. Winecoff, A., Clithero, J.A., Carter, R.M., Bergman, S.R., Wang, L.H., & Huettel, S.A. (2013). Ventromedial prefrontal cortex encodes emotional value. *Journal of Neuroscience, 33*(27), 11032–11039.
94. Motzkin, J.C., Philippi, C.L., Wolf, R.C., Koenigs, M., & Baskaya, M.K. (2015). Ventromedial prefrontal cortex is critical for the regulation of amygdala activity in humans. *Biological Psychiatry, 77*(3), 276–284.

95. Berkowitz, R.L., Coplan, J.D., Reddy, D.P., & Gorman, J.M. (2007). The human dimension: How the prefrontal cortex modulates the subcortical fear response. *Reviews in the Neurosciences, 18*(3–4), 191–208.
96. Stein, J.L., Wiedholz, L.M., Bassett, D.S., Weinberger, D.R., Zink, C.F., Mattay, V.S., et al. (2007). A validated network of effective amygdala connectivity. *NeuroImage, 36*(3), 736–745.
97. Greenberg, T., Carlson, J.M., Cha, J., Hajcak, G., & Mujica-Parodi, L.R. (2013). Ventromedial prefrontal cortex reactivity is altered in generalized anxiety disorder during fear generalization. *Depression and Anxiety, 30*(3), 242–250.

Chapter 11
Anxiety Disorders as Evolutionary Adaptations

Abstract The chapter examines the thesis, first advanced by clinical psychologists and psychiatrists in the 1970s and 1980s, that psychiatric symptoms are rooted in our evolution history. This premise has come to be called Evolutionary Psychiatry. Key among the early advocates of evolutionary psychiatry was the American psychiatrist Randolph M. Nesse who believed that many psychiatric disorders, particularly anxiety disorders, are expressions of proximate mechanisms that are adaptive for survival. This chapter explains how seven anxiety disorders reflect fears that evolved to protect us from different sources of dangers: acrophobia, agoraphobia, small animal phobias, general anxiety, society phobia (anxiety), panic attack, and obsessive compulsive disorder. The prevalence rates and age of onset of subclinical levels of these classes of psychiatric symptoms in the general public are presented wherever possible, and estimates are given regarding when some of the proximate mechanisms underlying these symptoms probably evolved in our animal or human ancestors. The chapter also explains that these proximate mechanisms are prone to making "false alarms," much as smoke alarms do, because they operate under the "better safe than sorry principle." A major point of the chapter is the same as the major premise of evolutionary psychiatry, i.e., that all people have subclinical levels of various psychiatric symptoms because the proximate mechanisms that produce them once were and may still be important for survival. The chapter also notes that the theoretical focus of evolutionary psychology on the last 1.8 million years of human existence is obviously inadequate for understanding how tens of millions and hundreds millions of years of evolution have molded human behavior.

Keywords Acrophobia • Age of onset • Agoraphobia • Anxiety disorders • Evolutionary Psychiatry • Fear • Fixed-action patterns • OCD • Panic attack • Prevalence • Proximate mechanisms • Psychiatric disorders • Threat of harm

K.J. Flannelly, *Religious Beliefs, Evolutionary Psychiatry, and Mental Health in America*, Religion, Spirituality and Health: A Social Scientific Approach 1,
DOI 10.1007/978-3-319-52488-7_11

11.1 Background

A handful of clinical psychologists and psychiatrists in the 1980s attempted to explain the evolutionary roots of specific classes of psychiatric symptoms, the first of whom was the American psychiatrist Randolph M. Nesse [1]. Nesse explained how certain psychiatric disorders [2], particularly the anxiety disorders, result from the operation of proximate brain mechanisms that are adaptive characteristics which helped our ancestors to survive [3–6]. Nesse's basic premise is that anxiety disorders are associated with fears that have evolved to protect us from different sources of danger [3, 4].

Two articles by Nesse described a dozen or so subtypes of anxiety and the types of harm they protect us from [3, 4]. Table 11.1 lists eight of these subtypes of anxiety and their corresponding threats of harm, according to Nesse.[1]

11.2 Fear of Small Animals

Nesse thought fear of small animals served an obvious survival function because many kinds of small animals can cause us harm. It is not surprising, therefore, that animal phobias are very common [7–9] and that they begin in childhood and persist through adulthood [10–13]. Fear of snakes and spiders are especially common, despite the fact that most snakes and spiders are not poisonous. Nevertheless, because some are dangerous, the simplest and safest thing to do is to avoid all snakes and spiders. As snakes and spiders are so different in their appearance, behaviors, and habitats, humans probably have evolved separate proximate brain mechanisms

Table 11.1 Anxiety subtypes and the threats they address in human evolutionary history

Subtype of anxiety	Type of threat posed
Small animal phobias	Possibility of physical harm posed by small animals
Acrophobia	Threat of injury from falling from a height
Panic attack	Imminent attack by a predator or human enemy
Agoraphobia	Environment in which an attack may occur
Society phobia (anxiety)	Threat to social status or group membership
Excessive cleaning[a]	Health threat posed by infectious diseases
Excessive hoarding[a]	Threat of lack of food or other resources
General anxiety	Unspecified threats

[a]Nesse actually used the terms "obsessive cleaning" and "obsessive hoarding," but his use of the term "obsessive" is not consistent with current usage in psychiatry, so I replaced "obsessive" with "excessive"

[1]The descriptions of the types of threat generally paraphrase Nesse's descriptions and take into account the different descriptions he used in his 1990 and 1998 papers, as well as descriptions offered by other theorists about some of these threats.

to avoid snakes and spiders, although a Swedish study found people who are afraid of snakes tend to be afraid of spiders and vice versa [7]. I am not aware of any research on fear of spiders in primates other than humans, but there is evidence that some primates share our innate fear of snakes [14]. It has been suggested that fear of snakes evolved in primates about 20 million years ago [14], whereas fear of small animals and insects evolved in humans about 70,000 years ago [15].

Even though most small animals are not poisonous, they can spread disease, so separate brain mechanisms may have evolved to avoid insects and rodents or other small animals. Such proximate mechanisms do not identify animals that are harmless (negative instances of potential harm); they only provide algorithms or rules for identifying animals that can cause harm (positive instances of potential harm). These mechanisms do not need to be very good at differentiating between harmless and dangerous animals, as it is better for survival to treat a harmless animal as if it is dangerous ("a false positive") than it is to treat a dangerous animal as if it is harmless ("a false negative"). Nesse called this defensive strategy the "smoke detector principle" (p. 402) [3], and the cognitive psychotherapist and evolutionary theorist, Paul Gilbert, called it the "better safe than sorry principle" (p. 147) [16]. As Gilbert explains, the proximate brain mechanisms to assess threats have "evolved to minimize the cost of mistakes, but not mistakes themselves" [17]. Thus, "warning alarms" may go off somewhat too often, or be too intense, but this is required to assure adequate protection from harm [3].

The 1990–1992 National Comorbidity Survey (NCS) found almost 6% of Americans (15–55 years old) met the criteria for a diagnosis of animal phobia at some time during their lives (i.e., the lifetime prevalence rate), making it the most common phobia among Americans [18]. More important, in my view, the study found that over 22% of the people surveyed said they had a fear of animals sometime during their lives, which did not meet the threshold for being a clinical diagnosis of animal phobia (i.e., they had subclinical symptoms) [18]. This indicates that the proportion of people who had a fear of animals sometime during their lifetime was nearly four times higher than the proportion of people who were diagnosed with animal phobia during their lifetime. Likewise, a 2011 Canadian survey found that the percentage of adults who had a fear of animals during the past 12 months (the 12-month prevalence rate), who did not meet the criteria for a clinical diagnosis of animal phobia, was roughly four times higher that the percentage who met the criterion for a clinical diagnosis of animal phobia during the past year [10].

I think these findings are very important because they show that symptoms of animal phobia are far more common among the general public than one might expect based on the relatively low rate of clinical cases of animal phobia. The reason why the prevalence rates of clinical cases of animal phobia is far less than the subclinical rates of fear of small animals is that a person must meet several stringent criteria to receive a clinical diagnosis for any psychiatric disorder. For cases of animal and other phobias, the criteria are that: (1) the fear is persistent and excessive; (2) the phobic stimulus always evokes anxiety; (3) the person recognizes the fear is unreasonable or excessive; (4) the phobic stimulus is avoided or endured with intense anxiety; and (5) avoiding the stimulus or distress from exposure to the stimulus significantly interferes with the individual's normal activity [2].

11.3 Acrophobia (Fear of Heights)

The function of acrophobia (fear of heights) is obvious, once you accept Nesse's perspective. The fear of heights is a mechanism for avoiding high places from which one could fall and suffer serious injury or death. If an individual experiences acrophobia when already in a high place, such as looking out the window of a tall building, s/he may freeze, just as many animals do when are frightened; in natural settings freezing could keep an individual from falling [6]. The survival value of acrophobia presumably accounts for the fact that acrophobia is the second most common phobia in the U.S [11, 18]. Like animal phobia, the NCS found the rate of Americans who had a fear of heights (20%) sometime during their lifetime was four times higher than the rate of Americans who qualified for a diagnosis of acrophobia (5%) sometime during their lifetime [18]. This is because the diagnosis of acrophobia is based on the same type of stringent criteria as those used for animal phobia. National surveys of adults in other Western countries have reported even higher lifetimes rates of nonclinical fear of heights: Germany = 28% [19]; Iceland = 41% [20].

11.4 Panic Attack and Agoraphobia

Panic attack entails the experience of extreme fear when no potential source of physical harm is present [1, 4, 5]. A person having a panic attack exhibits signs of fear like the behaviors Darwin described in *The Expression of Emotions* [21], including momentary immobility, or freezing [1, 5]. The most common symptoms are feeling one's heart pounding, sweating, difficulty breathing, and shacking and trembling; less common symptoms are a sensation of smothering, chest pain, tingling in the hands or feet, and feeling faint or dizzy [5, 22, 23]. Fear of dying or a sense of "unreality" also are common [5, 22, 23].

Many symptoms of panic attack are similar to the so-called "fight or flight" reaction to threat, which is produced by the autonomic component of the peripheral nervous system.[2] These bodily sensations are mainly superficial signs of fear, whereas the emotion of fear, itself, is produced by a brain structure called the amygdala (which is part of the central nervous system). The fact that panic attacks often

[2] The nervous system is divided into two parts: the central nervous system (which is located entirely within the skull and spinal cord), and the peripheral nervous system. The peripheral nervous system is further divided into two parts, the somatic and the autonomic nervous systems. The somatic nervous system controls the skeletal muscles and the autonomic nervous system regulates the internal organs and controls their related muscles.

involve "freezing," which is a common anti-predator behavior in mammals, suggests that it reflects a reaction to a non-existent predator. It also suggests that panic attack may reflect an adaptation to predatory threats that could have evolved in the early mammals that first appeared on earth roughly 280 million years ago [24], or in modern mammals, which appeared about 100 million years ago [25–27].

Individuals experience their first panic attack between their mid-teens and their early 30s [5, 22, 28], and the first attack usually occurs in a public place [4, 5, 29]. Most people quickly flee the site of the panic attack and go home [29]. Although panic attacks often occur during stressful times in a person's life, the attack seems to "come out of the blue," and the person cannot point to something that precipitated the attack [1, 5, 29]. A national survey of Americans between 15 and 54 years of age found roughly 15% had at least one panic attack in their lifetime and 4% had a series of repeated attacks within a month of their first attack [30].

Nesse thought panic attacks were normal in the sense that they represent evolutionary adaptive responses to a life-threatening danger, such as the imminent attack of a predator, but they were abnormal in that panic attacks occur when no such threat is actually present. He hypothesized that the threshold for perceiving situations as threatening was an inherited trait that was normally distributed among individuals (as any inherited trait is), and that individuals who suffer from panic attacks are at the extreme end of the distribution in which the threshold of what constitutes a threat of harm is very low. Nevertheless, he suspected that there must be something wrong with a proximate mechanism that triggers such intense defensive reactions when there is no immediate, identifiable threat of harm. Given that panic attacks mostly occur in public places and rarely occur at home, Lelliot et al. thought panic attacks might reflect a general fear of the dangers posed by being outside one's territory or home-range [29]. This might help explain why panic attacks occur when there is no obvious source of immediate danger.

Nesse initially thought agoraphobia was a learned fear of being in open spaces that developed because of repeated panic attacks [1, 5]. After each attack, an individual would avoid the place where the attack occurred and this would quickly generalize to become a fear of being outdoors. There is research to support Nesse's notion that individuals' avoid the locations in which they have had a panic attack [29], but there seems to be no research to support the notion that agoraphobia is a learned reaction to repeated panic attacks. Moreover, a large U.S. study found that half the individuals who had repeated panic attacks did not develop agoraphobia [30], and numerous studies of clinical and community samples have identified people who suffer from agoraphobia who have never had a panic attack [31]. Thus, agoraphobia may be a learned fear in some individuals, but an unlearned fear in others. If agoraphobia represents fear of being harmed when outside the safety of one's home-range or territory [6, 29], its evolutionary roots could be very ancient, as most lizards and many fish exhibit territoriality.

11.5 Social Phobia (Social Anxiety)

Social anxiety may represent fear of being rejected by a social group and the consequences of being rejected [32]. Like most primates, humans have evolved to live in close social groups, and close social relationships are important for providing protection from harm, child rearing, and acquiring and sharing food and other resources [33–36]. However, social groups inevitably entail social hierarchies [3, 16, 33, 34], which are created and maintained in sub-human primates and other vertebrates by agonistic behaviors, including threats of aggression and actual aggression by dominant animals in conjunction with submissive behaviors by subordinate animals [33, 36, 37]. Social hierarchies in humans are established along a number of dimensions, including ability, beauty, intelligence, and wealth, as well as formal hierarchies that exist within business, military, political, professional, religious organizations [16]. Higher status within a group is usually associated with more resources, be it money, power, or prestige, whereas lower status is associated with fewer resources. However, since expulsion from a group can completely bar access to resources, it usually is better to accept one's subordinate status and submit to the social norms of the group, which in humans, may include dress, speech, customs, beliefs, etc. [6, 38].

Americans primarily develop social anxiety sometime between their early teens and mid-20's [28] and its lifetime prevalence is roughly 13% [28, 39]. Social anxiety entails the fear of acting in ways and being in situations that will make us less attractive to, and/or more likely to be rejected by others [40]. Any type of social encounter can evoke social anxiety, from things that many people find stressful (e.g., public speaking, job interviews, or dealing with authority figures) to more mundane things (e.g., dating, returning an item to a store, or walking into a room in which people are already present) [40, 41]. Shyness, a key characteristic of social anxiety, generally helps one to win social acceptance, but it also tends to ensure that one has subordinate rank within a social group [6, 40].

Since the evolution of social groups has been particularly important for the success of primates [42], the evolutionary origin of social anxiety may date back to the evolution of monkeys over 50 million years ago, or at least back to the split between monkeys and apes around 20 million years ago [43, 44]. Whenever the brain mechanisms underlying social anxiety evolved, they surely had to arise before our human ancestral line diverged from the modern apes.

11.6 Obsessive-Compulsive Disorder

Nesse's anxiety subtypes of excessive cleaning and hoarding in humans fall within the broader psychiatric classification of obsessive-compulsive disorder (OCD) [45], which includes hoarding, sexual and religious obsessions, cleaning/washing associated with fears of contamination, and the fear that one has not done something that could cause severe harm [46, 47]. OCD consists of obsessive thoughts that harm will come if an individual does not perform certain behaviors, which are called compulsions or compulsive acts. The obsessive thoughts are associated with anxiety and the compulsive acts are performed to reduce anxiety [48]. Persons with OCD realize that their obsessive thoughts and compulsive acts are irrational but they cannot stop them. While some of the compulsive behaviors that were just mentioned may not have obvious survival value, cleaning and hoarding clearly do. In animals, grooming serves to reduce the likelihood of infections, and hoarding serves to refurbish stores of foods because of seasonal fluctuations in resources, as seen in squirrels and other small mammals that hoard food for the winter.

Although it has been suggested that compulsive hoarding and washing evolved in humans just 70,000 years ago [15], the psychiatrist Dan J. Stein saw a strong parallel between the pattern and functions of human and animal forms of hoarding and washing (also called self-cleaning and grooming) behaviors [49]. The psychiatrist Martin Brune also saw a parallel between human compulsive behavior acts and animal behavior from an ethological perspective. Research on ethology has described behaviors called "displacement activities," which are seemingly irrelevant fixed-action patterns that are exhibited when an animal is apparently faced with two competing motivations, such as fight or flight [50]. Niko Tinbergen gives the example of a seagull engaged in agonistic behavior with a male rival, which – apparently torn between attacking the rival or fleeing from it – exhibited fixed-action patterns related to nest-building [50, 51]. Other research has reported comparable displacement activities in rats, which have been observed to suspend fixed-action patterns related to territorial aggression, briefly, to engage in fixed-action patterns normally involved in self-grooming or digging. Brune proposed that at least some compulsive acts in humans are displacement activities, which would help explain why some compulsive acts have no immediately obvious survival value in relation to the situation in which they are exhibited. Though Brune did not suggest that OCD is related to aggression or social conflict, other psychiatrists have done so [52].

Other authors also have noticed the similarity between the repetitive nature of obsessive-compulsive acts, such as cleaning and washing, and the repetitiveness of fixed-action patterns used by many mammals to groom themselves and perform other functions [53–55]. Poliment et al. regard the fact that these fixed-action patterns evolved in mammals over 100 million years ago as evidence that the evolutionary roots of OCD extend far back in time [53].

The 2001–2003 National Comorbidity Survey Replication (NCS-R) found that symptoms of OCD usually begin in Americans between the mid-teens and late 20s. Although the lifetime rate of clinical cases of OCD in the U.S. is less than 3% [56, 57], close to 30% of Americans say they have experienced obsessions or compulsions sometime in their lives [47]. Checking is the most common symptom of OCD among Americans, closely followed by hoarding. Cleaning/washing is far less common [47].

11.7 General Anxiety

Marks and Nesse's suggestion that "General anxiety probably evolved to deal with threats whose nature cannot be defined very clearly" (p. 249), [6] is consistent with animal research which indicates that general anxiety is a response to ill-defined animate and inanimate threats of harm [58, 59]. It is, furthermore, very similar to Sigmund Freud's notion that anxiety is "free-floating fear" in which we cannot make a connection between a particular threat of danger and our sense of fear [60]. Christian Grillon of the National Institute of Mental Health recently defined fear as "a response to an impending identifiable danger" and anxiety "as a state of constant apprehension about future harm" (p. 422) [61]. One function of general anxiety or generalized anxiety disorder (GAD) seems to be to increase vigilance in order to recognize potential threats of harm in our surroundings [6].

The onset of the GAD in the U.S. commonly occurs when people are in their early teens through their late 30s, with the first onset of GAD being very rare after age 40 [56, 62]. The lifetime prevalence of GAD is typically estimated to be 4–6% based on national studies [39, 56], however, the lifetime rate is higher if the clinical criteria of a GAD diagnosis are less stringent. The estimates of 4–6% are based on GAD attacks that last at least 12 months; if attacks lasting only one month are included, the estimated lifetime prevalence is closer to 13% [62]. I am not aware of any estimates of the lifetime rate of symptoms of general anxiety among Americans who do not meet the clinical criteria of GAD.

11.8 Chapter Highlights and Comments

Randolph M. Nesse introduced the notion that psychiatric symptoms are evolutionary adaptations that involve proximate mechanisms that evolved to protect us from various sources of harm. Most proximate brain mechanisms underlying anxiety disorders activate specific or general fears that are commonly experienced by the general public, and the proportion of individuals who have symptoms of anxiety disorders far exceeds the proportion of individuals who are diagnosed with anxiety disorders.

Although evolutionary psychology views the last 1.8 million years as a critical period of evolution for understanding human behavior, evolutionary adaptations going back possibly 100's of millions of years have a great influence on human behavior today. For example, primates share our innate fear of snakes [14], which suggests that our fear of snakes may have evolved as a proximate mechanism to protect us from harm 20 million years ago. Social anxiety may represent the action of proximate mechanisms that evolved between 20 and 50 million years ago, and panic attack and agoraphobia may represent the action of proximate mechanisms that evolved in mammals between 100 and 280 million years ago. Given our common descent from animal predecessors, I think ethological research may provide unique insights into many types of anxiety symptoms, including general anxiety, agoraphobia, panic attack, and OCD.

References

1. Nesse, R.M. (1984). An evolutionary perspective on psychiatry. *Comprehensive Psychiatry, 25*(6), 575–580.
2. *Diagnostic and statistical manual of mental disorders*. (2013). (5th ed.). Washington, DC: American Psychiatric Association.
3. Nesse, R. (1998). Emotional disorders in evolutionary perspective. *British Journal of Medical Psychology, 71*(4), 397–415.
4. Nesse, R.M. (1990). Evolutionary explanations of emotions. *Human Nature, 1*(3), 261–289.
5. Nesse, R.M. (1987). An evolutionary perspective on panic disorder and agoraphobia. *Ethology and Sociobiology, 8*, 73S–83S.
6. Marks, I.M., & Nesse, R.M. (1994). Fear and fitness: An evolutionary analysis of anxiety disorders. *Ethology and Sociobiology, 15*(5–6), 247–261.
7. Fredrikson, M., Annas, P., Fischer, H., & Wik, G. (1996). Gender and age differences in the prevalence of specific fears and phobias. *Behaviour Research and Therapy, 34*(1), 33–39.
8. Kirkpatrick, D.R. (1984). Age, gender and patterns of common intense fears among adults. *Behaviour Research and Therapy, 22*(2), 141–150.
9. Merckelbach, H., de Jong, P.J., Muris, P., & van den Hout, M.A. (1996). The etiology of specific phobias: A review. *Clinical Psychology Review, 16*(4), 337–361.
10. Grenier, S., Schuurmans, J., Goldfarb, M., Préville, M., Boyer, R., O'Connor, K., et al. (2011). The epidemiology of specific phobia and subthreshold fear subtypes in a community-based sample of older adults. *Depression and Anxiety, 28*(6), 456–463.
11. LeBeau, R.T., Glenn, D., Liao, B., Wittchen, H.U., Beesdo-Baum, K., Ollendick, T., & Craske, M.G. (2010). Specific phobia: A review of DSM-IV specific phobia and preliminary recommendations for DSM-V. *Depression and Anxiety, 27*, 148–167.
12. Antony, M.M., Brown, T.A., & Barlow, D.H. (1997). Heterogeneity among specific phobia types in DSM-IV. *Behaviour Research and Therapy, 35*(12), 1089–1100.
13. Burstein, M., Georgiades, K., He, J.P., Schmitz, A., Feig, E., Khazanov, G.K., et al. (2012). Specific phobia among U.S. adolescents: Phenomenology and typology. *Depression and Anxiety, 29*(12), 1072–1082.
14. Isbell, L.A. (2009). *The fruit, the tree and the serpent*. Cambridge, MA: Harvard University Press.
15. Bracha, H.S. (2006). Human brain evolution and the "Neuroevolutionary time-depth principle:" Implications for the reclassification of fear-circuitry-related traits in DSM-V and for studying resilience to warzone-related posttraumatic stress disorder. *Progress in Neuro-Psychopharmacology and Biological Psychiatry, 30*(5), 827–853.
16. Gilbert, P. (1993). Defence and safety: Their function in social behaviour and psychopathology. *British Journal of Clinical Psychology, 32*(Pt 2), 131–153.
17. Gilbert, P. (1998). The evolved basis and adaptive functions of cognitive distortions. *British Journal of Medical Psychology, 71*(Pt 4), 447–463.
18. Curtis, G.C., Magee, W.J., Eaton, W.W., Wittchen, H.-U., & Kessler, R.C. (1998). Specific fears and phobias: Epidemiology and classification. *British Journal of Psychiatry, 173*, 212–217.
19. Huppert, D., Grill, E., & Brandt, T. (2013). Down on heights? One in three has visual height intolerance. *Journal of Neurology, 200*(2), 597–604.

20. Lindal, E., & Stefansson, J.G. (1993). The lifetime prevalence of anxiety disorders in Iceland as estimated by the US National Institute of Mental Health Diagnostic Interview Schedule. *Acta Psychiatrica Scandinavica,* 88(1), 29–34.
21. Darwin, C. (1872). *The expression of emotions in man and animals.* London: John Murray.
22. Von Korff, M.R., Eaton, W.W., & Keyl, P.M. (1985). The epidemiology of panic attacks and panic disorder results of three community surveys. *American Journal of Epidemiology,* 122(6), 970–981.
23. Meuret, A.E., White, K.S., Ritz, T., Roth, W.T., Hofmann, S.G., & Brown, T.A. (2006). Panic attack symptom dimensions and their relationship to illness characteristics in panic disorder. *Journal of Psychiatric Research,* 40(6), 520–527.
24. Kaas, J.H. (2011). Neocortex in early mammals and its subsequent variations. *Annals of the New York Academy of Sciences,* 1225, 28–36.
25. Kaas, J.H. (2011). Reconstructing the areal organization of the neocortex of the first mammals. *Brain, Behavior and Evolution,* 78(1), 7–21.
26. Seiffert, E.R. (2012). Early primate evolution in Afro-Arabia. *Evolutionary Anthropology,* 21(6), 239–253.
27. Luo, Z.-X. (2007). Transformation and diversification in early mammal evolution. *Nature,* 450(7172), 1011–1019.
28. Magee, W.J., Eaton, W.W., Wittchen, H.U., McGonagle, K.A., & Kessler, R.C. (1996). Agoraphobia, simple phobia, and social phobia in the national comorbidity survey. *Archives of General Psychiatry,* 53, 159–168.
29. Lelliott, P., Marks, I., McNamee, G., & Tobena, A. (1989). Onset of panic disorder with agoraphobia: Toward an integrated model. *Archives of General Psychiatry,* 46(11), 1000–1004.
30. Eaton, W.W., Kessler, R.C., Wittchen, H.U., & Magee, W.J. (1994). Panic and panic disorder in the United States. *American Journal of Psychiatry,* 151(3), 413–420.
31. Horwath, E., Lish, J.D., Johnson, J., Hornig, C.D., & Weissman, M.M. (1993). Agoraphobia without panic: Clinical reappraisal of an epidemiologic finding. *American Journal of Psychiatry,* 150(10), 1496–1501.
32. Moscovitch, D.A. (2009). What is the core fear in social phobia? A new model to facilitate individualized case conceptualization and treatment. *Cognitive and Behavioral Practice,* 16(2), 123–134.
33. Etkin, W. (1964). *Social behavior and organization among vertebrates.* Chicago: University of Chicago Press.
34. Mesterton-Gibbons, M., Gavrilets, S., Gravner, J., & Akcay, E. (2011). Models of coalition or alliance formation. *Journal of Theoretical Biology,* 274(1), 187–204.
35. Dunbar, R. (1997, April 10). The monkeys' defence alliance. *Nature,* 386, p. 555.
36. Nishida, T. (1983). Alpha status and agonistic alliance in wild chimpanzees (*Pan troglodytes* schweinfurthii). *Primates,* 24(3), 318–336.
37. Collias, N.E. (1944). Aggressive behavior among vertebrate animals. *Physiological Zoology,* 17(1), 83–123.
38. Gilbert, P. (2001). Evolutionary approaches to psychopathology: The role of natural defences. *The Australian and New Zealand Journal of Psychiatry,* 35(1), 17–27.
39. Kessler, R.C., McGonagle, K.A., Zhao, S., Nelson, C.B., Hughes, M., Eshleman, S., et al. (1994). Lifetime and 12-month prevalence of DSM-III-R psychiatric disorders in the United States: Results from the National Comorbidity Study. *Archives of General Psychiatry,* 51(1), 8–19.
40. Gilbert, P. (2001). Evolution and social anxiety. The role of attraction, social competition, and social hierarchies. *Psychiatric Clinics of North America,* 24(4), 72–51.
41. Stein, M.B., Torgrud, L.J., & Walker, J.R. (2000). Social phobia symptoms, subtypes, and severity: Findings from a community survey. *Archives of General Psychiatry,* 57(11), 1046–1052.

42. Boesch, C. (2012). The ecology and evolution of social behavior and cognition in primates. In J. Vonk, & T. K. Shackelford (Eds.), *The Oxford handbook of comparative evolutionary psychology* (pp. 489–503). Oxford: Oxford University Press.
43. Barras, C. (2013). Humanity's earliest cousin. *New Scientist,* 218(2920), 8–9.
44. Jaeger, J.-J., & Marivaux, L. (2005). Shaking the earliest branches of anthropoid primate evolution. *Science,* 310(5746), 244–245.
45. *Diagnostic and statistical manual of mental disorders.* (2000). (4th (Text Revision) ed.). Washington, DC: American Psychiatric Association.
46. McKay, D., Abramowitz, J.S., Calamari, J.E., Kyrios, M., Radomsky, A., Sookman, D., Taylor, S., et al. (2004). A critical evaluation of obsessive–compulsive disorder subtypes: Symptoms versus mechanisms. *Clinical Psychology Review,* 24(3), 283–313.
47. Ruscio, A.M., Stein, D.J., Chiu, W.T., & Kessler, R.C. (2010). The epidemiology of obsessive-compulsive disorder in the National Comorbidity Survey Replication. *Molecular Psychiatry,* 15(1), 53–63.
48. Brune, M. (2006). The evolutionary psychology of obsessive-compulsive disorder: The role of cognitive metarepresentation. *Perspectives in Biology and Medicine,* 49(3), 317–329.
49. Stein, D.J. (2000). Advances in the neurobiology of obsessive-compulsive disorder. Implications for conceptualizing putative obsessive-compulsive and spectrum disorders. *Psychiatric Clinics of North America,* 23(2), 545–562.
50. Tinbergen, N. (1968). *Curious naturalists.* Garden City: Anchor Books.
51. Tinbergen, N. (1972). *The animal in its world: Explorations of an ethologist* (1). Cambridge, MA: Harvard University Press.
52. Baxter, L.R., Jr. (2003). Basal ganglia systems in ritualistic social displays: Reptiles and humans; function and illness. *Physiology & Behavior,* 79451–460(3), 451–460.
53. Polimeni, J., Reiss, J.P., & Sareen, J. (2005). Could obsessive-complusive disorder have originated as a group-selective adaptive trait in traditional societies? *Medical Hypotheses,* 65(4), 655–664.
54. Baxter, L.R. (2003). Basal ganglia systems in ritualistic social displays: Reptiles and humans; function and illness. *Physiology & Behavior,* 79, 451–460.
55. Rapoport, J.L., & Fiske, A. (1998). The new biology of obsessive-complusive disorder: Implications for evolutionary psychology. *Perspectives in Biology and Medicine,* 41(2), 159–175.
56. Kessler, R.C., Berglund, P., Demler, O., Jin, R., Merikangas, K.R., & Walters, E.E. (2005). Lifetime prevalence and age-of-onset distributions of DSM-IV disorders in the National Comorbidity Survey Replication. *Archives of General Psychiatry,* 62(6), 593–602.
57. Eisen, J.L., & Rasmussen, S.A. (2002). Phenomenology of obsessive-compulsive disorder. In D. J. Stein, & E. Hollander (Eds.), *Textbook of anxiety disorders* (pp. 173–189). Washington, DC: American Psychiatric Publishing.
58. McNaughton, N., & Corr, P.J. (2004). A two-dimensional neuropsychology of defense: Fear/Anxiety anmd defensive distance. *Neuroscience and Behavioral Reviews,* 28, 285–305.
59. Blanchard, D.C., Griebel, G., & Blanchard, R.J. (2001). Mouse defensive behaviors: Pharamacological and behavioral assays for anxiety and panic. *Neuroscience and Behavioral Reviews,* 25, 205–218.
60. Freud, S. (1920). *A general introduction to psychoanalysis.* New York: Horace Liveright.
61. Grillon, C. (2008). Models and mechanisms of anxiety: Evidence from startle studies. *Psychopharmacology,* 199(3), 421–437.
62. Kessler, R.C., Brandenburg, N., Lane, M., Roy-Byrne, P., Stang, P.D., Stein, D.J., et al. (2005). Rethinking the duration requirement for generalized anxiety disorder: Evidence from the National Comorbidity Survey Replication. *Psychological Medicine,* 35(7), 1073–1082.

Chapter 12
Other Psychiatric Disorders as Evolutionary Adaptations

Abstract This chapter explores the evolutionary roots of three classes of psychiatric symptoms that are not anxiety disorders: depression, somatization, and paranoid ideation. Although depression might seem to be the least likely psychiatric disorder to be an evolutionary adaption, the chapter discusses over a half dozen theoretical articles that propose that it is. The chapter also describes how the proximate mechanisms underlying different types of paranoid delusions (i.e., persecutory and jealous delusions) may have evolved from different modes of evolution, Charles Darwin's "Natural Selection" and "Sexual Selection," respectively. The end of the chapter discusses why the proximate mechanisms underlying anxiety disorders and other psychiatric disorders, which evolved to protect us from harm, do not seem to be adaptive to us in everyday life, including the frequency, intensity, and duration of symptoms, and the fundamental problem that the mechanisms trigger fear and anxiety when no real threat of harm exists. Finally, the chapter highlights some of the shortcomings of evolutionary psychology, which is interested in only the last 1.8 million years of human evolution.

Keywords Depression • Evolution • Evolutionary Psychiatry • Paranoia • Prevalence • Proximate mechanisms • Psychiatric disorders • Somatization • Threat

A number of other psychiatric disorders, aside from the anxiety disorders, have been identified as being the product or byproduct of evolutionary adaptations or adaptive characteristics that have had survival value for our ancestors. These disorders include depression, somatization, and paranoid ideation.

12.1 Depression

Major depressive disorder (MDD) is defined as having five or more of nine types of symptoms during the same 2-week period [1]. In brief, the nine types of symptoms are: (1) feeling sad or empty most of the day or nearly every day; (2) markedly reduced interest or pleasure in anything; (3) unintentional significant weight loss or

K.J. Flannelly, *Religious Beliefs, Evolutionary Psychiatry, and Mental Health in America*, Religion, Spirituality and Health: A Social Scientific Approach 1,
DOI 10.1007/978-3-319-52488-7_12

weight gain; (4) insomnia or hypersomnia almost every day; (5) psychomotor agitation or retardation; (6) fatigue almost every day; (7) feelings of worthlessness or guilt; (8) inability to think or concentrate; and (9) frequently thinking about death.

Depression might seem to be the least likely psychiatric disorder to be an evolutionary adaption; yet over a half dozen theoretical articles have proposed that it is [2–9]. Most of these theories propose that depression mainly evolved to deal with social losses, including the loss of social status, social rejection, and the termination of social relationships [2–6, 10]. The American psychologist and neuroscientist Jaak Panksepp believes that depression is associated with an innate "GRIEF" system in the brain that evolved more than 100 million years ago to regulate social relationships, including infant-parent attachment, and that depressive symptoms are triggered when social bonds are broken [10].

Some theorists believe depression serves a more general purpose to deal with any kind of major loss, such as the loss of resources [4–6], whereas others believe it evolved to deal with any unfavorable circumstances, including unsatisfactory social relationships [8]. I suspect Panksepp is right that depression is related to a brain system that evolved for maintaining social bonds and was adaptive for dealing with social and other kinds of losses.

Those who hold the theoretical view that depression is a reaction to the loss of social status see it as part of the process of submission in social competition, which was originally an adaptation for maintaining group membership and reducing the risk of physical harm from combat [2–4, 9]. Others think its function is to provide a temporary respite to adjust to loss [6, 10]. Theorists who have a more cognitive perspective on the function of depression believe it is adaptive because it creates a useful, albeit painful, time-out to assess an apparently bad situation, recruit personal and social resources to address the situation and to develop a plan for future action [5, 6, 8]. Most theorists agree that depression is maladaptive for humans in the short-term partly because humans tend to ruminate about events, which probably prolongs depression and may contribute to recurring episodes of depression [11].

The chance of an American having an episode of MDD sometime during his or her lifetime is estimated to be between 17% and 19% [12, 13]. The first episode of MDD (which does not include bipolar disorder), usually occurs between the late teens and the late 30s. General anxiety tends to be comorbid with depression, with persons who suffer from depression being likely to suffer from anxiety [13].

12.2 Somatization

Two evolutionary theories have been proposed to explain somatization, which entails symptoms of pain, gastrointestinal and other somatic symptoms that cannot be traced to a physical cause. The term somatization was first applied to complaints of motor and sensory deficits of an unexplained origin that were initially called hysteria and hysterical neurosis [14, 15]. Somatization belongs to a class of psychiatric disorders that has been called "somatoform disorders" and more recently "somatic symptom disorders," which include pain disorder (feeling pain that does not have a medically identified cause) and hypochondriasis (excessive fear of having a serious disease), among other things [1]. Other related disorders that cannot be medically explained are chronic fatigue syndrome, fibromyalgia (widespread muscle pain and stiffness), and irritable bowel syndrome (chronic abdominal pain and related symptoms) [14, 16, 17].

To receive a diagnosis of somatization disorder, a person must have multiple somatic complaints that cannot be medically explained and first occurred before the age of 30. These include at least four pain-related symptoms, two gastrointestinal symptoms, one sexually related symptom, and one pseudoneurological symptom (a symptom that appears to have a neurological basis, e.g., paralysis or loss of sensation in some area of the body) [1, 18].

A review of research from 24 countries found the 12-month prevalence rate of somatization ranged from 0.8% to 2.9%, with a lifetime prevalence of 5.9% [17]. However, the prevalence rate was much higher when less stringent diagnostic criteria were used. Regional and national surveys in the U.S. in 1980s suggest that its lifetime prevalence is less than 1% or 2% [16, 19–21]. A large epidemiological study conducted in California also found a lifetime prevalence rate of less than 1% for somatization disorder. However, the lifetime prevalence rate was 4.4% for an abridged definition of somatization, which required the presence of fewer symptoms than those required for a clinical diagnosis of somatization disorder [22]. A later study using the same definition found that 22% of patients seeking primary healthcare at a health clinic in New Jersey had "abridged somatization" [23].

One evolutionary theory of somatization claims it is related to social competition [3]. Simply put, it says the competitor who de-escalates, or submits, in a social competition instinctively (and unconsciously) develops somatic complaints to reduce the chances of injury, in what may be considered the metaphorical equivalent of claiming: "I am too sick to retaliate" (p. 5) [3]. Interestingly, current psychoanalytic theories claim that somatization arises from internal emotional conflicts, and that somatic symptoms either lie outside the realm of cognitive control or reflect impaired cognitive functioning [24, 25].

The other evolutionary theory of somatization proposes that it is an adaptation to detect internal rather than external threats of harm. Although Isaac Marks and Randolph Nesse drew comparisons between the adaptiveness of psychiatric symptoms and immune responses, they did not think that any psychiatric symptoms were directly related to immune responses [26]. Yet, this is essentially the evolutionary interpretation of somatization proposed by American physician Professor Robert Dantzer, who thinks somatization reflects the malfunction of a brain system that monitors and assesses threats to the internal environment [27].

12.3 Paranoid Ideation

Paranoid ideation represents a basic distrust of people, which is typically expressed as the belief that people (or someone in particular) will deceive, exploit, or harm you, or that they are actively doing so, when there is no concrete evidence that this belief is true. Technically, false beliefs such as these are only called delusions when they demonstrate a clear break from reality [1, 18]. Before discussing paranoid ideation, generally, I should mention that there is a category of psychiatric disorders called delusional disorders, which as its names implies, specifically addresses delusions. This diagnostic category includes, among others, persecutory, jealous, grandiose, erotomatic, and nihilistic types of delusions. I will try to describe the essence of each one of these delusional disorders in a short sentence. Persecutory delusions are beliefs that a person or persons are trying to harm you in some way. Jealous delusions entail the belief that your spouse or lover is being unfaithful. Grandiose delusions encompass beliefs that you are exceptional in some way that other people fail to recognize. Erotomatic delusions are beliefs that someone of higher social status is in love with you. Nihilistic delusions are beliefs that something catastrophic will happen. The diagnosis of a delusional disorder assumes that the delusion reflects a severe form of psychosis other than schizophrenia [1, 28].

Apart from the diagnosis of delusional disorder, itself, delusions commonly occur in two types of psychiatric disorders: schizophrenia, which is a form of psychosis, and paranoid personality disorder, which is not. Both have lifetime prevalence rates of less than 4% among Americans [21, 29–31]. Other studies have found that the 12-month prevalence rates of non-psychotic paranoid ideation in the U.S. may be 2–3 times higher than the rate of diagnosed cases of paranoia [32, 33], and a nationwide U.K. survey found that the 12-month prevalence rate of sub-clinical paranoid ideation was nearly 19% [34]. However, since paranoid personality disorder is one of the least studied of the personality disorders [29], the lifetime prevalence rate of sub-clinical levels of paranoid ideation among Americans has not been investigated.

The two most common types of paranoid ideation are: (1) persecutory delusions, which entail beliefs about deceit, exploitation, and/or physical harm; and (2) jealousy delusions, which entail beliefs about sexual infidelity. At first glance, jealous delusions or ideation about sexual infidelity might seem only to involve deceit. However, from an evolutionary perspective, paranoid ideation about sexual infidelity may be a response to a perceived threat to one's reproductive success, which entails exploitation in the sense that one may be unintentionally committing one's own resources to increase someone else's reproductive success. Taken by itself, exploitation seems to correspond to the threat of cheating in social exchanges [35], and persecutory delusions could reflect a primitive mechanism for detecting such cheating. Refined measures of paranoid ideation may make it possible to differentiate among these different, but related, functions of paranoia.

Thus, paranoid ideation, in general, may represent the action of at least three different proximate brain mechanisms, which probably evolved in our primate ancestors: one mechanism for detecting potential physical harm by members of one's own species (conspecifics), one mechanism for detecting exploitation by cheating in social exchanges, generally, and one mechanism for specifically detecting exploitation by cheating in sexual relationships (i.e., infidelity). If so, one would expect that the first two mechanisms would have evolved by Natural Selection, and the last one would have evolved by sexual selection.

The social systems of non-human primates are far more complex than the social systems of many other animals, and some theorists believe that the complexity of primate social relationships drove the evolution of the cognitive abilities of primates [36–39]. As the social exchanges that occur within groups of monkeys and apes take many forms (e.g., cooperation in child rearing, foraging, grooming, territorial defense), one would expect that the evolution of proximate mechanisms to detect cheating in social exchanges would have occurred long before the evolution of modern humans or our immediate human ancestors, as evolutionary psychologists believe [35].

It seems to me, it is possible that one particular form of social exchange may underlie persecutory paranoid ideation; that is, the development of agonistic alliances or coalitions within social groups, which is unique to primate social groups [40–46]. These alliances have been observed among lower ranking males in groups of monkeys, baboons, and chimpanzees in natural situations. The apparent purpose of these alliances is twofold. One purpose of male alliances is to overthrow the dominant male within the group. As the social cognitive abilities of primates needed to form alliances to defeat a dominant male evolved, the cognitive ability to detect such alliances surely did too; hence, this detection mechanism may be the source of persecutory paranoid ideation.

The other related purpose of agonistic alliances in male primates is to gain reproductive access to females by defeating the dominant male. Therefore, the dominant male's need to recognize this threat to its reproductive success could likewise underlie paranoid jealousy. However, since female primates usually mate with multiple males within a group, and since restricting access to females is a common function of territoriality in many animals, the biological roots of sexual jealousy may date back beyond the evolution of primate social systems. On the other hand, paranoid jealousy may not have evolved until our primate ancestors evolved a system of male-female pair-bonding.

Finally, it is noteworthy that several European studies have found positive correlations between the prevalence and severity of social anxiety and paranoid symptoms in both clinical populations and the general public [47–51]. Hence, I think it is possible that the association between social anxiety and paranoid ideation is the result of their shared evolutionary heritage, in which social anxiety evolved to address the threat of rejection from one's social group and paranoia evolved to address the various types of threats posed by group members. One must keep in mind, however, that a presumably cohesive primate group may consist of two or more competing subgroups vying for power and resources, and paranoia may represent a mechanism that monitors threats posed by one subgroup to another subgroup (i.e., subgroup "insiders" and "outsiders").

12.4 Problems with Proximate Mechanisms

Of course, the fact that psychiatric disorders result from the operation of proximate brain mechanisms that are adaptive does not mean that psychiatric disorders themselves are adaptive [4, 52]. The symptoms may be adaptive for survival generally, but the fact that symptoms can become so frequent, so intense, or so prolonged that they interfere with a person's life is not an evolutionary adaptation.

The frequent occurrence of anxiety and related symptoms, such as paranoia, is a side effect of the operating characteristics of the brain mechanisms for detecting threats of harm. Since the detection and assessment of potential threats must be rapid to ensure protection from harm, decisions about what poses a threat are biased towards identifying danger even when none exists. Hence, threat assessment mechanisms produce many "false alarms," in that they identify something as potentially dangerous when it is not dangerous [53–60]. These repeated false alarms may seem to be malfunctions, even though the proximate mechanisms are operating properly, and they certainly can be distressing, but that is how the mechanisms work.

Similarly, the intensity level of reactions to threat (i.e., the symptoms) may be appropriate from an evolutionary perspective even though the level of intensity is disruptive. Two obvious examples of the disruptive effects of the intensity of response to potential threats are panic attack and agoraphobia.

The prolonged duration of symptoms may be attributed to at least two causes. I alluded to the first cause in connection to depression. Since proximate mechanisms for detecting threats have evolved to react to immediate short-term threats, their prolonged activation can be problematic [61]. For most animals, once a threat no longer exists the mechanism underlying the threat assessment returns to its normal baseline. However, because humans have the ability to think about the past and future, they can activate self-defense mechanisms when no potential threat exists [52, 62].

The other cause for the prolonged activation of some psychiatric symptoms may be that there is no "off-switch" for our threat detection mechanisms. Since assessments of threats are usually based on little tangible evidence and ambiguous stimuli [57], the proximate mechanisms of threat assessment systems rarely get definitive feedback that no threat actually exists, so anxiety tends to persist over time [53]. Indeed, a 2012 experimental study supports the notion that the persistence of OCD symptoms results from the inability of compulsive acts to provide definitive neural feedback that the source of potential harm has been eliminated [63].

Finally, it is possible that some proximate mechanisms that cause psychological distress are no longer adaptive, or are less important than they once were. Paul Gilbert suggests this might be the case for the mechanisms underlying social anxiety. Although humans evolved to live in small, relatively stable social groups, similar to many primates, our mechanisms for detecting social threats may not function well in larger societies in which we have more extensive social interactions [64–67]. Thus, our assessment of social threats may not be appropriate in the social systems in which we live now.

12.5 Chapter Highlights and Comments

Depression, somatization, and paranoid ideation are thought to be evolutionary adaptations, although paranoid ideation seems to me to fit more neatly into Nesse's conception of psychiatric disorders as adaptations that protect us from harm than do the other two. Whatever the adaptive value of depression, it appears to be an adaptation to social loss.

Evolutionary psychology, which is an outgrowth of cognitive psychology, assumes that the last two million years of human evolution encompass the critical period for understanding human nature. Thus, for example, it posits that a cognitive mechanism evolved in humans to detect cheating in social exchanges within the past two million years [35], while ignoring the fact that social exchanges within primate groups have been occurring for 30 million years or more. I suspect that primates evolved a proximate mechanism for detecting cheating in social exchanges long before humans evolved and that the operation of this mechanism and related mechanisms are manifested in paranoid ideation.

It is noteworthy that several studies have found positive correlations between the prevalence and severity of social anxiety and paranoid symptoms [47–51]. I think this correlation may reflect the shared evolutionary heritage of social anxiety and paranoia, in which social anxiety evolved as a result of the effects of potential rejection from one's social group and paranoia evolved as a result of the possible harm that can be caused by group membership.

Despite the adaptive value of psychiatric symptoms, this does not mean that psychiatric disorders themselves are adaptive, since the frequency, intensity, and/or the duration of symptoms are distressing and disrupt a person's life. The operating characteristics of the proximate mechanisms for detecting threats contribute to this distress, such as the frequency of "false alarms." In addition, the influence of cognition on these basically innate systems can further contribute to psychological distress. Finally, the fact that these proximate mechanisms were adaptive in the past does not mean that all of them are still adaptive today.

References

1. *Diagnostic and statistical manual of mental disorders.* (2013). (5th ed.). Washington, DC: American Psychiatric Association.
2. Price, J.S., Gardner Jr, R., Wilson, D.R., Sloman, L., Rohde, P., & Erickson, M. (2007). Territory, rank and mental health: The history of an idea. *Evolutionary Psychology, 5*(3), 531–554.
3. Price, J.S., Gardner, R., Jr., & Erickson, M. (2004). Can depression, anxiety and somatization be understood as appeasement displays? *Journal of Affective Disorders, 79*(1–3), 1–11.
4. Sloman, L., Gilbert, P., & Hasey, G. (2003). Evolved mechanisms in depression: The role of attachment and social rank in depression. *Journal of Affective Disorders, 74*(2), 107–121.
5. Watson, P.J., & Andrews, P.W. (2002). Toward a revised evolutionary adaptationist analysis of depression: The social navigation hypothesis *Journal of Affective Disorders, 72*(1), 1–14.

6. Welling, H. (2003). An evolutionary function of the depressive reaction: The cognitive map hypothesis. *New Ideas in Psychology, 21*(2), 147–156.
7. Nettle, D. (2004). Evolutionary origins of depression: A review and reformulation. *Journal of Affective Disorders, 81*(2), 91–102.
8. Nesse, R.M. (2000). Is depression an adaptation? *Archives of General Psychiatry, 57*(1), 14–20.
9. Gilbert, P. (2006). Evolution and depression: Issues and implications. *Psychological Medicine, 36*(3), 287–297.
10. Panksepp, J. (2010). Affective neuroscience of the emotional BrainMind: Evolutionary perspectives and implications for understanding depression. *Dialogues in Clinical Neuroscience, 12*(4), 533–544.
11. Lavender, A., & Watkins, E. (2004). Rumination and future thinking in depression. *British Journal of Clinical Psychology, 43*(2), 129–142.
12. Kessler, R.C., McGonagle, K.A., Zhao, S., Nelson, C.B., Hughes, M., Eshleman, S., et al. (1994). Lifetime and 12-month prevalence of DSM-III-R psychiatric disorders in the United States: Results from the National Comorbidity Study. *Archives of General Psychiatry, 51*(1), 8–19.
13. Kessler, R.C., Berglund, P., Demler, O., Jin, R., Merikangas, K.R., & Walters, E.E. (2005). Lifetime prevalence and age-of-onset distributions of DSM-IV disorders in the National Comorbidity Survey Replication. *Archives of General Psychiatry, 62*(6), 593–602.
14. Burton, C. (2003). Beyond somatisation: A review of the understanding and treatment of medically unexplained physical symptoms (MUPS). *British Journal of General Practice, 53*(488), 231–239.
15. Kanaan, R.A., Armstrong, D., & Wessely, S.C. (2011). Neurologists' understanding and management of conversion disorder. *Journal of Neurology, Neurosurgery & Psychiatry, 82*(9), 961–966.
16. Mai, F.O. (2004). Somatization disorder: A practical review. *Canadian Journal of Psychiatry, 49*(10), 652–662.
17. Haller, H., Cramer, H., Lauche, R., & Dobos, G. (2015). Somatoform disorders and medically unexplained symptoms in primary care. *Deutsches Ärzteblatt International, 112*, 279–287.
18. *Diagnostic and statistical manual of mental disorders.* (1994). (4th ed.). Washington, DC: American Psychiatric Association.
19. Swartz, M., Blazer, D., George, L., & Landerman, R. (1986). Somatization disorder in a community population. *American Journal of Psychiatry, 143*(11), 1403–1408.
20. Robins, L.N., Helzer, J.E., Weissman, M.M., Orvaschel, H., Gruenberg, E., Burke, J.D., et al. (1984). Lifetime prevalence of specific psychiatric disorders in three sites. *Archives of General Psychiatry, 41*(10), 949–958.
21. Rabins, P.V., Black, B., German, P., Roca, R., McGuire, M., Brant, L., et al. (1996). The prevalence of psychiatric disorders in elderly residents of public housing. *The Journals of Gerontology Series A: Biological Sciences and Medical Sciences, 51*(6), M319–M324.
22. Escobar, J.I., Golding, J.M., Hough, R.L., Karno, M., Burnam, M.A., & Wells, K.B. (1987). Somatization in the community: Relationship to disability and use of services. *American Journal of Public Health, 77*(7), 837–840.
23. Escobar, J.I., Waitzkin, H., Silver, R.C., Gara, M., & Holman, A. (1998). Abridged somatization: A study in primary care. *Psychosomatic Medicine, 60*(4), 466–472.
24. Taylor, G.J. (2003). Somatization and the conversion: Distinct or overlapping contructs? *The Journal of the American Academy of Psychoanalysis and Dynamic Psychiatry, 31*(3), 487–508.
25. Waller, E., & Schedit, C.E. (2006). Somatoform disorders of affect regulation: A development perspective. *International Review of Psychiatry, 18*(1), 13–24.
26. Marks, I.M., & Nesse, R.M. (1994). Fear and fitness: An evolutionary analysis of anxiety disorders. *Ethology and Sociobiology, 15*(5–6), 247–261.

27. Dantzer, R. (2005). Somatization: A psychoneuroimmune perspective. *Psycho-neuroendocrinology, 30*(10), 947–952.
28. Fennig, S., Fochtmann, L.J., & Bromet, E.J. (2005). Delusional disorder and shared psychotic disorder In B. J. Sadock, & V. A. Sadock, *Kaplan and Sadock's comprehensive textbook of psychiatry* (8th ed., 1525–1533). Philadelphia: Lippincott, Williams & Wilkins.
29. Triebwasser, J., Chemerinski, E., Roussos, P., & Siever, L.J. (2013). Paranoid personality disorder. *Journal of Personality Disorders, 27*(6), 795–805.
30. Bernstein, D.P., Useda, D., & Siever, L.J. (1993). Paranoid personality disorder: Review of the literature and recommendations for DSM-IV. *Journal of Personality Disorders, 7*(1), 53–62.
31. Kramer, M., Von Korff, M., & Kessler, L. (1980). The lifetime prevalence of mental disorders: Estimation, uses and limitations. *Psychological Medicine, 10*(3), 429–435.
32. Bazargan, M., Bazargan, S., & King, L. (2001). Paranoid ideation among elderly African American persons. *Gerontologist, 41*(3), 366–373.
33. Blazer, D.G., Hays, J.C., & Salive, M.E. (1996). Factors associated with paranoid symptoms in a community sample of older adults. *Gerontologist, 36*(1), 70–75.
34. Freeman, D., McManus, S., Brugha, T., Meltzer, H., Jenkins, R., & Bebbington, P. (2011). Concomitants of paranoia in the general population. *Psychological Medicine, 41*(5), 923–936.
35. Cosmides, L., & Tooby, J. (1992). Cognitive adaptations for social exchange. In J. Barkow, L. Cosmides, & J. Tooby (Eds.), *The adapted mind: Evolutionary psychology and the generation of culture*. New York: Oxford University Press.
36. Barrett, L., Henzi, P., & Rendall, D. (2007). Social brains, simple minds: Does social complexity really require cognitive complexity? *Philosophical Transactions of the Royal Society of London B Biological Sciences, 362*(1480), 561–575.
37. Rushworth, M.F.S., Mars, R.B., & Sallet, J. (2013). Are there specialized circuits for social cognition and are they unique to humans? *Current Opinion in Neurobiology, 23*(3), 436–442.
38. Cheney, D., Seyfarth, R., & Smuts, B. (1986). Social relationships and social cognition in nonhuman primates. *Science, 234*, 1361–1366.
39. Seyfarth, R.M., Cheney, D.L., & Bergman, T.J. (2005). Primate social cognition and the origins of language. *Trends in Cognitive Sciences, 9*(6), 264–266.
40. Chapais, B. (1995). Alliances as a means of competition in primates: Evolutionary, developmental, and cognitive aspects. *Yearbook of Physical Anthropology, 38*(S21), 115–136.
41. Mesterton-Gibbons, M., Gavrilets, S., Gravner, J., & Akcay, E. (2011). Models of coalition or alliance formation. *Journal of Theoretical Biology, 274*(1), 187–204.
42. Nishida, T. (1983). Alpha status and agonistic alliance in wild chimpanzees (*Pan troglodytes* schweinfurthii). *Primates, 24*(3), 318–336.
43. Dixson, A.F. (1997). Evolutionary perspectives on primate mating systems and behavior. *Annals of the New York Academy of Sciences, 807*(1), 42–61.
44. Higham, J.P., & Maestripieri, D. (2010). Revolutionary coalitions in male rhesus macaques. *Behaviour, 147*(13–14), 1889–1908.
45. Bercovitch, F.B. (1988). Coalitions, cooperation and reproductive tactics among adult male baboons. *Animal Behaviour, 36*, 1198–1209.
46. Widdig, A., Streich, W.J., & Tembrock, G. (2000). Coalition formation among male Barbary macaques (*Macaca sylvanus*). *American Journal of Primatology, 50*(1), 37–51.
47. Stopa, L., Denton, R., Wingfield, M., & Taylor, K.N. (2013). The fear of others: A qualitative analysis of interpersonal threat in social phobia and paranoia. *Behavioural and Cognitive Psychotherapy, 41*(2), 188–209.
48. Taylor, K.N., & Stopa, L. (2013). The fear of others: A pilot study of social anxiety processes in paranoia. *Behavioural and Cognitive Psychotherapy, 41*(1), 66–88.
49. Gilbert, P., Boxall, M., Cheung, M., & Irons, C. (2005). The relationship of paranoid ideation and socity anxiety in a minxed clinical population. *Clinical Psychology & Psychotherapy, 12*, 124–133.

50. Rietdijk, J., Van Os, J., Graaf, R.D., Delespaul, P., & Gaag, M.V.D. (2009). Are social phobia and paranoia related, and which comes first? *Psychosis, 1*(1), 29–38.
51. Schutters, S.I.J., Dominguez, M.D.G., Knappe, S., Lieb, R., van Os, J., Schrucrs, K.R.J., et al. (2012). The association between social phobia, social anxiety cognitions and paranoid symptoms. *Acta Psychiatrica Scandinavica, 125*(3), 213–227.
52. Gilbert, P. (2001). Evolutionary approaches to psychopathology: The role of natural defences. *Australian and New Zealand Journal of Psychiatry, 35*(1), 17–27.
53. Eilam, D., Izhar, R., & Mort, J. (2011). Threat detection: Behavioral practices in animals and humans. *Neuroscience and Biobehavioral Reviews, 35*(4), 999–1006.
54. Neuberg, S.L., Kenrick, D.T., & Schaller, M. (2011). Human threat management systems: Self-protection and disease avoidance. *Neuroscience and Biobehavioral Reviews, 35*(4), 1042–1051.
55. Stein, D.J., & Nesse, R.M. (2011). Threat detection, precautionary responses, and anxiety disorders. *Neuroscience & Biobehavioral Reviews, 35*(4), 1075–1079.
56. Woody, E., & Boyer, P. (2011). Threat-detection and precaution: Introduction to the special issue. *Neuroscience & Biobehavioral Reviews, 35*(4), 989–990.
57. Woody, E.Z., & Szechtman, H. (2011). Adaptation to potential threat: The evolution, neurobiology, and psychopathology of the security motivation system. *Neuroscience and Biobehavioral Reviews, 35*(4), 1019–1033.
58. Flannelly, K.J., Koenig, H.G., Galek, K., & Ellison, C.G. (2007). Beliefs, mental health, and evolutionary threat assessment systems in the brain. *Journal of Nervous and Mental Disease, 195*(12), 996–1003.
59. Leahy, R.L. (2002). Pessimism and the evolution of negativity. *Journal of Cognitive Psychotherapy, 16*, 295–316.
60. Nesse, R. (1998). Emotional disorders in evolutionary perspective. *British Journal of Medical Psychology, 71*(4), 397–415.
61. Panksepp, J. (1998). *Affective neuroscience: The foundations of human and animal emotions.* New York: Oxford University Press.
62. Beck, A.T., Emery, G., & Greenberg, R.L. (1985). *Anxiety disorders and phobias: A cognitive perspective*. New York: Basic Books.
63. Hinds, A.L., Woody, E.Z., Van Ameringen, M., Schmidt, L.A., & Szechtman, H. (2012). When too much is not enough: Obsessive-compulsive disorder as a pathology of stopping, rather than starting. *PLoS ONE, 7*(1), e30586.
64. Gilbert, P. (1998). Evolutionary psychopathology: Why isn't the mind designed better than it is? *British Journal of Medical Psychology, 71*(Pt 4), 353–373.
65. Gilbert, P. (1998). The evolved basis and adaptive functions of cognitive distortions. *British Journal of Medical Psychology, 71*(Pt 4), 447–463.
66. Gilbert, P. (2001). Evolution and social anxiety. The role of attraction, social competition, and social hierarchies. *Psychiatric Clinics of North America, 24*(4), 72–51.
67. Gilbert, P. (2002). Evolutionary approaches to psychopathology and cognitive therapy. *Journal of Cognitive Psychotherapy: An International Quarterly, 16*(3), 263–294.

Chapter 13
Beliefs and Psychiatric Symptoms

Abstract The chapter begins with an historical description of the nature of beliefs, including the philosophical perspective that beliefs represent linguistic propositions about the nature of the world that are either true or false, and the Platonic and Aristotelian concepts of *phantasia* and *doxa*. The first section of the chapter also: (a) connects *phantasia* and *doxa* to Lewis Wolpert's concepts of weak and strong causal beliefs, and describes human research findings indicating (b) that beliefs more commonly take the form of mental models than linguistic propositions, (c) that people are born with certain beliefs about the world, and (d) that individuals may simultaneously hold contradictory beliefs. The second section links Wolpert's strong causal beliefs to so-called folk beliefs about inanimate and animate objects, which are thought to be inherited. The third section describes how folk beliefs are thought to underlie certain religious beliefs and how folk beliefs about biology probably contributed to both the historical rejection and acceptance of the concept of organic evolution. The following section presents clinical and research evidence that negative beliefs about the world, including negative beliefs about people, underlie many psychiatric disorders, such as general anxiety, social anxiety, obsessive-compulsive disorder, and personality disorders. The final section discusses the processing of beliefs in the brain, particularly the role of the ventromedial area of the prefrontal cortex.

Keywords Aristotle • Brain • Causal beliefs • Dysfunctional beliefs • Evolution • Folk beliefs • Logic • Prefrontal cortex • Psychiatric symptoms

13.1 The Nature of Beliefs

Plato and Aristotle thought there were two types of beliefs: *phantasia* and *doxa* [1, 2]. *Phantasia* is the product of perception, whereas *doxa* is the product of abstract thought. Aristotle claimed that *doxa* is uniquely human, but that some animals are capable of *phantasia*. Although the beliefs that many people hold simply reflect the beliefs they were taught, Aristotle proposed a method to develop and evaluate

K.J. Flannelly, *Religious Beliefs, Evolutionary Psychiatry, and Mental Health in America*, Religion, Spirituality and Health: A Social Scientific Approach 1,
DOI 10.1007/978-3-319-52488-7_13

beliefs using syllogistic reasoning (or syllogisms[1]), which is the central element of deductive logic – i.e., the formal philosophical system for developing and testing rational beliefs [3–7].

Rcsearch on non-human primates (mainly monkeys and apes) indicates that some species may develop expectations (or beliefs) about the behavior of other members of their own species based on observational learning, but their level of reasoning is limited to their immediate observable situation [8, 9]. There is no concrete evidence that monkeys or apes hold beliefs about the world or engage in logical reasoning as we do [10]. Thus, Aristotle's presumption that *doxa* is unique to humans seems to be true, since even the great apes do not appear to engage in the kind of abstract reasoning that characterizes deductive logic or deduction.

The concepts of *phantasia* and *doxa* seem to be similar to the concepts of "weak" and "strong" causal beliefs discussed by the British evolutionary biologist Lewis Wolpert in 2007 [10]. Wolpert, like the American psychologist David Premack, said there are two types of perceived causal relationships: arbitrary causal relations and natural causal relationships. Wolpert called beliefs about such relationships, "weak and "strong" causal beliefs, respectively. Beliefs about arbitrary causal relationships are the product of associative learning processes that humans share with other animals (like *phantasia*). These weak causal beliefs arise from observing the repeated pairing of events that have no obvious connection. Strong causal beliefs, which are unique to humans (like *doxa*), "are preprogrammed into our brains so that we have evolved the ability to have a concept of forces acting on objects" (p. 27) [10]. These causal beliefs became critical for our survival [10].

Historically, beliefs have been considered to be propositions or statements about the nature of the world that can be true or false [11–16], and it was considered irrational for a person to hold two contradictory beliefs simultaneously [13, 16–18]. Although deductive logic was long regarded to be the mechanism through which rational beliefs are developed [6, 16, 19], traditional conceptions about beliefs have changed. First, beliefs are now regarded by many scholars and researchers be to mental representations [12, 13, 20–23], or mental models of the world that are not necessarily linguistic [14, 23, 24]. Second, it is now recognized that individuals may rationally hold contradictory beliefs. This is so because beliefs are not absolute, and the truth or falseness a belief often is not evident [16, 17, 25]. Hence, as extensive research has shown, individuals may hold multiple contradictory beliefs with varying degrees of certainty [11, 18, 25–29]. Moreover, individuals are able to assign numerical values to express their degree of certainty in a particular personal belief that they have [10, 25, 26, 28], just as one can express one's certainty in the belief that something will happen, such as your belief that you will get a promotion, or win the lottery, or that your favorite baseball team will win the World Series.

---

[1] Irving Copi's *Introduction to Logic* provides a number of examples of syllogisms, including the following one:

All citizens are residents.
All voters are citizens.
Therefore: All voters are residents.

13.1.1 Folk Beliefs

Folk beliefs are essentially what Professor Lewis Wolpert called strong causal beliefs [10]. Research since the 1980's has shown that very young children have implicit mental models or basic beliefs about the nature of world. One conclusion that may be drawn from this research, which Wolpert emphasized, is that we inherit beliefs about the nature of animate and inanimate objects [10, 30]. Since beliefs help us deal with the world under conditions of uncertainly, including gaps in our knowledge [10, 12, 30, 31], it obviously would be adaptive for us to be born with basic conceptions about the characteristics of objects [10, 30].

These innate mental models, which include beliefs about physical, psychological, and biological phenomena, have come to be known as "naïve beliefs" or "folk beliefs," including folk physics, psychology, and biology, respectively [32–34]. Wolpert proposed that strong causal beliefs began to evolve when humans began to use and manufacture tools,[2] so folk physics presumably evolved in humans before other folk beliefs did [10]. Folk physics includes beliefs about the physical characteristics of objects, the motion of objects, and most importantly, the concept that one thing can be the cause of another thing [30, 32, 34–37].

After early humans developed causal beliefs about tool use, according to Wolpert [10], they developed causal beliefs about other things, especially after the evolution of language, which led the human brain to develop a need to understand the causes of everything we observe in our world. Folk psychology, for example, includes our a propensity to believe that other beings have beliefs and desires that are similar, in a general sense, to our own [32–34, 38–40], and that other humans and animals have the power of agency, i.e., the ability to perform intentional acts [38, 40]. In short, we believe that people and animals are conscious, and that they think the way we do and act for the same reasons we do.

Research has identified a number of different types of human beliefs about animals (called folk biology) [30, 32]. For instance, we are strongly inclined to hold the three related beliefs that (a) each species or genus of animal is an unchanging "natural kind," (b) that no kind of animal can become another kind of animal, and (c) that the offspring of any natural kind of animal are the same natural kind as their parents [30, 34]. These three beliefs probably contributed to the reluctance of naturalists in the 18th and 19th Centuries to reject the concept of the mutability of species (regardless of their religious beliefs) and, therefore, to reject the concept of organic of evolution.

The belief that each animal represents its own "natural kind" implies that each kind of animal has a unique essence that makes it what it is in terms of its appearance, behavior, and lifestyle, even though individual animals of the same kind differ from one another and individual animals may change in their appearance, behaviors, etc., over the course of their lifespan [30, 34]. This belief seems to me to be much like Plato's concept of forms that said each thing is a reflection of its universal

[2]Although some primates and other animals use tools, Wolper suggested that tool use may have been acquired through associative learning.

essence. These three beliefs collectively suggest that certain kinds of animals can be grouped into intuitive natural hierarchies ("folk-biological categories') of similar animals [30]. Taken together, they also provide a framework for making inferences about expected similarities in the characteristics of similar natural kinds and expected differences in the characteristics of different natural kinds [30].

These beliefs may have spurred Natural Theologians like John Ray to try to establish natural taxonomic systems within the context of the *Book of Genesis*, whereas they spurred naturalists like Buffon, Lamarck, Erasmus Darwin, and Charles Darwin to seek natural explanations for these intuitive hierarchies, which led them to the concept of descent from a common ancestor. Hence, these folk beliefs about biology probably posed barriers to accepting the concept of organic evolution, itself, but these same beliefs may have facilitated accepting the theory of evolution by common descent once Charles Darwin clearly described how evolution could occur.

13.1.2 Religious Beliefs as Folk Beliefs

Wolpert claimed that "once causal beliefs evolved in relation to tools, and once language evolved, it was inevitable that people would want to understand the causes of all the events that affected their lives, from illness, to changes in climate, to death itself … and this could have led to religious beliefs" (*p.* 118) [10]. He also suggested that religious beliefs "provide answers to difficult questions and can give order and meaning to situations even when explanations are absent" (*p.* 120). Moreover, they can offer "an explanation of evil events" which "helps to maintain religious observance" (*p.* 120) [10].

Several anthropologists and psychologists have proposed that many religious beliefs reflect a natural human tendency to presume that actions or events are caused by agents, even when no agent is apparent [33, 34, 41, 42]. These naïve or folk beliefs about agency tend to assume that harmful supernatural agents (e.g., angry ancestors, evil gods, or demons) are the cause of negative life events, and beneficent supernatural agents (e.g., supportive ancestors or gods) are the cause of positive life events [33, 34, 41]. Such beliefs are facilitated by the fact that humans tend to create causal explanations (or beliefs) based on very little information about the actual causes of events [33, 34]. Gods and demons are typically believed to be human-like beings, just as our deceased ancestors are human beings [34, 43, 44]. Thus, some people will attribute natural disasters to Gods' anger and some survivors of natural disasters will attribute their survival to God's grace. Other people believe that the devil is the cause of human evil, so some people demonize members of other social groups, especially if they are competitors.

The anthropologist Pascal Boyer and his colleagues generally link belief in supernatural agency to the principle that it is "better to be safe than sorry" in saying that we have a "agency-detection system" that is biased towards the "over-detection of agency" [43, 45]. I would call this concept the "over-attribution" rather than the "over-detection" of agency in that we attribute a cause to an agent even though there may be no causal connection, or even an actual agent. The anthropologist Scott

Atran and psychologist Ara Norenzayan also link the "better safe than sorry principle" to the attribution of evil to humans, especially outsiders. They see the attribution of evil as a cognitive manifestation of this principle, which they believe evolved in humans because the members of our genus (Homo[3]) probably posed a greater threat of harm than that posed by predators during human evolution [33]. Thus, Atran and Norenzayan claim it was adaptive to evolve a proximate mechanism to make us wary of other "humans," just as it was adaptive to evolve a mechanism to make us wary of predators [33, 34]. However, what these theorists apparently fail to recognize is that such an "agency-detection system" simply represents the overlaying of a cognitive system upon preexisting emotional and instinctive "threat detection" or "threat assessment" systems that arose in animals eons before the evolution of cognition or humans [33, 34, 41, 45].

Another religious belief that has been cast as a folk belief is belief in life-after-death, which I will discuss in Chaps. 15, 16, 17, and 18. A central point of the social scientists who have linked religious beliefs to folk beliefs is that all supernatural beliefs are intuitive rather than rational; thus, they cannot be refuted by the rules of logical reasoning that normally govern explanations of causation [33, 34, 45].

13.2 Beliefs and Psychiatric Symptoms

Aaron T. Beck, the founder of cognitive therapy, published a book in 1985 that claimed, based on clinical evidence, that anxiety disorders are associated with beliefs about the dangerousness of the world, and that patients' excessive thoughts about potential harm are a crucial element in anxiety disorders [46]. Other authors have also characterized the key feature of general anxiety to be the belief that the world is a dangerous place (e.g., [47])

Beck and his co-authors said that "The anxious patient is so sensitive to any stimulus that might be taken as indicating an imminent disaster or harm that he is constantly warning himself, as it were, about the potential dangers" (p. 31) [46]. Because virtually any stimulus may be perceived as dangerous or threatening, Beck and his colleagues thought a perceived threat can trigger an alarm, which causes anxious individuals to experience frequent "false alarms" that keep them in a constant state of emotional distress. The book proposed that the preoccupation with danger that anxious patients exhibit is the product of the rules (or beliefs) they use to evaluate situations. These rules, which often seem to operate outside of conscious awareness, include such beliefs as:

> "Any strange situation should be regarded as dangerous."
> "A situation or a person is unsafe until proven to be safe."
> "It is always best to assume the worst."[46, p. 63]

---

[3] The earliest known species that is considered to be sufficiently similar to us (*Homo sampiens*) to be placed in the same genus (*Homo*) as us is *Homo* habilis. In all, there are seven species that have been classified as belonging to the genus Homo, including our own species.

Beck et al. also described different beliefs held by patients with agoraphobia, all of which reflect the core belief held by individuals with agoraphobia that a catastrophe can occur at any time when they are outside their homes [46]. The association between agoraphobia and panic attack is reflected in the observation that individuals with panic disorder believe that ordinary physical and emotional experiences are harbingers of catastrophic events [48, 49].

Other beliefs that Beck et al. [46] mention are specifically about people (e.g., "Strangers despise weakness") and personal responsibility (e.g., "My security and safety depend on anticipating and preparing myself at all times for any possible danger"; "My survival depends on my always being competent and strong"). In their later writings, Beck and his colleagues called these kinds of beliefs "dysfunctional beliefs."

A subsequent book by Beck and Freeman [50] described the "dysfunctional beliefs" underlying different personality disorders. For example, individuals with narcissistic personalities believe "I don't have to be bound by the rules that apply to other people," whereas people with paranoid personalities believe "Other people will try to use me or manipulate me if I don't watch out." These and other dysfunctional beliefs held by people with various personality disorders were confirmed in subsequent research on clinical samples by Beck and his associates [51–54].

Borderline personality disorder is more complex, consisting of three different dimensions of beliefs [51, 53]: dependency (hopelessness, weakness, and neediness), distrust of others, and the belief that one should act preemptively to thwart a threat. The latter includes the specific belief that "People will get me if I don't get them first." Distrust of others is expressed in a number of ways that imply that people pose a threat of some kind, for example [53, p. 171]:

> "People will take advantage of me if I give them the chance."
> "I have to be on my guard at all times."
> "If people get close to me, they will discover the real me and reject me."

The first two of these three beliefs are expressions of paranoid ideation [55, 56]. Similar paranoid beliefs occur in persecutory paranoid ideation: e.g., "I cannot trust anyone"; "People talk about me behind my back"; Someone has it in for me"; and "Someone is trying to steal my ideas" [56]. Other dysfunctional beliefs underlie other forms of paranoid ideation, such as jealousy ideation in which a person believes his/her sexual partner is being unfaithful [57].

Research and clinical observations indicate that dysfunctional beliefs are associated with many other psychiatric disorders. These include bipolar disorder [58], eating disorders [59], hypochondriasis [60, 61], social anxiety [62–64], obsessive-compulsive disorder [65, 66], and post-traumatic stress disorder [67].

Like borderline personality disorder, social anxiety disorder and obsessive-compulsive disorder (OCD) are associated with multiple dimensions of beliefs. The dysfunctional beliefs in social anxiety have been categorized in several ways, including beliefs about oneself and beliefs about others [68–71]. Some researchers think OCD involves up to six dimensions of concerns and related beliefs [65, 72]. First and foremost, however, are the beliefs that world is unsafe and that some serious harm is going to occur [65, 66, 73, 74]. Two other key features of OCD entail an exaggerated belief that one is responsible for causing whatever harm might occur and intolerance of uncertainty, i.e., the belief that it is necessary to be certain about future events [65, 66].

As early as 1967, Beck introduced a cognitive model that explained how depression was the result of three types of negative beliefs [75]. These are beliefs about one's self (e.g., "I am completely useless"), beliefs about the world, especially one's life (e.g., "My life is a mess"), and beliefs about the future (e.g., "Things will never get better"). The basic tenets of Beck's theoretical model of depression are widely accepted and supported by research [76–79].

13.3 Beliefs and the Brain

The brain has been called a belief-generating machine [34, 80]. Obviously, the brain does not just generate beliefs; it must store them someplace [5, 25, 81]. Yet, is not clear where beliefs are stored. Memories of personal experiences and knowledge are thought to distributed throughout the brain's neocortex [82, 83]. However, researchers view beliefs and knowledge as separate forms of memory [84–86]. Knowledge is said to be stored in explicit memory, which is conscious and primarily verbal, whereas beliefs are said to be stored in implicit memory, which may be unconscious, non-verbal, and emotional in nature [84]. Unfortunately, very little research has been done on the storage or processing of beliefs in the brain [87].

Even though memories seem to be stored throughout the neocortex [82, 83], two areas of the neocortex – the medial temporal lobe and the prefrontal area of the frontal lobe – are specifically involved in storing and retrieving long-term memories [82, 83]. Although it is not evident whether these two cortical areas also participate in the storage and retrieval of beliefs to and from long-term memory, recent neuroimaging studies indicate that a part of the frontal cortex called the prefrontal cortex (PFC) is active in processing some types of beliefs in working memory [88–91].

Three recent neuroimaging studies have investigated the activity of the ventromedial area of the PFC (the vmPFC) while individuals performed a task in which they had to decide whether a statement expressing a belief (which was visually presented) was true or false [89–91]. The three studies included some religious beliefs, and two of the studies included participants who were non-religious persons and religiously committed Christians. All three studies found the vmPFC was active during the processing of beliefs, but none of them found differences in vmPFC activity between religious and non-religious beliefs or between religious and non-religious study participants. However, one of the studies found that other areas of the brain, including some involved in emotions, were activated more when participants agreed with the religious beliefs that were presented [89]. Other research suggests that beliefs can influence the functioning of the vmPFC, as will be discussed in Chap. 14 [92].

13.4 Chapter Highlights and Comments

I drew a parallel in the beginning of the chapter between the Greek concepts of *phantasia* and *doxa* [1, 2] and the concepts of "weak" and "strong" causal beliefs advanced by the British evolutionary biologist Lewis Wolpert [10]. Wolpert proposed that animals and humans both have weak causal beliefs (as Aristotle claimed for *phantasia*), but strong causal beliefs were unique to humans (as Aristotle claimed for *doxa*). Wolpert traced the origin of strong causal beliefs to the evolution of tool-making in humans, and he claimed that strong causal beliefs are preprogrammed in the human brain [10].

Though beliefs were historically thought of as propositions about the nature of the world that must be true or false, research has found: (a) that individuals can hold multiple contradictory beliefs at the same time, and (b) beliefs often consist of mental models of the world rather that statements about it. Other research indicates that people may inherit basic beliefs about animate and inanimate objects, commonly called folk beliefs, which appear to be essentially what Wolpert called strong causal beliefs. Some folk beliefs appear to underlie religious beliefs regarding the attribution of causation to supernatural forces and attitudes towards other humans.

Research and clinical evidence has demonstrated that anxiety and other psychiatric disorders are associated with beliefs about the dangerousness of the world, and that these beliefs often lie outside of consciousness. Such dysfunctional beliefs have been identified in cases of depression, general anxiety, social anxiety, bipolar disorder, eating disorders, hypochondriasis, obsessive-compulsive disorder, and post-traumatic stress disorder.

Finally, recent research has discovered areas of the brain that are involving in processing beliefs, particularly the vmPFC. This findings is quite important because, as discussed in earlier and later chapters, the vmPFC is involved in modulating fear, which underlies many psychiatric symptoms.

References

1. Gronroos, G. (2013). Two kinds of belief in Plato. *Journal of the History of Philosophy, 51*(1), 1–19.
2. McCready-Flora, I. (2013). Aristotle's cognitive science: Belief, affect and rationality. *Philosophy and Phenomenological Research, 89*(2), 394–435.
3. Hudry, J. L. (2013). Aristotle on deduction and inferential necessity. *Review of Metaphysics, 67*(1), 29–54.
4. Andrade, E. J., & Becerra, E. S. (2008). Establishing connections between Aristotle's natural deduction and first-order logic. *History and Philosophy of Logic, 29*(4), 309–325.
5. Grimaltos, T., & Hookway, C. (1995). When deduction leads to belief. *Ratio, 8*(1), 24–41.
6. Gärdenfors, P. (1990). An epistemic analysis of explanations and causal beliefs. *Topoi, 9*(2), 109–124.
7. Copi, I. M. (1969). *Introduction to logic* (3rd ed.). London: MacMillan.

8. Martin, A., & Santos, L. R. (2014). The origins of belief representation: Monkeys fail to automatically represent others' beliefs. *Cognition, 130*(3), 300–308.
9. Povinelli, D. J., & Giambrone, S. (2001). Reasoning about beliefs: A human specialization? *Child Development, 72*(3), 691–695.
10. Wolpert, L. (2007). *Six impossible things before breakfast: The evolutionary origins of beliefs.* New York: W.W. Norton & Co.
11. Curley, S. P., & Golden, J. I. (1994). Using belief functions to represent degrees of belief. *Organizational Behavior and Human Decision Processes, 58*, 271–303.
12. Smith, G. F., Benson, P. G., & Curley, S. P. (1991). Belief, knowledge, and uncertainty: A cognitive perspective on subjective probability. *Organizational Behavior and Human Decision Processes, 48*(2), 291–321.
13. Gilbert, D. T. (1991). How mental systems believe. *American Psychologist, 46*(2), 107–119.
14. Leben, D. (2014). When psychology undermines beliefs. *Philosophical Psychology, 27*(3), 328–350.
15. McKinsey, M. (1999). The semantics of belief ascriptions. *Nous, 33*(4), 519–557.
16. Egan, A. (2008). Seeing and believing: Perception, belief formation and the divided mind. *Philosophical Studies, 140*(1), 47–63.
17. Priest, G. (1985–1986). Contradiction, belief and rationality. *Proceedings of the Aristotelian Society, 86*, 99–116.
18. Leitgeb, H. (2014). The stability theory of belief. *Philosophical Review, 123*(2), 131–171.
19. Evans, J. S. B. T., & Over, D. E. (2013). Reasoning to and from belief: Deduction and induction are still distinct. *Thinking and Reasoning, 19*(3–4), 267–283.
20. Nichols, S. (2006). Just the imagination: Why imagining doesn't behave like believing. *Mind & Language, 21*(4), 459–474.
21. Green, D. W. (1993). Mental models: Rationality, representation and process. *Behavioral and Brain Sciences, 16*(2), 352–353.
22. Johnson-Laird, P. N., & Byrne, R. M. J. (1993). Precis of deduction. *Behavioral and Brain Sciences, 16*(2), 323–380.
23. Malt, B. C. (1990). Features and beliefs in the mental representation of categories. *Journal of Memory and Language, 29*(3), 289–315.
24. Bara, B. G. (1993). Toward a developmental theory of mental models. *Behavioral and Brain Sciences, 16*(2), 336.
25. Koriat, A., & Adiv, S. (2012). Confidence in one's social beliefs: Implications for belief justification. *Consciousness and Cognition, 21*, 1599–1616.
26. Kyburg, H. E. (2003). Are there degrees of belief? *Journal of Applied Logic, 1*(3), 139–149.
27. Enoch, D., & Schechter, J. (2008). How are basic belief-forming methods justified? *Philosophy and Phenomenological Research, 76*(3), 547–579.
28. Over, D. (1993). Deduction and degrees of freedom. *Behavioral and Brain Sciences, 16*(2), 361–362.
29. Zynda, L. (2000). Representation theorems and realism about degrees of belief. *Philosophy of Science, 67*(1), 45–69.
30. Atran, S. (1998). Folk biology and the anthropology of science: Cognitive universals and cultural particulars. *The Behavioral and Brain Sciences, 21*(4), 547–609.
31. Fox, J. (2003). Probability, logic and the cognitive foundations of rational belief. *Journal of Applied Logic, 1*, 197–224.
32. Wellman, H. M., & Gelman, S. A. (1992). Cognitive development: Foundational theories of core domains. *Annual Review of Psychology, 43*, 337–375.
33. Atran, S., & Norenzayan, A. (2004). Religion's evolutionary landscape: Counterintuition, commitment, compassion, communion. *Behavioral and Brain Sciences, 27*(6), 713–730.
34. Boyer, P. (2001). *Religion explained: The evolutionary origins of religious thought.* New York: Basic Books.
35. Bertamini, M., & Casati, R. (1993). False beliefs and naive beliefs: They can be good for you. *Behavioral and Brain Sciences, 16*(2), 512–513.

36. Reiner, M., Slotta, J. D., Michelene, T. H. C., & Resnick, L. B. (2000). Naive physics reasoning: A commitment to substance-based conceptions. *Cognition and Instruction, 18*(1), 1–34.
37. Markman, K. D., & Guenther, C. L. (2007). Psychological momentum: Intuitive physics and naive beliefs. *Personality and Social Psychology Bulletin, 33*(6), 800–812.
38. Arico, A., Fiala, B., Nichols, S., & Goldberg, R. F. (2011). The folk psychology of consciousness. *Mind & Language, 26*(3), 327–352.
39. Greenwood, D. J. (Ed.). (1991). *The future of folk psychology*. Cambridge: Cambridge University Press.
40. Christensen, S. M., & Turner, D. R. (Eds.). (1993). *Folk psychology and the philosophy of mind*. Hillsdale: Lawrence Erlbaum.
41. Rossano, M. J. (2006). The religious mind and the evolution of religion. *Review of General Psychology, 10*(4), 346–364.
42. Bloom, P. (2007). Religion is natural. *Developmental Science, 10*(1), 147–151.
43. Boyer, P., & Bergstrom, B. (2008). Evolutionary perspectives on religion. *Annual Review of Anthropology, 37*, 111–130.
44. Noss, J. B. (1969). *Man's religions* (5th ed.). New York: MacMillan Publishing.
45. Baumard, N., & Boyer, P. (2013). Religious beliefs as reflective elaborations on intuitions: A modified dual-process model. *Current Directions in Psychological Science, 22*(4), 295–300.
46. Beck, A. T., Emery, G., & Greenberg, R. L. (1985). *Anxiety disorders and phobias: A cognitive perspective*. New York: Basic Books.
47. Wells, A. (2000). *Emotional disorders and metacognition: Innovative cognitive therapy*. New York: Wiley.
48. Wenzel, A., Sharp, I. R., Brown, G. K., Greenberg, R. L., & Beck, A. T. (2006). Dysfunctional beliefs in panic disorder: The panic belief inventory. *Behaviour Research and Therapy, 44*(6), 819–833.
49. Hoppe, L. J., Ipser, J., Gorman, J. M., & Stein, D. J. (2012). Panic disorder. In T. E. Schaepfer, & C. B. Nemeroff (Eds.), *Handbook of clinical neurolology: Neurobiology of psychiatric disorders* (Vol. 106, pp. 363–374). Amsterdam: Elsevier.
50. Beck, A. T., & Freeman, A. (1990). *Cognitive therapy of personality disorders*. New York: Guilford Press.
51. Butler, A. C., Brown, G. K., Beck, A. T., & Grisham, J. R. (2002). Assessment of dysfunctional beliefs in borderline personality disorder. *Behaviour Research and Therapy, 40*(10), 1231–1240.
52. Beck, A. T., Butler, A. C., Brown, G. K., Dahlsgaard, K. K., Newman, C. F., & Beck, J. S. (2001). Dysfunctional beliefs discriminate personality disorders. *Behaviour Research and Therapy, 39*(10), 1213–1225.
53. Bhar, S. S., Brown, G. K., & Beck, A. T. (2008). Dysfunctional beliefs and psychopathology in borderline personality disorder. *Journal of Personality Disorders, 22*(2), 165–177.
54. Fournier, J. C., DeRubeis, R. J., & Beck, A. T. (2012). Dysfunctional cognitions in personality pathology: The structure and validity of the Personality Belief Questionnaire. *Psychological Medicine, 42*(4), 795–805.
55. Fenigstein, A. (1984). Self-consciousness and the overperception of self as a target. *Journal of Personality and Social Psychology, 47*(4), 860–870.
56. Fenigstein, A., & Vanable, P. A. (1992). Paranoia and self-consciousness. *Journal of Personality and Social Psychology, 62*(1), 129–138.
57. Mueser, K. T. (2000). Paranoia or delusional disorder. In *Encyclopedia of psychology* (Vol. 6, pp. 35–39). New York: Oxford University Press.
58. Alatiq, Y., Crane, C., Williams, J. M. G., & Goodwin, G. M. (2010). Dysfunctional beliefs in bipolar disorder: Hypomanic vs. depressive attitudes. *Journal of Affective Disorders, 122*(3), 294–300.
59. Jones, C., Leung, N., & Harris, G. (2007). Dysfunctional core beliefs in eating disorders: A review. *Journal of Cognitive Psychotherapy, 21*(2), 156–171.

60. Marcus, D. K., & Church, S. E. (2003). Are dysfunctional beliefs about illness unique to hypochondriasis? *Journal of Psychosomatic Research, 54*, 543–547.
61. Weck, F., Neng, J. M. B., Richtberg, S., & Stangier, U. (2012). Dysfunctional beliefs about symptoms and illness in patients with hypochondriasis. *Psychosomatics, 53*(2), 148–154.
62. Gumley, A., O'Grady, M., Power, K., & Schwannauer, M. (2004). Negative beliefs about self and illness: A comparison of individuals with psychosis with or without comorbid social anxiety disorder. *The Australian and New Zealand Journal of Psychiatry, 38*(11/12), 960–964.
63. Moscovitch, D. A. (2009). What is the core fear in social phobia? A new model to facilitate individualized case conceptualization and treatment. *Cognitive and Behavioral Practice, 16*(2), 123–134.
64. Gilbert, P. (2001). Evolution and social anxiety. The role of attraction, social competition, and social hierarchies. *Psychiatric Clinics of North America, 24*(4), 72–51.
65. Taylor, S., Abramowitz, J. S., McKay, D., Calamari, J. E., Sookman, D., Kyrios, M., et al. (2006). Do dysfunctional beliefs play a role in all types of obsessive-compulsive disorder? *Journal of Anxiety Disorders, 20*(1), 85–97.
66. Moulding, R., Anglim, J., Nedeljkovic, M., Doron, G., Kyrios, M., & Ayalon, A. (2011). The Obsessive Beliefs Questionnaire (OBQ): Examination in nonclinical samples and development of a short version. *Assessment, 18*(3), 357–374.
67. Vogt, D. S., Shipherd, J. C., & Resick, P. A. (2012). Posttraumatic maladaptive beliefs scale: Evolution of the personal beliefs and reactions scale. *Assessment, 19*(3), 308–317.
68. Clark, D. M., & Wells, A. (1995). A cognitive model of social phobia. In R. G. Heimberg, M. R. Leibowitz, D. A. Hope, & F. R. Schneier (Eds.), *Social phobia: Diagnosis, assessment, and treatment* (pp. 69–93). New York: Guilford Press.
69. Boden, M. T., John, O. P., Goldin, P. R., Werner, K., Heimberg, R. G., & Gross, J. J. (2012). The role of maladaptive beliefs in cognitive-behavioral therapy: Evidence from social anxiety disorder. *Behaviour Research and Therapy, 50*(5), 287–291.
70. Wong, Q. J. J., & Moulds, M. L. (2011). A new measure of the maladaptive self-beliefs in social anxiety: Psychometric properties in a non-clinical sample. *Journal of Psychopathology and Behavioral Assessment, 33*(2), 273–284.
71. Clark, D. M. (2001). A cognitive perspective on social phobia. In W. R. Crozier, & L. E. Alden (Eds.), *International handbook of social anxiety: Concepts, research and interventions relating to the self and shyness* (pp. 405–430). New York: Wiley
72. Group, O.-C. C. W. (1997). Cognitive assessment of obsessive-compulsive disorder. *Behaviour Research and Therapy, 35*(7), 667–681.
73. Taylor, S., McKay, D., & Abramowitz, J. S. (2005). Hierarchical structure of dysfunctional beliefs in obsessive-compulsive disorder. *Cognitive Behaviour Therapy, 34*(4), 216–228.
74. Chik, H. M., Calamari, J. E., Rector, N. A., & Riemann, B. C. (2010). What do low-dysfunctional beliefs obsessive-compulsive disorder subgroups believe? *Journal of Anxiety Disorders, 24*, 837–846.
75. Beck, A. T. (1967). *Depression: Causes and treatment*. Philadelphia: University of Pennsylvania Press.
76. Haaga, D. A., Dyck, M. J., & Ernst, D. (1991). Empirical status of cognitive theory of depression. *Psychological Bulletin, 110*(2), 215–236.
77. Clark, D. A., Beck, A. T., & Alford, B. A. (1999). *Scientific foundations of the cognitive theory of depression*. New York: Wiley.
78. Zauszniewski, J. A., & Rong, J. R. (1999). Depressive cognitions and psychosocial functioning: A test of Beck's cognitive theory. *Archives of Psychiatric Nursing, 13*(6), 286–293.
79. Crews, W. D., Jr., & Harrison, D. W. (1995). The neuropsychology of depression and its implications for cognitive therapy. *Neuropsychology Review, 5*(2), 81–123.
80. Alcock, J. E. (1995). The belief engine. *The Skeptical Inquirer, 19*(3), 14–18.
81. Piazza, T. (2009). Evidentialism and the problem of stored beliefs. *Philosophical Studies, 145*(2), 311–324.
82. Arnold, M. B. (2013). *Memory and the brain*. East Sussex: Psychology Press.

83. Tulving, E. (Ed.). (2013). *Memory, consciousness and the brain: The Tallinn Conference*, Psychology Press.
84. Damasio, A. R. (2001). Thinking about beliefs: Concluding remarks. In D. L. Schacter, & E. Scarry (Eds.), *Memory, brain, and belief* (pp. 325–334). Cambridge, MA: Harvard University Press.
85. Eichenbaum, H., & Bodkin, J. A. (2001). Beliefs and knowledge as distinct forms of memory. In D. L. Schacter, & E. Scarry (Eds.), *Memory, brain, and belief* (pp. 176–207). Cambridge, MA: Harvard University Press.
86. Westbury, C., & Dennett, D. C. (2001). Mining the past to construct the future: Memory and belief as forms of knowledge. In D. L. Schacter, & E. Scarry (Eds.), *Memory, brain, and belief* (pp. 11–34). Cambridge, MA: Harvard University Press.
87. Sacks, O., & Hirsch, J. (2008). A neurology of belief. *Annals of Neurology, 63*(2), 129–130.
88. Xue, G., He, Q., Lu, Z.-L., Levin, I. P., Dong, Q., & Bechara, A. (2013). Agency modulates the lateral and medial prefrontal cortex responses in belief-based decision making. *PloS One, 8*(6), e65274–e65274.
89. Harris, S., Kaplan, J. T., Curiel, A., Bookheimer, S. Y., Iacoboni, M., & Cohen, M. S. (2009). The neural correlates of religious and nonreligious belief. *PloS One, 4*(10), e0007272–e0007272.
90. Harris, S., Sheth, S. A., & Cohen, M. S. (2008). Functional neuroimaging of belief, disbelief, and uncertainty. *Annals of Neurology, 63*(2), 141–147.
91. Han, S., Mao, L., Gu, X., Zhu, Y., Ge, J., & Ma, Y. (2008). Neural consequences of religious belief on self-referential processing. *Social Neuroscience, 3*(1), 1–15.
92. Evans, J. S. B. T. (2003). In two minds: Dual-process accounts of reasoning. *Trends in Cognitive Sciences, 7*(10), 454–459.

Chapter 14
Evolutionary Threat Assessment Systems Theory

Abstract The first section of the chapter provides an overview of theoretical articles supporting Evolutionary Threat Assessment Systems Theory (ETAS Theory). The second section summarizes the results of an extensive review of research on the brain areas that have been implicated in seven classes of psychiatric disorders: small animal phobias, depression, general anxiety, social anxiety, panic attack, paranoia, and obsessive-compulsive disorder. The next two sections provide evidence that partially confirms the association predicted by ETAS Theory between these classes of psychiatric symptoms and several areas of the brain (the brain stem, the basal ganglia, the limbic system, and prefrontal cortex) and graphically depict these associations to illustrate four possible models of possible ETAS. The rest of the chapter explains how ETAS operate and covers a number of topics that are important for understanding the operation of ETAS. These include the role of the ventromedial prefrontal cortex (vmPFC) in deductive reasoning and threat assessment, the influence of beliefs on the vmPFC's decision-making, the degree to which a sense of safety affects threat assessments, and the vmPFC's sensitivity to safety cues, as well as sources of safety, including supportive social relationships, familiar places, self-esteem, and self-efficacy.

Keywords Aversive amplification circuit • Beliefs • Brain • ETAS Theory • Evolution • Logic • Psychiatric disorders • Safety • Self-esteem • Self-efficacy • Social support • Threat • Threat assessment

14.1 Background

A 2007 theoretical article by me and my colleagues proposed that the proximate mechanisms underlying many psychiatric disorders involve neural circuits connecting the basal ganglia, the limbic system, and prefrontal cortex (PFC), which we called "Evolutionary Threat Assessment Systems" [1]. Figure 14.1 shows the model of ETAS that the article proposed. The figure shows that the PFC, the limbic system, and the basal ganglia are inter-connected, as described in Chaps. 9 and 10, that each of them receives separate sensory input and input from other cortical areas, and that the threat assessments of each brain area is influenced by past experience. Beliefs,

K.J. Flannelly, *Religious Beliefs, Evolutionary Psychiatry, and Mental Health in America*, Religion, Spirituality and Health: A Social Scientific Approach 1,
DOI 10.1007/978-3-319-52488-7_14

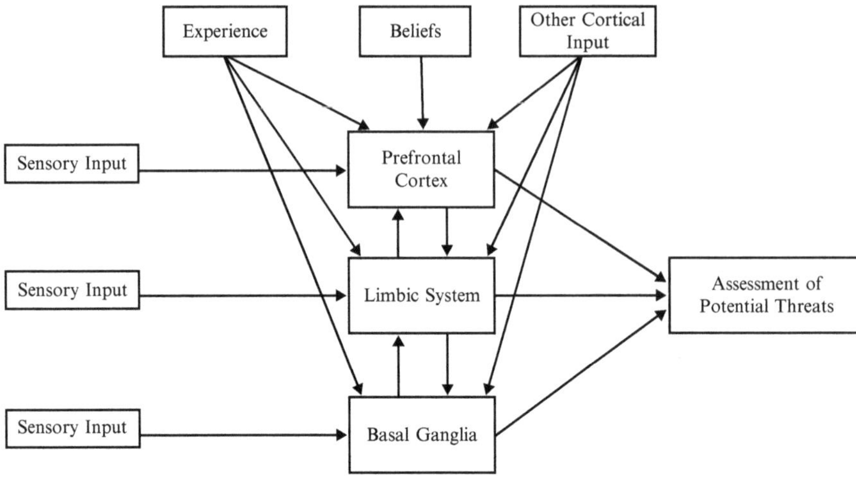

Fig. 14.1 Original model of Evolutionary Threat Assessment Systems presented in the 2007 theoretical article by Flannelly et al. in the *Journal of Nervous and Mental Disease*; see reference list for citation; reproduced by permission

however, only have a direct effect on the PFC, which evaluates the threat assessments of the limbic system and basal ganglia. The article did not provide evidence about the degree of involvement of these brain regions in different psychiatric disorders and we did not include the brain stem in our theoretical model. However, the 2007 article did explain that multiple brain mechanisms or systems for threat assessment obviously are needed to detect the many different kinds of threats that we and other animals face, and that different classes of psychiatric symptoms represent the reaction of these systems to various kinds of potential threats of harm.

Since the publication of our 2007 paper, a number of theoretical articles have been published that endorse the basic premise of ETAS Theory that psychiatric symptoms in patients with mental illness and the general public are the product of threat assessment systems that evolved for self-protection [1–11]. Most of these articles as well as other articles [12–17] support the theory's proposition that regions of the PFC, limbic system, basal ganglia, and brain stem are involved in threat assessments. Different authors have discussed different types of threat assessment systems in the brain, including systems that address the threat of predators, conspecifics (members of one's own species), and disease [3, 4, 6, 9, 17], but numerous other threat assessment systems certainly must exist [1, 18].

The unique feature of ETAS Theory, which differentiates it from other theoretical models of threat assessment systems, is that ETAS Theory explains how beliefs influence psychiatric systems by influencing the brain systems that make threat assessments. I will return to this point, shortly.

Table 14.1 Involvement of different brain regions in psychiatric disorders that are thought to be the product of evolutionary adaptations

Psychiatric disorder	Prefrontal cortex	Limbic system	Basal ganglia	Brain stem
Panic attack	✔	✔	✓	✔
Social anxiety	✔	✔	✔	✓
Major depression	✔	✔	✔	✓
Paranoid ideation	✔	✔	✔	
General anxiety	✔	✔		
Animal phobia	✔	✔		
Obsession-compulsion	✔	✓	✔	✔

14.2 Brain Regions Involved in Different Psychiatric Disorders

I recently conducted an exhaustive literature review of studies that have examined the potential involvement of the PFC, limbic system, basal ganglia, and the brain stem in different classes of psychiatric disorders. My review was limited to those disorders I discussed in Chaps. 11 and 12 about psychiatric symptoms being evolutionary adaptations. Unfortunately, there are so few studies on acrophobia, agoraphobia (without panic attack), and somatization that the existing evidence is insufficient to determine what brain regions may be involved in them, and thus, they are not included in Table 14.1. Substantial evidence of involvement is indicated in the table by a large checkmark ("✔") and limited evidence of involvement is indicated by a small checkmark ("✓").

The review found that all four brain regions are involved in panic attack, social anxiety, and major depression to some degree. A quick glance at the table shows that the PFC is implicated in all the disorders and the limbic system is strongly implicated in all the disorders except obsessive-compulsive disorder (OCD). The amygdala is implicated in every disorder in which the limbic system is involved except OCD, although the research does not identify if different regions of the amygdala are active in different disorders.

The evidence is strong that the brain stem (particularly the periaqueductal gray - PAG) is involved in panic attack, but the evidence is weak that it is involved in social anxiety and major depression. On the other hand, the evidence is strong that the basal ganglia are involved in social anxiety and major depression, but weak that the basal ganglia are involved in panic attack. The areas of the limbic system that are most consistently implicated in social anxiety and major depression are the amygdala, the anterior cingulate cortex (ACC), and the insula. Research also consistently implicates the ventromedial area of the PFC (the vmPFC) in panic attack, social anxiety, and major depression, and there is recent evidence that the dorsomedial PFC (dmPFC) may be involved in social anxiety [19].

There is solid evidence that the PFC, the limbic system, and the basal ganglia are involved in paranoid ideation, although what specific parts of these brain regions are involved is not clear. There has been less research than one might expect on the brain structures underlying generalized anxiety disorder, but what research there is strongly implicates the PFC and limbic system. There is also strong evidence that the vmPFC and the amygdala play a role in general anxiety, and some evidence that the dmPFC may be involved as well [19].

Extensive research has been conducted on small animal phobia, especially fear of snakes and spiders. This research strongly implicates the PFC and the limbic system in the fear of snakes and spiders, but none of this research implicates the basal ganglia or the brain stem in either of these phobias. The latter finding aligns with the notion that fear of small animals is a relatively recent adaptation, having developed long after the evolution of the brain stem and basal ganglia. For example, it has been suggested that fear of snakes evolved in primates about 20 million years ago [20], whereas fear of small animals and insects evolved in humans about 70,000 years ago [21]. The part of the limbic system most often implicated in all the research is the amygdala; I found one study that implicated the bed nucleus [22]. There is some evidence that the vmPFC and the dorsolateral PFC also play a role in both phobias.

Although there is some evidence that OCD involves limbic structures (namely, the ACC and insula), it is the only disorder listed in Table 14.1 that does not involve the amygdala. The fact that the amygdala is not involved in OCD may seem odd, since OCD is classified as an anxiety disorder and the amygdala is thought to be the primary source of anxiety/fear in humans. The basal ganglia have long been implicated in OCD, and research confirms the involvement of the striatum and the palladium of the basal ganglia in OCD. There is also strong evidence that the brain stem plays some part in OCD. Although the PFC is active in OCD, there is no evidence, to date, that the vmPFC is involved.

14.3 ETAS in the Brain

The extensive inter-connections among the PFC, the limbic system, the basal ganglia, and the brain stem, including the specific structures I have mentioned [23–28], are thought to form overlapping neural circuits that comprise ETAS and produce psychiatric symptoms. However, few neuro-anatomical models of different classes of psychiatric symptoms have been developed. To date, conceptual models of structural connections have only been presented for social anxiety and OCD, to the best of my knowledge [13, 14, 29–31]. Those models are more detailed than the ones I present below, and they include brain structures associated with sensory processing, which I have ignored.

Figure 14.2 updates the model of ETAS presented in Fig. 14.1 by including the brain stem, but it greatly simplifies the model by eliminating the sources of input used by the different brain regions (the PFC, limbic system, basal ganglia, and brain stem) to make their threat assessments. Instead, Fig. 14.2 merely illustrates the basic interconnections among these four brain regions. Collectively, the four regions are proposed to create a number of threat assessment systems that make the evaluations that underlie psychiatric symptoms. The model is hierarchical with respect to the historical evolution of each region and the top-down control that higher brain

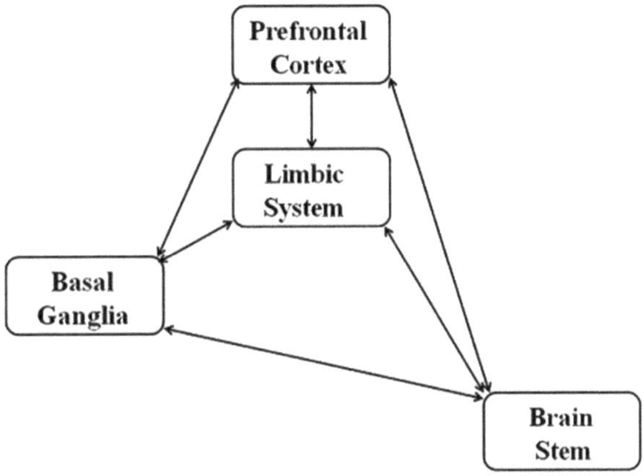

Fig. 14.2 Schematic general model of ETAS, showing the theoretical involvement of four key brain areas in psychiatric symptoms

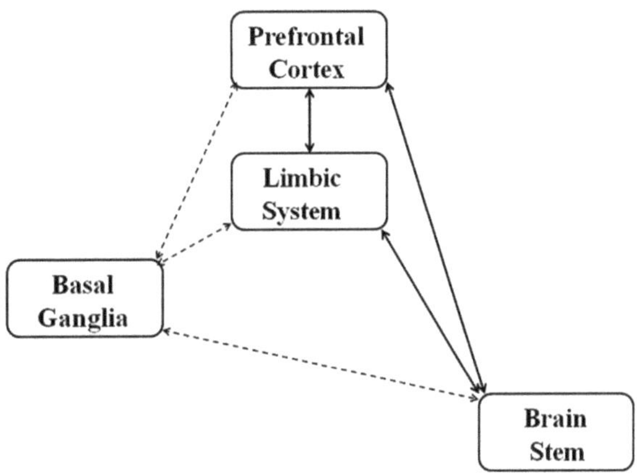

Fig. 14.3 Schematic ETAS model of panic attack, indicating the actual involvement of four key brain areas based on current evidence

regions exert on the activity of the lower brain regions. The other three ETAS models are based on the best evidence that currently exists about the association between the four brain regions and different classes of psychiatric symptoms.

The model for panic attack (Fig. 14.3) is identical to the general model shown in Fig. 14.2, except that it indicates the weak evidence for basal-ganglia involvement in panic attack by showing weaker connections (dashed lines) between the basal ganglia and the other brain regions. Likewise, the model for both social anxiety disorder (SAD) and major depressive disorder (MDD), which is shown in Fig. 14.4, illustrates the weak evidence for brain stem involvement in these disorders by showing weaker connections between the brain stem and the other regions. Given the current state of the evidence, a model for paranoid ideation would eliminate the connections with the brain stem, and models for general anxiety and small animal phobia would also eliminate connections with the basal ganglia.

Finally, the ETAS model for obsessive compulsive disorder (Fig. 14.5) illustrates the fact that I could find relatively little evidence that the limbic system is involved in OCD, and I could find no evidence that the amygdala is involved in OCD. This

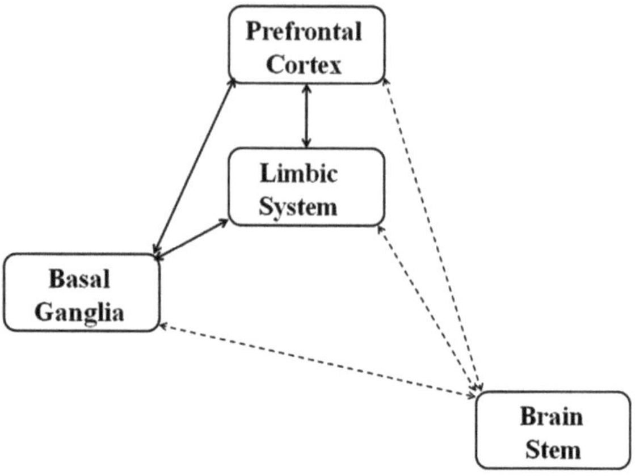

Fig. 14.4 Schematic ETAS model of SAD and MDD, indicating the actual involvement of four key brain areas based on current evidence

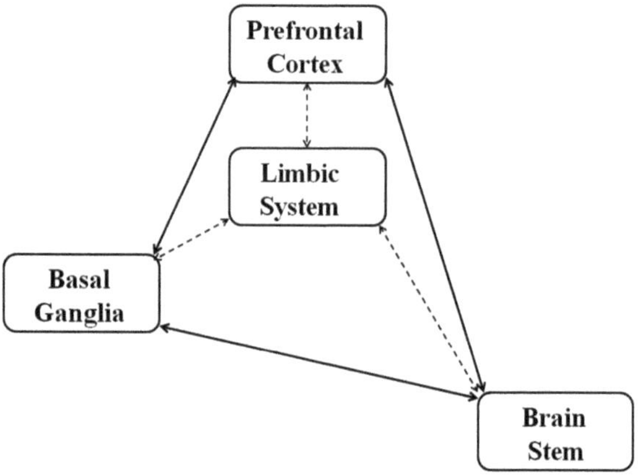

Fig. 14.5 Schematic ETAS model of OCD, indicating the actual involvement of four key brain areas based on current evidence

seems odd at first, because the amygdala, which is considered to be the nexus of fear in the brain, does not seem to be involved in the anxious thoughts that are a critical component of OCD. The limbic system (which includes the amygdala) may not be involved in OCD because the basal ganglia are much older than the limbic system. Thus, the sense of fear associated with OCD may be generated by the basal ganglia themselves or possibly by the brain stem's periaqueductal gray, different portions of which have been implicated in assessing different types of threats [32]. However, there is no reason to think that the "fear" generated by the basal ganglia or the PAG is the same "fear" that is generated by the amygdala, if such different sources of "fear" exist.

The repetitive behaviors exhibited in OCD are an obvious hallmark of a problem with the basal ganglia, which control repetitive ritualized behaviors (i.e., fixed-action patterns) in animals. Since the basal ganglia evolved long before cognition, the anxious thoughts in OCD seem to reflect the overlaying of cognition upon a disturbance in a much older brain region that is associated with instinctive behaviors serving self-protection and other survival functions.

14.4 The Operation of ETAS

Before describing how ETAS function, we must consider related avenues of research about the PFC, especially the vmPFC, that I have not touched on yet. I summarize these limited but important research results about the vmPFC in the next three sections.

14.4.1 *The vmPFC in Deductive Reasoning and the Influence of Beliefs*

Research has established that the PFC is involved in inductive logic and deductive logic (or reasoning) [33–37]. The dorsolateral PFC (dlPFC) seems to be mainly involved in inductive reasoning [33, 36], which is the generation or extrapolation of rules or hypotheses from specific instances [33, 36, 38, 39]. Researchers have proposed that there are two brain systems involved in deductive logic in humans [39, 40]. One system, which uses language and abstract reasoning [40] seems to be comparable to Aristotle's concept of *doxa* [41, 42]. The other system, which may be comparable to Aristotle's concept of *phantasia* [41, 42], is shared by humans and some other animals [40]. This second deductive system, which does not rely on language [43, 44], involves areas of the PFC [43, 44], including the vmPFC [45].

The second system of deductive reasoning is not strictly logical and it can be influenced by beliefs [40, 46, 47]. Research indicates that the deductions of the vmPFC are particularly prone to being influenced by beliefs about the world [40, 47]. Unlike the traditional view of deductive logic as a binary decision about whether a belief or statement is true or not, this second system is probabilistic in its decision-making [39], which is consistent with the suggestion that the vmPFC assigns valences to stimuli when assessing if they pose a threat [48]. Within the context of deductive decision-making, I interpret the notion of the vmPFC assigning a valence to a stimulus as the vmPFC assigning a probability of the degree to which a stimulus poses a threat of harm. The assignment of such probabilities is influenced by beliefs about the world.

14.4.2 *Threat, Safety, and the vmPFC*

A 1993 article by Paul Gilbert, the British clinical psychologist and evolutionary theorist, proposed that safety is not just the absence of threat, and that the human brain contains both a threat system and a safety system, the latter of which evolved in the context of social relationships, especially mother-infant relationships [49]. Gilbert's idea of a safety system is based on John Bowlby's concept of an attachment system that underlies mother-infant bonding and close adult relationships, which will be described in Chap. 21. In short, Gilbert believes that relationships with people who are supportive and helpful promote a sense of safety [49]. As Gilbert explained in a later paper, a sense of safety alters the processing of potential threats, such that "one can feel relatively safe even in the presence of threat stimuli" (p. 110) [50]. Whether or not a specific safety system exists is not critical to ETAS Theory, but the concept of safety is, as is Gilbert's notion that social relationships can provide a sense of safety.

Research has shown that attachment relationships can reduce a sense of threat [51, 52], that the vmPFC is responsive to safety cues [52], and that the vmPFC and other areas of the PFC are involved in attachment and social emotion [51, 53–58]. Just as the vmPFC may assign probabilities about the threat posed by a stimulus, it may assign probabilities about safety, which are also influenced by beliefs.

Like Gilbert, the Canadian psychologist Stanley Rachman has theorized about the interplay between safety and threat across the spectrum of anxiety disorders, especially general anxiety disorder and agoraphobia [59, 60]. Rachman believes a sense of safety is provided not only by social relationships, but also by situations and other aspects of human experience. A person's home, for example, is a source of safety that inhibits fear in persons with agoraphobia, just as an animal's territory seems to provide a sense of safety or security [61].

Although there has been very little research on the association between psychiatric disorders and "a sense of safety," per se, there is substantial evidence that positive social relationships have a salutary association with mental health. For example, a large national survey of American adults conducted in 2001–2005 found that people's perceptions that they have supportive social relationships had a salutary association with general anxiety, social anxiety, major depression, panic attack, and specific phobias, such as fear of small animals [62].

This study and many others like it have confirmed, what is called, the "stress buffering effect" of supportive social relationships (called "social support") on mental health. Based on the theoretical framework of psychologists Richard Arnold and Susan Folkman, stress buffering refers to the hypothesis that the perceived availability of social resources (i.e., perceived social support) reduces one's assessment of the severity of threats posed by adverse events in one's life [63]. Many large-scale surveys in America, Europe, and elsewhere have found that emotional support (believing that people care about you) is as least as important for one's mental health as tangible or instrumental support (believing that people will help you financially or do something that you need to be done) [e.g., 64–67]. I suspect that survey findings of the salutary association between social support and mental health are linked to neural coding of safety, although this type of social research does not provide evidence for that connection. However, a 2011 study of 100 community-dwelling American adults provides evidence for such a connection in that it demonstrated the association between amygdala activity and trait anxiety was mediated by perceived social support [68]. The study's results showed that social support was associated with lower amygdala activity, which in turn, was associated with lower anxiety.

Psychological characteristics of individuals, such as self-esteem and self-efficacy, also provide a sense of personal safety because they enhance the belief that an individual has the personal resources to deal with adverse life events effectively. Thus, like social support, self-esteem and self-efficacy should buffer against the anxiety produced by various threats of harm encountered in the world. Indeed, a 2001 study by Chris Ellison and his colleagues [69] demonstrated that social support, self-esteem, and self-efficacy each had unique salutary effects on psychological well-being and psychological distress that countered the pernicious effects of adverse life events.

Though the brain and behavioral mechanisms that I have considered here regarding threat and safety may be directly involved only in psychiatric symptoms and their relationship to beliefs about the world, I strongly suspect that psychiatric symptomology, especially anxiety, influences the effects of religious and other beliefs on positive emotions. I provide limited evidence that this is so in Part IV of this book. Based on this evidence, it appears that ETAS play a role in the control of positive emotions as well as the negative emotions associated with psychiatric symptoms. The reader should see the literature review by Burgdorf and Panksepp about the brain structures involved in positive emotions [70].

14.4.3 The Role of the vmPFC in Threat Assessment

The vmPFC plays a critical role in threat assessment, according to the research results described in the preceding sections of this chapter and earlier chapters. First, the vmPFC independently assesses safety as well as threats. Thus, if the vmPFC arrives at a different threat assessment than the subcortical areas of the brain, it can override their threat assessments and suppress the activity of the amygdala, thereby reducing fear and psychiatric symptoms related to fear. As there seem to be other subcortical areas that generate fear or anxiety, it presumably suppresses their activity as well.

Second, the vmPFC is involved in the processing of beliefs [71, 72] and deductive logic [40, 45, 47], and the deductions of the vmPFC are influenced by beliefs about the world [40, 47]. Therefore, its decisions about the degree that something poses a threat of harm are influenced by beliefs about the world.

14.4.4 The Role of Other PFC Regions in Threat Assessment

I focus attention on the vmPFC because the best evidence indicates that it is involved in threat assessment and the processing of both fear and beliefs. However, other areas of the PFC appear to play a role in all three of these brain activities. The orbitofrontal portion of the PFC (the OFC) is a case in point. There is limited evidence that the OFC, like the vmPFC, may regulate the activity of the amygdala [73, 74] and that the OFC may be involved in threat assessment [74, 75]. The OFC also is associated with optimism, and it may underlie the ability of optimism to reduce anxiety [76]. Since optimism reflects positive beliefs about present or future conditions, the OFC also could be involved in processing beliefs that influence amygdala activity. Thus, the OFC might serve functions that are similar or complementary to the functions of the vmPFC in threat assessment.

Recent findings about the dorsomedial PFC (dmPFC) are particularly important for ETAS Theory. A series of related studies have found that the human dmPFC enhances the activity of the amygdala as part of an "aversive amplification circuit" [19, 77], which was originally discovered in research on fear conditioning in laboratory rats [78]. The circuit includes the amygdala, the dorsomedial PFC, and the anterior cingulate cortex (ACC), which is part of the limbic system. As mentioned in Chap. 10, the ACC is activated during the cognitive assessments of threats [79–82]. Human research shows that the circuit "is associated with elevated threat processing" (p. 295) [19]. The findings of two studies are of special interest. One is that the "aversive amplification circuit" was more active in healthy adults during the "threat" condition (compared to a "safety" condition) of an experiment designed to induce anxiety under the threat condition [77]. The second is that the circuit was more active in adults with general anxiety disorder or social anxiety disorder than it was in healthy adults [19]. Thus, whereas the vmPFC is able to suppress fear generated by the amygdala, the dmPFC (in conjunction with the ACC) appears to be able to enhance fear. The researchers concluded that the "aversive amplification circuit" enhances fear by priming the amygdala to be more sensitive to potential threats [77].

The ACC, the vmPFC, the dorsolateral PFC, and other areas of the PFC have been found to be involved in processing beliefs [71, 83, 84], yet I do not know of any evidence that implicates the dmPFC in processing beliefs. Nevertheless, it is quite possible that it is. If so, one would expect that beliefs about the dangerousness of the world would increase the activity of the "aversive amplification circuit," thereby increasing anxiety-related symptoms in healthy adults and adults with various kinds of psychiatric disorders.

14.4.5 Description of ETAS Functioning

The brain stem, the basal ganglia, the limbic system, and the PFC are all thought to be involved in threat assessments that underlie psychiatric symptoms. Structures in each of these regions are thought to assess threats as part of their functions. As they evolved at different points in time, the brain stem and basal ganglia operate at an instinctive level, whereas limbic structures operate at an emotional level [1, 3, 32], and the PFC operates at a cognitive level [1, 3, 7]. The threat assessments of the brain stem, basal ganglia, and limbic structures are automatic and made outside of awareness, for the most part [1, 3, 79]. The exceptions are the anterior cingulate cortex (ACC) and the insula (or insular cortex) of the limbic system, which are involved in the conscious processing of threats [79–82].

Subcortical structures, most prominently the amygdala, make automatic assessments about whether a situation, or an animate or inanimate object, poses a threat of harm [1, 3, 85–87]. These brain areas are biased toward deciding a stimulus poses a threat even when it may not be a threat. The amygdala even treats unpredictability, lack of control over current events and uncertainty about future events as forms of threat [88–94].

The PFC integrates information from subcortical structures and any cortical areas that are activated by the subcortical structures [3, 12], while making its own threat assessments based on cognition. The cognitive threat assessments made by the vmPFC are particularly important because the vmPFC can override the amygdala's threat assessments by inhibiting its activity [95, 96], and thereby reducing the level of fear that it generates. On the other hand, the "aversive amplification circuit," which includes the dmPFC, appears to increase amygdala activity by making it more sensitive to possible threats, thereby increasing fear.

When the vmPFC makes its threat assessments, it takes beliefs about the world into account in assigning a probability that a stimulus poses a threat. It also takes personal safety into account, including social support, situations, and beliefs that provide a sense of safety. If the vmPFC decides a stimulus does not pose a threat of harm, based on all the information available to it, including sensory input, subcortical input, memory, and beliefs, it decreases the activity of the amygdala, which decreases anxiety and related symptoms. Since the vmPFC decisions are probabilistic, this is not an all-or-none process, so it may modulate amygdala activity in terms of the degree of threat posed by the stimulus, thereby modulating anxiety and related symptoms. Thus, the vmPFC acts as a gating system that sets a threshold for what is and what is not a threat of harm. Generally, given its ability to reduce the activity of the amygdala, the vmPFC appears to raise the threshold of what constitutes a threat. The dmPFC, on the other hand, which is a major component of the "aversive amplification circuit," may lower the threshold of what constitutes a threat by priming the amygdala to be more sensitive to potential threats.

14.5 Chapter Highlights and Comments

Many researchers and clinicians agree that psychiatric symptoms in patients and the general public are the product of neural systems that evolved to provide self-protection by assessing the threat of harm posed by objects and situations. These neural systems involve specific brain areas that have been implicated in various psychiatric disorders. ETAS Theory explains how these systems work and how they cause psychiatric symptoms.

According to ETAS Theory, subcortical structures, including the brain stem, basal ganglia, and the limbic system unconsciously assess potential threats and convey this information (which is biased toward deciding something is a threat) to the PFC. The vmPFC plays a critical role in threat assessment because it is involved in deductive reasoning and processing beliefs, its deductive decisions are influenced by beliefs about the world, and it is particularly sensitive to safety cues. Based on the existing evidence, ETAS Theory proposes that the vmPFC employs input from subcortical areas along with its own assessment to determine the degree to which a stimulus (an object or situation) poses a threat of harm. In doing so, it takes safety, beliefs, and other information into account.

If thc vmPFC decides a stimulus does not pose a threat, based on all the information available to it (including information about personal safety), it decreases the activity of the amygdala, which decreases anxiety and related symptoms. Since the vmPFC decisions are probabilistic, this is not an all-or none process, so it may modulate amygdala activity in terms of the degree of threat posed by the stimulus, thereby modulating anxiety and related symptoms. Thus, the vmPFC acts as a gating system that sets a threshold for what is and what is not a threat of harm. However, the dmPFC, and perhaps, other areas of the PFC may process beliefs that are capable of increasing anxiety and other psychiatric symptoms by increasing amygdala activity.

References

1. Flannelly, K. J., Koenig, H. G., Galek, K., & Ellison, C. G. (2007). Beliefs, mental health, and evolutionary threat assessment systems in the brain. *Journal of Nervous and Mental Disease, 195*(12), 996–1003.
2. Marshall, R. D., Bryant, R. A., Amsel, L., Suh, E. J., Cook, J. M., & Neria, Y. (2007). The psychology of ongoing threat: Relative risk appraisal, the September 11 attacks, and terrorism-related fears. *American Psychologist, 62*(4), 304–316.
3. Eilam, D., Izhar, R., & Mort, J. (2011). Threat detection: Behavioral practices in animals and humans. *Neuroscience and Biobehavioral Reviews, 35*(4), 999–1006.
4. Canteras, N. S., Mota-Ortiz, S. R., & Motta, S. C. (2012). What ethologically based models have taught us about the neural systems underlying fear and anxiety. *Brazilian Journal of Medical and Biological Research, 45*, 321–327.
5. Fiddick, L. (2011). There is more than the amygdala: Potential threat assessment in the cingulate cortex. *Neuroscience and Biobehavioral Reviews, 35*(4), 1007–1018.
6. Neuberg, S. L., Kenrick, D. T., & Schaller, M. (2011). Human threat management systems: Self-protection and disease avoidance. *Neuroscience and Biobehavioral Reviews, 35*(4), 1042–1051.
7. Stein, D. J., & Nesse, R. M. (2011). Threat detection, precautionary responses, and anxiety disorders. *Neuroscience & Biobehavioral Reviews, 35*(4), 1075–1079.
8. Woody, E., & Boyer, P. (2011). Threat-detection and precaution: Introduction to the special issue. *Neuroscience & Biobehavioral Reviews, 35*(4), 989–990.
9. Woody, E. Z., & Szechtman, H. (2011). Adaptation to potential threat: The evolution, neurobiology, and psychopathology of the security motivation system. *Neuroscience and Biobehavioral Reviews, 35*(4), 1019–1033.
10. Graeff, F. G. (2011). Defense-related emotions in humans. *Psychology & Neuroscience, 4*(2), 183–189.
11. Brune, M., Belsky, J., Fabrega, H., Feierman, H. R., Gilbert, P., Glantz, K., et al. (2012). The crisis of psychiatry – Insights and prospects from evolutionary theory. *World Psychiatry, 11*(1), 55–57.
12. Price, J. S., Gardner, R., Jr., & Erickson, M. (2004). Can depression, anxiety and somatization be understood as appeasement displays? *Journal of Affective Disorders, 79*(1–3), 1–11.
13. Li, D., Chokka, P., & Tibbo, P. (2001). Toward an integrative understanding of social phobia. *Journal of Psychiatry and Neuroscience, 26*(3), 190–202.

14. Baxter, L. R. (2003). Basal ganglia systems in ritualistic social displays: Reptiles and humans; function and illness. *Physiology & Behavior, 79*, 451–460.
15. Mathew, S. J., Coplan, J. D., & Gorman, J. M. (2001). Neurobiological mechanisms of social anxiety disorder. *American Journal of Psychiatry, 158*(10), 1558–1567.
16. Price, J. S. (2003). Evolutionary aspects of anxiety disorders. *Dialogues in Clinical Neuroscience, 5*(3), 223–236.
17. Gross, C. T., & Canteras, N. S. (2012). The many paths to fear. *Nature Reviews Neuroscience, 13*(9), 651–658.
18. Ohman, A., Carlsson, K., Lundqvist, D., & Ingvar, M. (2007). On the unconscious subcortical origin of human fear. *Physiology & Behavior, 92*, 180–185.
19. Robinson, O. J., Krimsky, M., Lieberman, L., Allen, P., Vytal, K., & Grillon, C. (2014). Towards a mechanistic understanding of pathological anxiety: The dorsal medial prefrontal-amygdala "aversive amplification" circuit in unmedicated generalized and social anxiety disorders. *The Lancet Psychiatry, 1*(4), 294.
20. Isbell, L. A. (2009). *The fruit, the tree and the serpent*. Cambridge, MA: Harvard University Press.
21. Bracha, H. S. (2006). Human brain evolution and the "Neuroevolutionary Time-depth Principle:" Implications for the Reclassification of fear-circuitry-related traits in DSM-V and for studying resilience to warzone-related posttraumatic stress disorder. *Progress in Neuro-Psychopharmacology and Biological Psychiatry, 30*(5), 827–853.
22. Munsterkotter, A. L., Notzon, S., Redlich, R., Grotegerd, D., Dohm, K., Arolt, V., et al. (2015). Spider or no spider? Neural correlates of sustained and phasic fear in spider phobia. *Depression and Anxiety, 32*(9), 656–663.
23. Groenewegen, H. J., Wright, C. I., & Uylings, H. B. M. (1997). The anatomical relationships of the prefrontal cortex with limbic structures and the basal ganglia. *Journal of Psychopharmacology, 11*(2), 99–106.
24. Groenewegen, H. J., Berendse, H. W., & Wolters, J. G. (1990). The anatomical relationship of the prefrontal cortex with the striatopallidal system, the thalamus and the amygdala: Evidence for parallel organization. *Progress in Brain Research, 85*, 95–116.
25. Masterman, D. L., & Cummings, J. L. (1997). Frontal-subcortical circuits: The anatomic basis of executive, social and motivated behaviors. *Journal of Psychopharmacology, 11*(2), 107–114.
26. Groenewegen, H. J., & Uylings, H. B. M. (2000). The prefrontal cortex and the integration of sensory, limbic and autonomic information. *Progress in Brain Research, 126*, 3–28.
27. Gray, T. S. (1999). Functional and anatomical relationships among the amygdala, basal forebrain, ventral striatum, and cortex. An integrative discussion. *Annals of the New York Academy of Sciences, 29*, 439–444.
28. Price, J. L. (2003). Comparative aspects of amygdala connectivity. *Annals of the New York Academy of Sciences, 985*, 50–58.
29. Nakao, T., Okada, K., & Kanba, S. (2014). Neurobiological model of obsessive-compulsive disorder: Evidence from recent neuropsychological and neuroimaging findings. *Psychiatry and Clinical Neurosciences, 68*(8), 587–605.
30. Huey, E. D., Zahn, R., Krueger, F., Moll, J., Kapogiannis, D., Wassermann, E. M., et al. (2008). A psychological and neuroanatomical model of obsessive-compulsive disorder. *Journal of Neuropsychiatry and Clinical Neurosciences, 20*(4), 390–408.
31. Bruhl, A. B., Delsignore, A., Komossa, K., & Weidt, S. (2014). Neuroimaging in social anxiety disorder – A meta-analytic review resulting in a new neurofunctional model. *Neuroscience and Biobehavioral Reviews, 47*, 260–280.
32. Sokolowski, K., & Corbin, J. G. (2012). Wired for behaviors: From development to function of innate limbic system circuitry. *Frontiers in Molecular Neuroscience, 5*(55), 1–15.
33. Jia, X., Liang, P., Lu, J., Yang, Y., Zhong, N., & Li, K. (2011). Common and dissociable neural correlates associated with component processes of inductive reasoning. *NeuroImage, 56*, 2292–2299.

34. Bunge, S. A., Wendelken, C., Badre, D., & Wagner, A. D. (2005). Analogical reasoning and prefrontal cortex: Evidence for separable retrieval and integration mechanisms. *Cerebral Cortex, 15*(3), 239–249.
35. Fuster, J. (2008). *The prefrontal cortex*. London: Academic Press.
36. Goel, V., & Dolan, R. J. (2004). Differential involvement of left prefrontal cortex in inductive and deductive reasoning. *Cognition, 93*(3), B109-B121.
37. Waltz, J. A., & Knowlton, B. J. (1999). A system for relational reasoning in human prefrontal cortex. *Psychological Science, 10*(2), 119.
38. Patalano, A. (2005). Inductive reasoning. In N. Salkind (Ed.), *Encyclopedia of human development* (pp. 696–697). Thousand Oaks: SAGE Publications.
39. Evans, J. S. B. T., & Over, D. E. (2013). Reasoning to and from belief: Deduction and induction are still distinct. *Thinking and Reasoning, 19*(3–4), 267–283.
40. Evans, J. S. B. T. (2003). In two minds: Dual-process accounts of reasoning. *Trends in Cognitive Sciences, 7*(10), 454–459.
41. Gronroos, G. (2013). Two kinds of belief in Plato. *Journal of the History of Philosophy, 51*(1), 1–19.
42. McCready-Flora, I. (2013). Aristotle's cognitive science: Belief, affect and rationality. *Philosophy and Phenomenological Research, 89*(2), 394–435.
43. Monti, M. M., Osherson, D. N., Martinez, M. J., & Parsons, L. M. (2007). Functional neuroanatomy of deductive inference: A language-independent distributed network. *NeuroImage, 37*, 1005–1016.
44. Kroger, J. K., Nystrom, L. E., Cohen, J. D., & Johnson-Laird, P. N. (2008). Distinct neural substrates for deductive and mathematical processing. *Brain Research, 1243*, 86–103.
45. Houde, O., Zago, L., Crivello, F., Moutier, S., Pineau, A., Mazoyer, B., et al. (2001). Access to deductive logic depends on a right ventromedial prefrontal area devoted to emotion and feeling: Evidence from a training paradigm. *NeuroImage, 14*(6), 1486–1492.
46. Trippas, I., Handley, S. J., & Verde, M. F. (2014). Fluency and belief bias in deductive reasoning: New indices for old effects. *Frontiers in Psychology, 5*(June), 631.
47. Goel, V., & Dolan, R. J. (2003). Explaining modulation of reasoning by belief. *Cognition, 87*(1), B11-B22.
48. Winecoff, A., Clithero, J. A., Carter, R. M., Bergman, S. R., Wang, L. H., & Huettel, S. A. (2013). Ventromedial prefrontal cortex encodes emotional value. *Journal of Neuroscience, 33*(27), 11032–11039.
49. Gilbert, P. (1993). Defence and safety: Their function in social behaviour and psychopathology. *The British Journal of Clinical Psychology, 32*(Pt 2), 131–153.
50. Gilbert, P. (2007). Evolved minds and compassion in the therapeutic relationship. In P. Gilbert, & R. L. Leahy (Eds.), *The therapeutic relationship in cognitive behavioural psychotherapies* (pp. 107–142). London: Routledge.
51. Coan, J. A. (2010). Adult attachment and the brain. *Journal of Social and Personal Relationships, 27*(2), 210–217.
52. Eisenberger, N. I., Master, S. L., Inagaki, T. K., Taylor, S. E., Shirinyan, D., Lieberman, M. D., et al. (2011). Attachment figures activate a safety signal-related neural region and reduce pain experience. *Proceedings of the National Academy of Sciences, 108*(28), 11721–11726.
53. Coria-Avila, G. A., Manzo, J., Garcia, L. I., Carrillo, P., Miguel, M., & Pfaus, J. G. (2008). Neurobiology of social attachments. *Comparative Biochemistry and Physiology. Toxicology & Pharmacology, 148*(4), 401–410.
54. Minagawa-Kawai, Y., Matsuoka, S. D.I, ., Naoi, N., Nakamura, K., & Kojima, S. (2009). Prefrontal activation associated with social attachment: Facial-emotion recognition in mothers and infants. *Cerebral Cortex, 19*(2), 284–292.
55. Moutsiana, C., Fearon, P., Murray, L., Cooper, P., Goodyer, I., Johnstone, T., et al. (2014). Making an effort to feel positive: Insecure attachment in infancy predicts the neural underpinnings of emotion regulation in adulthood. *Journal of Child Psychology & Psychiatry, 55*(9), 999–1008.

56. Noriuchi, M., Kikuchi, Y., & Senoo, A. (2008). The functional neuroanatomy of maternal love: Mother's response to infant's attachment behaviors. *Biological Psychiatry, 63*(4), 415–423.
57. Vrticka, P., Sander, D., Vuilleumier, P., & Bondolfi, G. (2012). The neural substrates of social emotion perception and regulation are modulated by adult attachment style. *Social Neuroscience, 7*(5), 473–493.
58. Vrticka, P., & Vuilleumier, P. (2012). Neuroscience of human social interactions and adult attachment style. *Frontiers in Human Neuroscience, 6,* 212, *Retrieved from* http://journal.frontiersin.org/article/10.3389/fnhum.2012.00212/full
59. Rachman, S. (1984). Agoraphobia-A safety-signal perspective. *Behaviour Research and Therapy, 22*(1), 59–70.
60. Woody, S., & Rachman, S. (1994). Generalized anxiety disorder (GAD) as an unsuccessful search for safety. *Clinical Psychology Review, 14*(8), 743–753.
61. Flannelly, K. J., Flannelly, L., & Blanchard, R. J. (1984). Adult experience and the expression of aggression: A comparative analysis. In K. J. Flannelly, R. J. Blanchard, & D. C. Blanchard (Eds.), *Biological perspectives on aggression*. New York: Alan R. Liss.
62. Moak, Z. B., & Agrawal, A. (2009). The association between perceived interpersonal social support and physical and mental health: Results from the national epidemiological survey on alcohol and related conditions. *Journal of Public Health, 32*(2), 191–201.
63. Lazarus, R. S., & Folkman, S. (1984). *Stress, appraisal, and coping*. New York: Springer.
64. Dinenberg, R. E., McCaslin, S. E., Bates, M. N., & Cohen, B. E. (2014). Social support may protect against development of posttraumatic stress disorder: Findings from the heart and soul study. *American Journal of Health Promotion, 28*(5), 294–297.
65. Falcon, L. M., Todorova, I., & Tucker, K. (2009). Social support, life events, and psychological distress among the Puerto Rican population in the Boston area of the United States. *Aging & Mental Health, 13*(6), 863–873.
66. Grav, S., Hellzen, O., Romild, U., & Stordal, E. (2012). Association between social support and depression in the general population: The HUNT study, a cross-sectional survey. *Journal of Clinical Nursing, 21*(1–2), 111–120.
67. Santini, Z. I., Koyanagi, A., Tyrovolas, S., Mason, C., & Haro, J. M. (2015). The association between social relationships and depression: A systematic review. *Journal of Affective Disorders, 175,* 53–65.
68. Hyde, L. W., Gorka, A., Manuck, S. B., & Hariri, A. R. (2011). Perceived social support moderates the link between threat-related amygdala reactivity and trait anxiety. *Neuropsychologia, 49,* 651–656.
69. Ellison, C. G., Boardman, J. D., Williams, D. R., & Jackson, J. S. (2001). Religious involvement, stress, and mental health: Findings from the 1995 Detroit area study. *Social Forces, 80*(1), 215–249.
70. Burgdorf, J., & Panksepp, J. (2006). The neurobiology of positive emotions. *Neuroscience and Biobehavioral Reviews, 30*(2), 173–187.
71. Harris, S., Kaplan, J. T., Curiel, A., Bookheimer, S. Y., Iacoboni, M., & Cohen, M. S. (2009). The neural correlates of religious and nonreligious belief. *PloS One, 4*(10), e0007272-e0007272.
72. Harris, S., Sheth, S. A., & Cohen, M. S. (2008). Functional neuroimaging of belief, disbelief, and uncertainty. *Annals of Neurology, 63*(2), 141–147.
73. Timbie, C., & Barbas, H. (2014). Specialized pathways from the primate amygdala to posterior orbitofrontal cortex. *The Journal of Neuroscience, 34*(24), 8106–8118.
74. Shiba, Y., Kim, C., Santangelo, A. M., & Roberts, A. C. (2015). Lesions of either anterior orbitofrontal cortex or ventrolateral prefrontal cortex in marmoset monkeys heighten innate fear and attenuate active coping behaviors to predator threat. *Frontiers in Systems Neuroscience, 21*. Retrieved from http://journal.frontiersin.org/article/10.3389/fnsys.2014.00250/full
75. Coccaro, E. F., McCloskey, M. S., Fitzgerald, D. A., & Phan, K. L. (2007). Amygdala and orbitofrontal reactivity to social threat in individuals with impulsive aggression. *Biological Psychiatry, 62*(2), 168–178.

76. Dolcos, S., Hu, Y., Iordan, A. D., Moore, M., & Dolcos, F. (2016). Optimism and the brain: Trait optimism mediates the protective role of the orbitofrontal cortex gray matter volume against anxiety. *Social Cognitive and Affective Neuroscience, 11*(2), 263–271.
77. Vytal, K. E., Overstreet, C., Charney, D. R., Robinson, O. J., & Grillon, C. (2014). Sustained anxiety increases amygdala-dorsomedial prefrontal coupling: A mechanism for maintaining an anxious state in healthy adults. *Journal of Psychiatry & Neuroscience, 39*(5), 321.
78. Sotres-Bayon, F., Sierra-Mercado, D., Pardilla-Delgado, E., & Quirk, G. J. (2012). Gating of fear in prelimbic cortex by hippocampal and amygdala inputs. *Neuron, 76*(4), 804–812.
79. Öhman, A. (2005). The role of the amygdala in human fear: Automatic detection of threat. *Psychoneuroendocrinology, 30*(10), 953–958.
80. Bishop, S. J., Duncan, J., & Lawrence, A. D. (2004). State anxiety modulation of the amygdala response to unattended threat-related stimuli. *Journal of Neuroscience, 24*(46), 10364–10368.
81. Klumpp, H., Angstadt, M., Phan, K. L., & Nathan, P. J. (2010). Amygdala reactivity to faces at varying intensities of threat in generalized social phobia: An event-related functional MRI study. *Psychiatry Research: Neuroimaging, 183*(2), 167–169.
82. Alvarez, R. P., Chen, G., Bodurka, J., Kaplan, R., & Grillon, C. (2011). Phasic and sustained fear in humans elicits distinct patterns of brain activity. *NeuroImage, 55*(1), 389–400.
83. Sommer, M., Donnel, K., Sodian, B., Meinhardt, J., Thoermer, C., & Hajak, G. (2007). Neural correlates of true and false belief reasoning. *NeuroImage, 35*(3), 1378–1384.
84. Knutson, K. M., Mah, L., Manly, C. F., & Grafman, J. (2007). Neural correlates of automatic beliefs about gender and race. *Human Brain Mapping, 28*(10), 915–930.
85. Harris, J. A. (1996). Descending antinociceptive mechanisms in the brainstem: Their role in the animal's defensive system. *Journal of Physiology, 90*(1), 15–25.
86. Mobbs, D., Petrovic, P., Marchant, J. L., Hassabis, D., Weiskopf, N., Seymour, B., et al. (2007). When fear is near: Threat imminence elicits prefrontal-periaqueductal gray shifts in humans. *Science, 317*(5841), 1079–1083.
87. Zald, D. H. (2003). The human amygdala and the emotional evaluation of sensory stimuli. *Brain Research Reviews, 41*(1), 88–123.
88. Sarinopoulos, I., Grupe, D. W., Mackiewicz, K. L., Herrington, J. D., Lor, M., Steege, E. E., et al. (2010). Uncertainty during anticipation modulates neural responses to aversion in human insula and amygdala. *Cerebral Cortex, 20*(4), 929–940.
89. Grupe, D. W., & Nitschke, J. B. (2013). Uncertainty and anticipation in anxiety: An integrated neurobiological and psychological perspective. *Nature Reviews Neurology, 14*(7), 488–501.
90. Thompson, S. C. (1981). Will it hurt less if I can control it? A complex answer to a simple question. *Psychological Bulletin, 90*(1), 89–101.
91. Williams, L. E., Oler, J. A., Fox, A. S., McFarlin, D. R., Rogers, G. M., Jesson, M. A. L., et al. (2015). Fear of the unknown: Uncertain anticipation reveals amygdala alterations in childhood anxiety disorders. *Neuropsychopharmacology, 40*(6), 1428–1435.
92. Rosen, J. B., & Donley, M. P. (2006). Animal studies of amygdala function in fear and uncertainty: Relevance to human research. *Biological Psychology, 73*(1), 49–60.
93. Morriss, J., Christakou, A., & van Reekum, C. M. (2015). Intolerance of uncertainty predicts fear extinction in amygdala-ventromedial prefrontal cortical circuitry. *Biology of Mood & Anxiety Disorders, 5*(1), 1–13.
94. Hsu, M., Bhatt, M., Adolphs, R., Tranel, D., & Camerer, C. F. (2005). Neural systems responding to degrees of uncertainty in human decision-making. *Science, 310*(5754), 1680–1683.
95. Greenberg, T., Carlson, J. M., Cha, J., Hajcak, G., & Mujica-Parodi, L. R. (2013). Ventromedial prefrontal cortex reactivity is altered in generalized anxiety disorder during fear generalization. *Depression and Anxiety, 30*(3), 242–250.
96. Cha, J., Greenberg, T., Hajcak, G., Mujica-Parodi, L. R., Carlson, J. M., & DeDora, D. J. (2014). Circuit-wide structural and functional measures predict ventromedial prefrontal cortex fear generalization: Implications for generalized anxiety disorder. *Journal of Neuroscience, 34*(11), 4043–4053.

Part IV
Religious Beliefs and Mental Health

Chapter 15
Belief in God and Life-After-Death Among American Adults

Abstract The chapter summarizes the findings of large national surveys of U.S. adults and studies of convenience samples of American college students about their belief in God and life-after-death. This research shows that most Americans believe in God and that the percentage of people in the U.S. who believe in God is higher than the percentage in almost every other country in the world. However, Americans hold many different beliefs about the nature of God, some of which are overlapping and some of which are contradictory. Moreover, some beliefs about the nature of God are rooted in the Old Testament, some are rooted in the New Testament, and some have no Biblical connection at all. The most commonly held beliefs about God among Americans are that God is ever-present, just, kind, loving, forgiving, and fatherly; less commonly held beliefs are that God is critical, punishing, severe, and wrathful. The chapter also presents results showing that most Americans believe in life-after-death, but these beliefs take various forms. The most common American beliefs about the afterlife are that it entails peace and tranquility, union with God, and reunion with loved ones.

Keywords Afterlife • Belief about God • Belief in God • Christianity • God • Islam • Judaism • Life-after-death • Nature of God

15.1 Background

The 2008 "American Religious Identification Survey" interviewed a random sample of over 54,000 American adults to ascertain the religion to which they belonged. The question was simple: "What is your religion, if any?" [1]. Of those who said they belonged to a religion, nearly 98% belonged to one of the three Abrahamic religious faiths: Christianity (95.6%), Islam (0.7%), and Judaism (1.5%). The Abrahamic religions share a common history and belief in the same God; the God of Abraham is not only the God of Judaism, it is the God of Islam and Christianity [2, 3]. They also share a second theological belief, to some degree, belief in an after-life. Belief in life-after-death is a major tenet of both Christianity and Islam [4, 5], but it is far less important in Judaism. The *Torah* (the first five books of the *Hebrew Bible)* does not mention or imply the possibility of immortality, yet the concept of

K.J. Flannelly, *Religious Beliefs, Evolutionary Psychiatry, and Mental Health in America*, Religion, Spirituality and Health: A Social Scientific Approach 1,
DOI 10.1007/978-3-319-52488-7_15

life-after-death appears in the *Book of Job,* and the notion that the dead will be resurrected is introduced in the *Book of Ezekiel* [6, 7]. Buddhism, a religion that is on the rise in the U.S., does not entail belief in God [2, 3], but it does teach there is life-after-death in the form of reincarnation [4, 5].

This chapter presents survey results about Americans' belief in God and life-after-death to provide basic background information that is useful for understanding the results of studies in the next several chapters, which examine the association of mental health with beliefs about God and the afterlife. Other religious beliefs are discussed separately in subsequent chapters.

15.2 Americans' Belief in God

More than 90% of Americans say "Yes" when asked "Do you believe in God," according to a 2011 telephone survey of a random sample of over 1000 adults in all 50 states and Washington, D.C. [8]. Moreover, the percent of Americans who say they believe in God has been consistently higher than 90% since the 1940's, when the Gallop Poll began to ask Americans about their religious beliefs [9]. However, it is not necessarily clear what people mean when they say they believe in God [10]. A simple "Yes" may encompass a more complicated range of potential responses [8–11]. When pressed, some people say they do not believe in "God," per se, but they believe in a "Higher Power." Others say they believe in God, but they have doubts about God's existence [8, 11].

Nevertheless, more than 60% of Americans "strongly agreed" with following statement posed in a 2008 survey by the National Opinion Research Center: "I know God really exists and I have no doubts about it" [12]. The same survey, which was conducted in 42 countries throughout the word, found that only four countries had higher rates of "strong agreement" with the same statement than the U.S. sample; they were the Philippines, Chile, Israel, and Poland [12].

The Baylor Religion Survey asked random samples of U.S. adults several related questions regarding their belief about God in 2007 and 2010. The main question, which was designed to better understand what Americans mean when they say they believe in God, was: "Which one of these statements comes closest to your personal belief about God?" The response options were: (1) I have no doubt that God exists; (2) I believe in God but with some doubts; (3) I sometimes believe in God; (4) I believe in a higher power or cosmic force; (5) I don't know and there is no way to find out; (6) I am an atheist; and (7) I have no opinion. These are labeled in Fig. 15.1 as: No Doubt; Some Doubts; Sometimes; Higher Power; Don't Know; Atheist; and No Opinion. Other questions on the Baylor Survey asked about God's involvement in the world and specific beliefs about the nature of God.[1]

[1] The 2007 and 2010 Baylor Religion Surveys each sampled over 1500 American adults. The findings reported below regarding beliefs about God are based on my own analyses of the data from

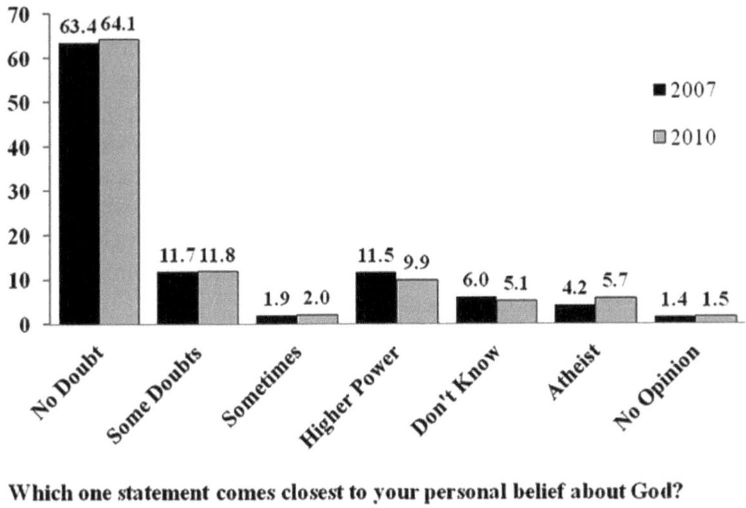

Fig. 15.1 Percent of U.S. adults who believe in God or a Higher Power, according to the 2007 and 2010 Baylor Religion Surveys

Close to two thirds of the 2007 and 2010 survey respondents said they had no doubt that God exists (No Doubt), whereas somewhat more than 11% believed in God, but had some doubts about God's existence (Some Doubts). It was relatively rare for people to say they only believed in God sometimes (Sometimes). Approximately 10–12% of the survey participants said they believed in a higher power or cosmic force (Higher Power), and 5–6.0% said they did not know and there was no way of knowing if God exists (Don't Know). All in all, roughly 88% of the Americans who participated in either of the Baylor surveys said they believed in God or a Higher Power.

15.3 Americans' Beliefs About God

Before returning to the Baylor Survey, I would like to mention two early studies that explored American beliefs about God [13, 14], as well as some related research. The two studies asked high school and/or college students to evaluate more than 60 adjectives describing hypothetical attributes of God. The adjectives encompassed a variety of beliefs, including the fundamental theological concepts in the Old Testament (the Hebrew Bible) that God is just, merciful, the creator of the world, omnipotent (all powerful), omniscient (all knowing), and omnipresent (present everywhere) [15, 16]. Related adjectives used in the studies included absolute, divine, eternal, and unchanging. Other adjectives conveyed images of God's actions against sinners and the wicked

---

these 2007 and 2010 surveys. The 2007 dataset was downloaded from The Association of Religious Data Archives; the 2010 dataset was obtained from the Baylor Institute for Studies of Religion.

in the Old Testament, such as, angry, punishing, and wrathful [16]. New Testament Christian beliefs about God included fatherly, loving, and forgiving [16]. Still other adjectives had no connection to either the Old Testament or the New Testament.

Both studies employed a statistical procedure called factor analysis to group the students' evaluations of the adjectives into categories. The first study, which was conducted by Bernard Spilka and his colleagues, identified six factors [14], which the authors called a kindly father, a stern father, a vindictive God, an impersonal allness, an impersonal supreme being, and an impersonal distant God. The second study, which was conducted by Richard Gorsuch, identified a similar set of factors [13], which were refined in later research [17].

Subsequent studies that grew out of this research, which mainly surveyed U.S. college students, found that deistic beliefs about God (e.g., all powerful, creator, and judge) and anthropomorphic beliefs about God from the Old and New Testament (e.g., angry, fatherly, kind, loving, and vindictive) are common among Americans [18 – 21]. Christians tend to hold these beliefs more strongly than Jews do [22], and devout Christians are much less inclined than other people to believe God is distant or disengaged from the world [19, 23, 24]. The most commonly held beliefs among American college students appear to be that God is close, loving, and forgiving [18, 25]. The belief that God is the creator and judge are also fairly common among U.S. college students [18, 21].

The 2007 Baylor Religion Survey also asked participants: "How well do you feel that each of the following words describe God in your opinion?" The question was followed by these 15 adjectives: Absolute, Critical, Distant, Ever-present, Fatherly, Forgiving, Friendly, Just, Kind, Kingly, Loving, Motherly, Punishing, Severe, and Wrathful. The response options were "not at all well," "not very well," "somewhat well," and "very well."[2]

Of those survey participants who believed in God at least to some degree, 94.0% or more believed Ever-present, Fatherly, Friendly, Forgiving, Just, Kind, and Loving described God "somewhat well" or "very well." Four of the most common beliefs about God were predominantly associated with the New Testament: Fatherly (94.5%), Forgiving (97.9%), Kind, (96.7%), and Loving (97.0%). Although God can certainly be considered to be the Father of Israel in the Old Testament, God is not a personal father figure in the Old Testament, whereas the universal fatherhood of God is both implicit and explicit in the New Testament [26].

Ever-present, which was the second most commonly held belief about God (97.5%), is one of the three related theological attributes of God in the Old Testament (omnipotent, omniscient, and omnipresent) [15]. Previous research suggests that Americans who hold one of these three beliefs about God hold all three of these beliefs [13, 18, 27]. The belief that God is Just, which is another major attribute of God in the Old Testament, was held by 96.5% of the participants in the 2007 Baylor Religion Survey who believed in God to some extent. Other national studies have found that many U.S. adults see God as the creator and, to a lesser extent, as a judge, but these adjectives were not included in the Baylor Survey [20, 22].

[2]The 2010 Baylor Religion Survey only listed eight adjectives describing God.

Belief in the negative attributes of God that are associated with the Old Testament were far less common among respondents to the Baylor Survey " i.e., Punishing (46.4%), Wrathful (36.7%), Critical (31.7%), and Severe (31.9%). The belief that God is Distant was very rare among the respondents (14.5%).

15.4 Americans' Belief in Life-After-Death

Belief in an afterlife is a central tenant of the world's major religions, including Buddhism [28, 29], Christianity [4, 30], Hinduism [31, 32], and Islam [33]. Belief in life-after-death is particularly common in America. The percentage of people in the U.S. who believe in an afterlife is comparable to the percentages reported in the predominantly Catholic countries of Ireland and Poland, and the percent of Americans who believe in life-after-death has been increasing slightly over the years, according to the General Social Service (GSS) [34 – 37]. Roughly 78–79% of all American adults said they believed in life-after-death in the 1970s and 1980s, and the percentage has been closer to 82% since the 1990s.

The sociologists Andrew Greeley and Michael Hout compared the percentages of U.S. adults surveyed by the GSS between 1973 and 1998,[3] who said they believed in life-after-death, by their religious affiliation: Protestant, Catholic, Jewish, and no religious affiliation (None) [35]. They grouped the percentages into six time-periods, which I have collapsed into three time-periods in Fig. 15.2.

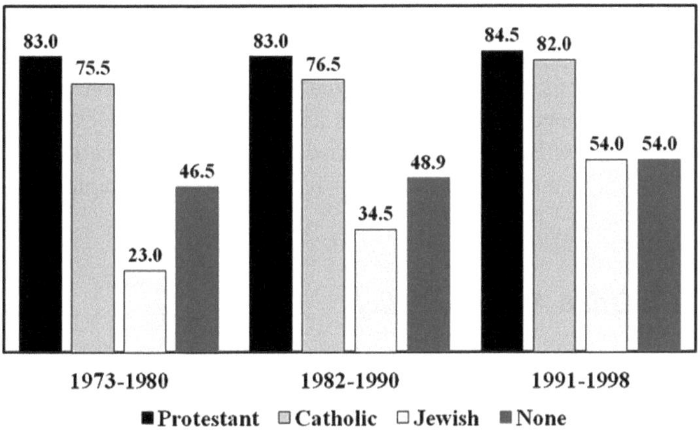

Fig. 15.2 Percent of U.S. adults of different religions who believe in life-after-death, as of 1998, according to the General Social Survey

[3] The General Social Survey (GSS) is conducted every two years by the National Opinion Research Center of the University of Chicago. The GSS randomly samples adults from the contiguous 48 states of the U.S. All the data are collected by face-to-face interviews.

As seen in Fig. 15.2, the proportion of Protestants who believe in life-after-death has been consistently higher than the proportion of Catholics across time. Jews are much less likely to believe in life-after-death than Christians are, although the data suggest that belief in an afterlife is increasing gradually among American Jews. I find it particularly interesting how many people with no religious affiliation say they believe in life-after-death.

15.5 Afterlife Beliefs of Several Major Religions

15.5.1 Jewish Afterlife Beliefs

The Hebrew Bible says very little about the fate of individuals when they die [5, 6, 38], but the Israelites are known to have shared the Babylonian belief that the dead went to an underground "land of no return," where they led a shadowy kind of existence. The Hebrew Bible calls this place Sheol, and refers to it as "the pit," and "the land of darkness," among other things [6, 7, 39].

The Bible includes the 6th Century (BCE) writings of Ezekiel that mention the restoration of the nation of Israel and the resurrection of the dead [6, 7, 39]. However, the concept of personal resurrection is first stated clearly in the 2nd Century (BCE) [6, 7, 39], in association with the theological concept that the dead will be united with their bodies at the "end-of-time" to live in a divine kingdom on earth [6, 7] – the "Olam Ha-Ba" or "world to come" [6, 40]. Some Jewish writings around this time redefined the concept of Sheol from being a neutral place for all the dead to a place for the wicked.

Other Jewish writings, called the Apocrypha, extensively described heaven and hell, but they were not included or "canonized" in the Hebrew Bible [6], so they had relatively little influence on Jewish beliefs about the afterlife. Despite the limited material in the Hebrew Bible about life-after-death and the resurrection of the physical body ("Tehiyat Hametim"), these beliefs became part of Rabbinic theology [41].

15.5.2 Christian Afterlife Beliefs

The New Testament repeatedly assures the faithful that there is life-after-death, although the Gospels do not state what that life will be like [42]. The early concepts of heaven and hell depicted in the Apocrypha evolved over time in Christianity. One of these concepts was that heaven was an incredibly pleasant and beautiful paradise that was reserved for the righteous. The wicked, on the other hand, were destined for hell. Although various images of heaven and hell emerged during the Middle Ages, the central theme remained that heaven was a place of eternal reward for the faithful and hell was a place of eternal punishment for sinners [4, 30]. Beyond that, however, going to heaven meant being in God's presence and being reunited with loved ones who had died [4, 30]. Though current Christian denominations have somewhat different conceptions of heaven, there is a general consensus that it is a place of peace and happiness in communion with God [30].

15.5.3 Islamic Afterlife Beliefs

The day of resurrection and judgment by God is a major theme of the Qur'ān or Koran [33]. Although the Qur'ān describes two phases of judgment, the first of which occurs immediately after death, the final judgment is the most important one. At the final judgment, the body will be resurrected and reunited with its soul and everyone will be held accountable for how they lived their lives. The good will enter the "Garden" and the bad will enter the "Fire" for all eternity [33, 43]. The Garden is the general term for paradise, where the faithful will be rewarded with the image of God, peace, and physical rewards and pleasures [33]. Some Islamic traditions teach that families will be re-united in the Garden, but this is not mentioned in the Qur'ān. Historically, some Islamic sects believed in re-incarnation, but this belief has never been a widely held belief in Islam [33, 43].

15.5.4 Hindu and Buddhist Beliefs

Hinduism encompasses a diverse collection of beliefs, not all of which are ascribed to by those who follow Hinduism. Indeed, there are even non-theistic and theistic forms of Hinduism; the former dating back to 1500 BCE, while the latter emerged around the 2nd century (BCE) [31]. The concept of re-incarnation or transmigration as part of the cycle of life, birth, death and rebirth, emerged around 800 BCE and became the central element of Hinduism [31, 32]. The goal of humankind in Hinduism is to escape the cycle of life (samasÃ£ra) and the suffering that it entails. Like Hinduism, Buddhism seeks liberation from the cycle of life and the pain and suffering that goes with it [28, 29]. Some Buddhist sects also teach that one's own actions in this life dictate one's circumstances in the next life. This is achieved by keeping oneself from fueling the desires that contribute to the cycle of birth, death, and rebirth. Though few humans achieve freedom from the cycle of life and death, and end their worldly existence, all are capable of doing so.

15.6 Different Afterlife Beliefs Among Americans

Greeley and Hout [35] provide limited information about the proportion of American adults who hold various beliefs about life-after-death, based on data from the 1983 and 1984 GSS. They found "nearly all Christians think that union with God, peace and tranquility, and reunion with relatives are very likely or likely to await them in the afterlife (p. 833)." In contrast, very few people endorsed the belief that life-after-death would be "a paradise of pleasures and delights," "a pale shadowy form of life, hardly life at all," or "reincarnation into another form." Greeley and Hout reported that "Jews rank most of the[se] images the same way Christians do (p. 833)," but they are less likely to endorse any of these beliefs.

Interestingly, Greeley and Hout reported that Orthodox and Conservative Jews were more likely to believe in life-after-death than Reform Jews were, although the data were limited [35]. They also noted that Jewish survey participants were more likely than Christian participants to express uncertainty about the possibility of an afterlife, rather than saying they did or did not believe in it.

15.7 Chapter Highlights and Comments

The percent of people in the U.S. who believe in God is higher than the percentage in almost any other country in the world. Americans, however, have various overlapping beliefs about the nature of God, some of which are rooted in the Old Testament, some of which are rooted in the New Testament, and some of which have no Biblical connection. The most commonly held beliefs are that God is ever-present, just, kind, loving, forgiving, and fatherly; less commonly held beliefs are that God is critical, punishing, severe, and wrathful. Most Americans also believe in life-after-death, and there is some evidence that belief in an afterlife may be increasing in the U.S. Like their beliefs about God, Americans' beliefs about the afterlife take various forms. These include the commonly held beliefs that the afterlife entails peace and tranquility, union with God, and reunion with loved ones. In contrast, relatively few Americans believe the afterlife entails a paradise of pleasures, a shadowy form of life, or reincarnation.

References

1. Kosmin, B. A., & Keysar, A. (2008). *American religious identification survey: Summary report*. Hartford: Trinity College.
2. Noss, J. B. (1969). *Man's religions* (Fifth ed.). New York: MacMillan Publishing.
3. Smith, H. (2009). *The world's religions*. New York: Harper Collins.
4. Obayashi, H. (Ed.). (1992). *Death and afterlife: Perspective of world religions* (Contributions to the study of religion). New York: Greenwood Press.
5. Segal, A. F. (2004). *Life after death: A history of the afterlife in the religions of the West*. New York: Doubleday.
6. Raphael, S. P. (1996). *Jewish views of the afterlife*. Northvale: Jason Aronson Inc.
7. Sonsino, R., & Syme, D. B. (1990). *What happens after I die? Jewish views of life after death*. New York: VAHC Press.
8. Newport, F. (2011). More than 9 in 10 Americans continue to believe in God. Princeton: Gallup. Retrieved from http://www.gallup.com/poll/147887/americans-continue-believe-god.aspx

9. Piazza, T., & Glock, C. Y. (1979). Images of God and their social meanings. In R. Wuthnow (Ed.), *The religious dimension: New directions in quantitative research.* New York: Academic Press.
10. Cranney, S. (2013). Do people who believe in God report more meaning in their lives? The existential effects of belief. *Journal for the Scientific Study of Religion* 52(3), 638–646.
11. Sherkat, D. E. (2008). Beyond belief: Atheism, agnosticism, and theistic certainty in the United States. *Sociological Spectrum,* 28(5), 438–459.
12. Smith, A. (2008). *Beliefs about God across time and countries.* Chicago: National Opinion Research Board.
13. Gorsuch, R. L. (1968). The conceptualization of God as seen in adjective ratings. *Journal for the Scientific Study of Religion,* 7(1), 56–64.
14. Spilka, B., Armatas, P., & Nussbaum, J. (1964). The concept of God: A factor analytic approach. *Review of Religious Research,* 6(1), 28–36.
15. Kaplan, A. (1984). The Judaic view of God. *Judaism,* 33(4), 402–415.
16. *King James Holy Bible* (1611/1999). Dayton: Greyden Press.
17. Schaefer, C. A., & Gorsuch, R. L. (1992). Dimensionality of religion: Belief and motivation as predictors of behavior. *Journal of Psychology and Christianity,* 11(3), 244–254.
18. Foster, R. A., & Keating, J. P. (1992). Measuring androcentrism in the Western God-concept. *Journal for the Scientific Study of Religion,* 31(3), 366–375.
19. Hammersla, J. F., Andrews-Qualls, L. C., & Frease, L. G. (1986). God concepts and religious committment among Christian university students. *Journal for the Scientific Study of Religion,* 25(4), 424–435.
20. Nelsen, H. M., Cheek, N. H., & Au, P. (1985). Gender differences in images of God. *Journal for the Scientific Study of Religion,* 24(4), 396–402.
21. Tamayo, A., & Desjardines, L. (1976). Belief systems and conceptual images of parents and God. *Journal of Psychology: Interdisciplinary and Applied,* 92(1), 131–140.
22. Roof, W. C., & Roof, J. L. (1984). Review of the polls: Images of God among Americans. *Journal for the Scientific Study of Religion,* 23(2), 201–205.
23. Froese, P., & Bader, C. D. (2010). *America's four Gods.* New York: Oxford Univeristy Press.
24. Noffke, J. L. M. S. H. (2001). Denominational and age comparisons of God concepts. *Journal for the Scientific Study of Religion,* 40(4), 747–756.
25. Hoffman, L., Hoffman, J. L., Dillard, K., Clark, J., Acoba, R., Williams, F., et al. (2008). Diversity and the God image: Examining ethnic differences in the experience of God for a college-age population. *Journal of Psychology & Theology,* 36(1), 26–41.
26. The fatherhood of God. (1903). *The Biblical World, 22*(3), 236–237.
27. Kunkel, M. A., Cook, S., Meshel, D. S., Daughtry, D., & Hauenstein, A. (1999). God images: A concept map. *Journal for the Scientific Study of Religion,* 38(2), 193–202.
28. Klein, A. C. (1998). Buddhism. In C. J. Johnson, & M. G. McGee (Eds.), *How different religions view death and afterlife.* (pp. 47–63). Philadelphia: The Charles Press.
29. Reynolds, F. E. (1992). Death as threat, death as achievement: Buddhist perspectives with particular reference to the Theravada tradition. In H. Obayashi (Ed.), *Death and afterlife: Perspectives of the world religions.* (pp. 157–167). New York: Greenwood Press.
30. Johnson, C. J., & McGee, M. G. (Eds.). (1998). *How different religions view death & afterlife.* Philadelphia: The Charles Press.
31. Hopkins, T. J. (1992). Hindu views of death and afterlife. In H. Obayashi (Ed.), *Death and afterlife: Perspectives of the world religions.* (pp. 143–155). New York: Greenwood Press.
32. Pearson, A. M. (1998). Hinduism. In J. C. Johnson, & M. G. McGee (Eds.), *How different religions view death and afterlife.* (pp. 109–131). Philadelphia: The Charles Press.
33. Smith, J. L., & Haddad, Y. Y. (2002). *The Islamic understanding of death and resurrection.* Oxford: Oxford University Press.
34. Davis, J. A., Smith, T. W., & Marsden, P. V. (2006). *General Social Survey cumulative codebook, 1972–2006.* Storrs: Roper Center.

35. Greeley, A. M., & Hout, M. (1999). Americans' increasing belief in life after death: Religious competition and acculturation. *American Sociological Review,* 64(6), 813–835.
36. Harley, B., & Firebaugh, G. (1993). Americans' belief in an afterlife: Trends over the past two decades. *Journal for the Scientific Study of Religion,* 32(3), 269–278.
37. Schwadel, P. (2011). Age, period, and cohort effects on religious activities and beliefs. *Social Science Research,* 40, 181–192.
38. Lamm, M. (1988). *The Jewish way in death and mourning*. New York: Jonathan David Publishers.
39. Routledge, R. L. (2008). Death and afterlife in the Old Testament. *Journal of European Baptist Studies,* 9(1), 22–39.
40. Werblowsky, R. J. Z., & Wigoder, G. (1966). *The encyclopedia of the Jewish religion*. New York: Holt, Rinehart and Winston, Inc.
41. Adler, J. J. (1994). The Bible and Life after death. *Jewish Bible Quarterly,* 22(2), 85–90.
42. Mitton, C. L. (1965). Life after death: The after-life in the New Testament. *Expository Times,* 76(11), 332–337.
43. Chittick, W. C. (1992). Your sight today is piercing: The Muslim understanding of death and afterlife. In H. Obayashi (Ed.), *Death and afterlife: Perspectives of the world religions*. (pp. 125–139). New York: Greenwood Press.

Chapter 16
Religion and Death Anxiety

Abstract The chapter reviews research findings on the degree to which religion faith, including religious beliefs, are associated with death anxiety (i.e., fear of death and the unknown after death). The research shows that Americans who practice their faith as an end in itself (internal religious motivation) have less fear of death than those who view religion as a means to achieve social goals (external religious motivation), and that the salutary association between internal religiosity and fear of death is mediated by the fact that individuals who have internalized their religious faith are more likely to believe in life-after-death. The findings of numerous, relatively small U.S. studies, which primarily surveyed Christians, indicate that belief in life-after-death tends to be negatively associated with death anxiety/fear of death. The results of four large-scale studies that specifically examined the positive and negative association of other religious beliefs with death anxiety also are described. However, research indicates that people have various fears about death, some of which are not affected by their belief in an afterlife and some of which seem to be affected more by other aspects of religious faith.

Keywords Death anxiety • *Denial of Death* • Extrinsic religious orientation • Fear of death • Intrinsic religious orientation • Life-after-death • Terror Management Theory

16.1 Denying Death

Ernst Becker's Pulitzer Prize winning book *The Denial of Death* argues that the central quandary of human beings is that we, unlike any other animal, are aware that we will inevitably die [1]. According to Becker, a cultural anthropologist, the fear of death pervades our lives and it is so intense that he called it terror rather than mere fear. It is the terror of facing our own non-existence, or as the German philosopher Martin Heidegger put it: "the terror into which the abyss of Nothing plunges us" (p. 192). [2]

Much of Becker's book is devoted to dismantling psychoanalytical interpretations of our fear of death as manifestations of repressed sexuality and showing it for what is: fear of death. Fear of death has long been called death anxiety in the field

K.J. Flannelly, *Religious Beliefs, Evolutionary Psychiatry, and Mental Health in America*, Religion, Spirituality and Health: A Social Scientific Approach 1,
DOI 10.1007/978-3-319-52488-7_16

of psychoanalysis, and though it is not a psychiatric disorder, it has received considerable attention in the psychoanalytic literature [3]. The remainder of Beck's book explores the societal mechanisms that are designed to suppress thoughts about death from becoming conscious. Oddly, Becker pays remarkably little attention to the role of religion in addressing the existential dilemma of living in the shadow of death, given that many scholars believe this is a major function of religion [e.g., 4, 5, 6].

In the late 1980s and early 1990s, Terror Management Theory (TM Theory) picked up where *The Denial of Death* left off in the 1970s, claiming that humans are terrified by their awareness of the inevitability of their own death, and that reminders of death induce death anxiety [7–9]. TM Theory specifically claims the primary function of religion is to reduce fear of death by offering a sense of security and the possibility of immortality through life-after-death [10, 11].

The publication of *The Denial of Death* coincided with heightened research interest in the fear of death, beginning with the publication of the Death Anxiety Scale in 1970 [12]. Studies conducted in the U.S. during the 1970s and 1980s suggested that death anxiety decreases across the life-span, from its peak in the late teens and early 20s, through old age [13]. A review of the research on older adults by Fortner and Neimeyer [14] found the main exception to this pattern were older adults with serious health or psychological problems. Other research supports the general assertion that religious beliefs and practices are inversely related to death anxiety in older adults [e.g., 15, 16].

However, studies have found an inverse relationship between religion and death anxiety less often than one might expect. A 2013 literature review by social scientists Lee Ellis and Eshah Wahab identified 84 studies on religion and death anxiety in 17 countries that were published between 1959 and 2010 [17]. Just 47% of them reported the expected inverse relationship between religion and death anxiety. Most of the other studies reported no relationship or a positive relationship between religion and death anxiety, and a few reported a curvilinear relationship [17]. The latter finding means that people who are very religious and people who are not at all religious have the lowest levels of death anxiety.

16.2 Intrinsic and Extrinsic Religious Orientation and Death Anxiety

The concepts of intrinsic religious orientation and extrinsic religious orientation or motivation were proposed by the American psychologist Gordon Allport, who observed that frequent church "attenders" seemed to place "intrinsic" value on their religion and accept "its total creed (including love for his neighbor) …as part of the fabric of [their] personality" (p. 131) [18]. Irregular church attenders, on the other hand, seemed to think "religion is more of an 'extrinsic' value" (p. 131) [18], in which religion serves them, they do not serve it. Allport concluded that irregular attenders go to church to maintain a communal connection and the social benefits

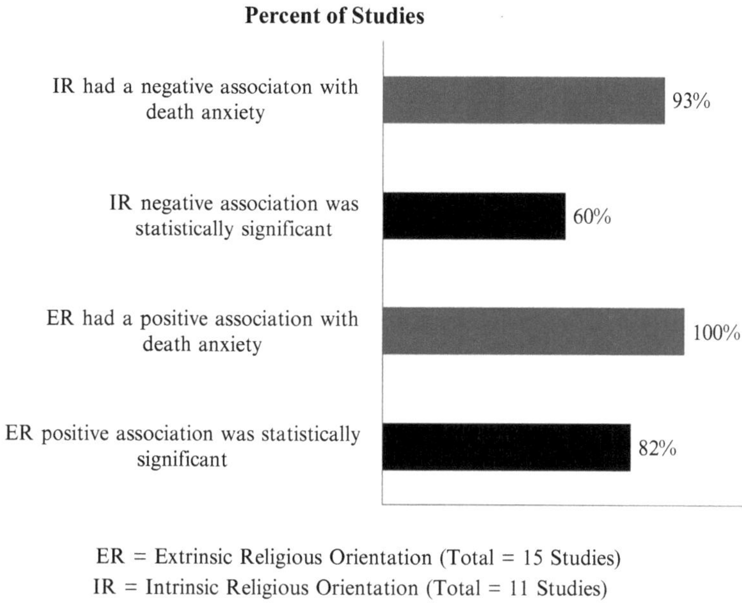

Fig. 16.1 Percent of studies reporting positive and negative correlations between religious orientation and death anxiety and the percent of studies reporting statistically significant correlations

that derive from it. For individuals who have an extrinsic religious orientation, this "communal type of [church] membership, supports and serves other, nonreligious ends" (p. 454) [19]. For individuals who have an intrinsic religious orientation, "religion is an end in itself – a final, not an instrumental goal" (p. 454) [19].

This conception of religious experience inspired the development of several scales to measure intrinsic and extrinsic religious orientation, the first two of which were nearly identical [20, 21]. The scales do not measure religious beliefs, per se, such as beliefs about God or an afterlife, but beliefs or attitudes about religion.

I found 16 studies in Ellis and Wahab's review on the association between death anxiety and intrinsic religious orientation and/or extrinsic religious orientation [17].[1] Fourteen of the 16 studies were conducted in the U.S., one was conducted in Canada, and one was conducted in Hong Kong.

Of these 16 studies, five measured only intrinsic religious orientation, one measured only extrinsic religious orientation, and ten measured both religious variables. Hence, as seen in Fig. 16.1, 15 studies measured the relationship between intrinsic religious orientation and death anxiety, and 11 studies measured the relationship between extrinsic religious orientation and death anxiety. Figure 16.1 shows that 93% (14 of 15) of the studies of intrinsic religiosity reported a negative association

[1] The studies were grouped into tables by whether they reported a statistically significant inverse (or negative) association, a statistically significant direct (or positive negative) association, or no statistically significant association between religious motivation and death anxiety. The term "statistically significant" means that the observed result is very unlikely to have occurred by chance.

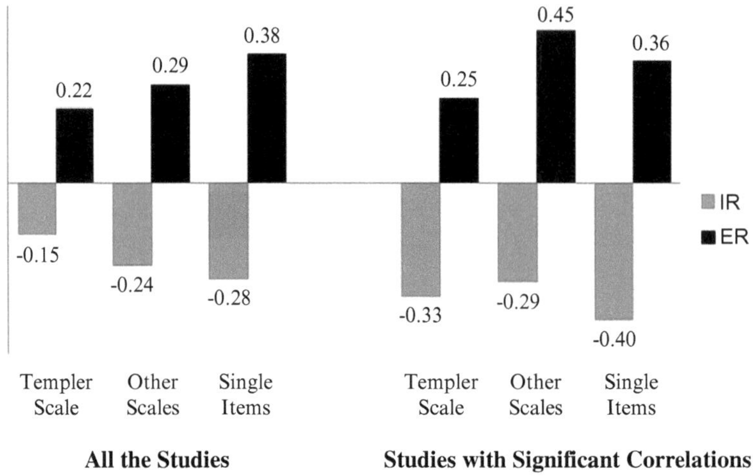

Fig. 16.2 Mean correlations of intrinsic religious (*IR*) and extrinsic religious (*ER*) orientation with different measures of death anxiety in all studies and in those studies reporting significant correlations

between intrinsic religiosity and death anxiety, and 100% of the studies of extrinsic religiosity reported a positive association between extrinsic religiosity and death anxiety. In all, 60% of the studies of intrinsic religiosity reported a significant[2] negative association between intrinsic religiosity and death anxiety, and 82% of the studies of extrinsic religiosity reported a significant positive association between extrinsic religiosity and death anxiety. These results illustrate that intrinsic religious orientation has a consistently negative or inverse association with death anxiety, whereas extrinsic religious motivation has a consistently positive or direct association with death anxiety.

Before taking a closer look at the association between religious orientation and death anxiety, I added one study to the sample that was not included in the Ellis and Wahab review [17], and excluded three studies for different reasons,[3] which left 14 studies that were conducted in North America. The majority of studies surveyed convenience samples of high school and/or college students, two surveyed older adults, and two surveyed church congregants. Half the studies used the Templer Death Anxiety Scale, four used other death anxiety scales, and four studies used a single item about fear of death or fear of the unknown after death.

Figure 16.2 shows the average or mean correlation coefficients of extrinsic and intrinsic religious orientation with each type of measure of death anxiety for all the studies and for those reporting significant correlations.[4] As seen in Fig. 16.2, intrin-

[2] The term "significant" is often used as shorthand for "statistically significant."

[3] Two studies were excluded because they did not report bivariate correlations and the third study was excluded because it was conducted in Hong Kong.

[4] Correlation is a statistical procedure that measures the degree of association between two numerical variables. A positive correlation means that when one variable increases in magnitude the other variable also increases in magnitude. A negative correlation means that when one variable increases

sic religion orientation had a negative correlation with death anxiety and extrinsic religion orientation had a positive correlation with death anxiety, regardless of the measure of death anxiety used in the studies. Naturally, the mean correlations are larger, in either direction, for those studies in which the correlations were statistically significant.

To summarize the findings in Fig. 16.2, people who viewed their religious faith as being a central part of their lives and practiced their religion as an end in itself were less afraid of death, whereas people who viewed their religious faith as a means to achieve their own social goals were more afraid of death. It should be kept in mind, that these findings are mainly based on U.S. Christian samples.

16.3 Belief in Life-After-Death and Death Anxiety

Two studies of U.S. adults and college students suggest that the salubrious association between intrinsic religiosity and death anxiety may be attributable to the fact that persons who are intrinsically religious are more likely to believe in life-after-death than persons who are extrinsically religious [22, 23]. A third study of U.S. high school and college students provides more definitive evidence that the salutary association between intrinsic religiosity and death anxiety is at least partially mediated by the direct effect of belief in life-after-death on death anxiety [24].

My inspection of Ellis and Wahab's tables identified 12 studies that specifically examined the relationship between belief in life-after-death and fear of death, which included 16 analyses [17]. The results of the twelve studies, which were conducted in the U.S. using convenience samples, are summarized in Fig. 16.3.

Although belief in life-after-death generally had a negative association with fear of death, this finding was not unanimous. The left side of Fig. 16.3 shows that nine of the twelve studies (75.0%) reported a negative association between belief in life-after-death and death anxiety, as one might expect, two (16.7%) reported a positive relationship, and one (8.3%) reported both negative and positive associations, depending on the measures of death anxiety. The right side of the Fig. 16.3 shows that six of the twelve studies found a statistically significant negative correlation (50.0%) between belief in life-after-death and death anxiety, four did not find any significant association (Neither, 33.3%), and two reported significant positive association (16.7%). The findings of these twelve U.S. studies indicate that belief in life-after-death tends to have a salutary association with death anxiety in convenience samples that are primarily Christian.[5]

---

the other variable decreases. Pearson's correlation coefficient is the most commonly used correlation measure; its coefficient is symbolized as r. A positive correlation coefficient ranges between 0 and 1; a negative correlation coefficient ranges between 0 and -1.

[5] I took a closer look at the U.S. samples to see if the differences in the findings might be attributable to differences in the samples or other features of the study. Based on their differences in methodology, four general factors might have accounted for the different results: the dependent variables, the independent variables, the sample size, and the sample composition with respect to

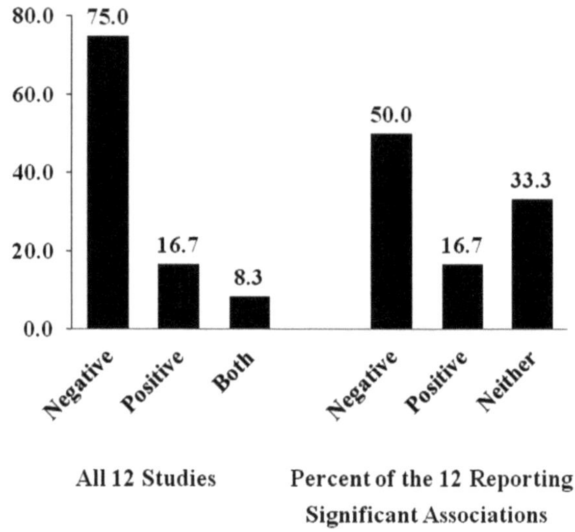

Fig. 16.3 Percent of U.S. studies reporting positive and negative associations between belief in life-after-death and death anxiety and the percent of those studies reporting statistically significant associations (N = 12)

16.4 Other Religious Beliefs and Death Anxiety

Other religious beliefs and aspects of religious faith have been found to be associated with death anxiety, including the belief that a person collaborates with God (which is discussed in detail in Chap. 20), the belief that one has been forgiven by God (which is discussed in Chap. 24), religious beliefs that the future will be better (which has been called "religious hope"), and having doubts about one's religious faith and beliefs (which is examined in Chap. 23). Four large-scale U.S. studies have examined the relationship of each of these variables with death anxiety, the essential results of which are presented in Fig.16.4.

The first two studies were based on data from national probability samples of older Americans who were practicing Christians [25, 26],[6] and both of them controlled for frequency of church attendance, frequency of private prayer, and demographic characteristics using regression analysis.[7] The two studies found, respectively, that believing one collaborates with God ($\beta = -.15$) [25],[8] and believ-

religion. Statistical analyses of these four factors found no evidence that any of them affected the proportion of studies reporting significant correlations, or the direction or size of the correlations.

[6] The first three studies used probability (i.e., randomly selected) samples. The sample sizes of the first two studies were N = 1211 and N = 1154 (N is the number of persons in a sample from a population.).

[7] The first two studies analyzed the data with Ordinary Least Squares (OLS) regression; the demographic variables in both studies were age, education, gender, and race. Regression is a statistical procedure that measures the degree of association of one numerical variable with one or more other numerical variables.

[8] The belief that one collaborates with God was measured with three items:"I rely on God to help me control my life"; "I can succeed with God's help"; and "All things are possible when I work together with God."

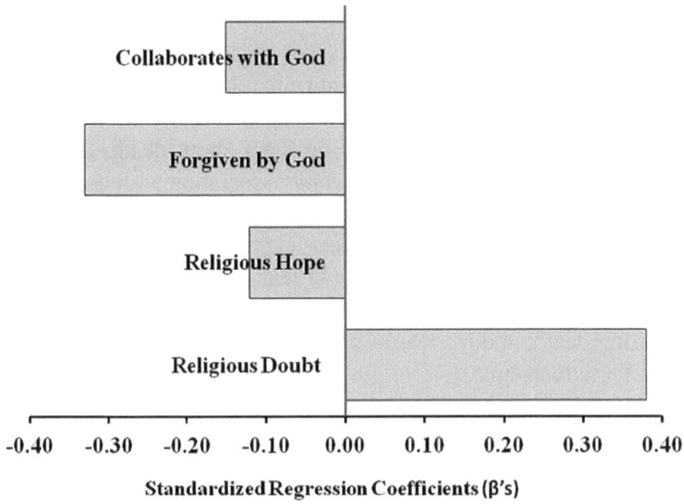

Fig. 16.4 Association of death anxiety with various religious beliefs and religious doubt in four studies

ing one has been forgiven by God ($\beta = -.33$)[9] [26] had significant negative associations with death anxiety. The third study, which used a large national sample of American adults of all religions[10] to investigate the degree to which positive religious beliefs about the future ("religious hope"[11]), showed that such beliefs also were significantly and negatively associated with death anxiety ($\beta = -.12$) [27].[12] The fourth study used a convenience sample of mainly college students of various religious denominations to examine the association between doubting one's religious beliefs ("religious doubt") and death anxiety [28].[13] That study revealed a significant positive relationship between death anxiety and religious doubt ($\beta = .38$).

[9] Beta (β) is a measure of association that is very similar to Pearson's r, and it is identical to *r* when there are only two variables in an OLS regression analysis.

[10] The data came from the 2013–2014 "Landmark Spirituality and Health Survey," which was conducted by the National Opinion Research Center (NORC). The sample size for this study was 2783. The NORC also conducts the biennial "General Social Survey."

[11] Religious hope was measured by three items: "My religious or spiritual beliefs help me see that things will turn out well in the future"; "My religious or spiritual beliefs help me see that the future will bring opportunities for a better life"; and "My religious or spiritual beliefs help me see that the future looks bright for me."

[12] The third and fourth studies analyzed their data using structural equation modeling (SEM), which combines OLS regression with factor analysis. The third study controlled for the same variables controlled in the first and second studies.

[13] N = 634; The study used OLS regression, controlling for age, gender, and multiple measures of religion. Religious doubt was measured with a 15-item scale, which included items about questioning the existence of God, wondering why God allows suffering and evil to exist in the world, dissatisfaction with clergy and church leaders, and the disparate viewpoints of the world offered by science and religion.

16.5 Religious Beliefs and Specific Fears About Death

All the findings I have discussed to this point were related to the association between belief in life-after-death and global measures of death anxiety. Though researchers have recognized a number of more specific fears about death, few studies have examined if belief in an afterlife has a salutary association with them. The sociologist Jon Hoelter's classification of death fears [29] is the most exhaustive classification, which includes eight dimensions of fear: (1) fear of the dying process; (2) fear of the dead; (3) fear of being destroyed; (4) fear for the well-being of significant others after your death; (5) fear of the unknown; (6) fear of conscious death; (7) fear for the body after death; and (8) fear of premature death. It is not known how common many of these fears are.

A study by Jon Hoelter and Rita Eply is the only study of which I am aware that has examined the relationship between these fears and various measures of religion [30]. The study used a sample of 375 college students in the U.S. Midwest to determine the correlation of each fear with five religious variables: current church attendance, childhood church attendance, self-perceived religiosity, religious orthodoxy, and belief in a supreme being. Of the 40 bivariate analyses performed, only five significant correlations were found between the fear of death and religion: fear of the unknown was negatively correlated with church attendance ($r = -.41$), self-perceived religiosity ($r = -.21$), religious orthodoxy ($r = -.64$), and belief in a supreme being ($r = -.51$), and fear of being destroyed was negatively correlated with church attendance ($r = -.10$).

A study by psychologist Nava Silton and her colleagues [31] that examined four fears about death yielded findings that are more congruent with the view that religion provides protection against fear of death. The four fears, which are comparable to four of Hoelter's eight fears, were used as dependent or outcome variables: fear of the unknown after death, fear of dying in pain, fear of dying alone, and fear of leaving loved ones' behind. The study, based on a 2002 survey of 935 members and elders of the Presbyterian Church (USA), is one of the relatively few studies on religion and fear of death to use multivariate statistical analyses instead of simple bivariate correlations.

Four measures of religion were used as independent variables: church attendance, church involvement, private devotion, and belief in life-after-death. Higher levels of church attendance and private religious devotion (i.e., private prayer and Bible reading) may be considered measures of intrinsic motivation. Church involvement, which measured church-related social activities apart from religious services, may be considered a measure of extrinsic religious motivation.

Logistic regression was used to analyze the associations between the four fears and the four religious variables. The results of logistic regression are reported as odds ratios in which values closer to 1 represent weaker associations and values farther away from 1 represent stronger associations.[14] For the sake of simplicity,

[14] This is different from the measure of association in correlation (e.g., Pearson's r) and the measure of association in OLS regression (β), in which values closer to 1 represent stronger associations and values farther away from 1 represent weaker associations.

Table 16.1 Odd ratios for the inverse associations between religious variables and fears about death

Religious variable	Unknown after death	Dying in pain	Leaving loved ones
Church attendance	.57	.82	.83
Church involvement	.65		.76
Private devotion	.67	.72	
Belief in an afterlife	.59		

Silton et al., 2011 [31]

only statistically significant associations are shown in Table 16.1; no significant associations were found between any of the of religious measure and fear of dying alone.

Table 16.1 shows that all four measures of religion had significant negative associations with fear of the unknown after death (OR's between .57 and .67), which is consistent with the idea that religion reduces one's fear of what happens after death because Christianity promises the faithful will have a life-after-death in Heaven. It is notable that belief in life-after-death (or afterlife) had one of the strongest negative associations with fear of the unknown (OR = .59), as one would expect, but it was not significantly associated with any of the other dependent variables.

Dying in pain had a salubrious association with church attendance (OR = .82) and private devotion (OR = .72). Both church attendance (OR = .83) and church involvement (OR = .76) had salubrious associations with fear of leaving loved ones behind, although church involvement had a somewhat stronger association.

When all four fears were analyzed simultaneously, fear of the unknown was most strongly associated with belief in life-after-death, fear of dying in pain was most strongly associated with private prayer, and fear of leaving loved ones was most strongly associated with church involvement. The reason for the salubrious association of belief in life-after-death and fear of the unknown is obvious. The unique net effect of private devotion with fear of dying in pain may be because private prayer involves a conversation with a personal God, which may help to reduce this concern. The singular salubrious association of church involvement with fear of leaving loved ones behind may represent an effect of extrinsic religious motivation. All church members presumably expect social support from their co-congregants for the loved ones they leave behind, but extrinsically motivated congregants may feel more certain that they have secured the social connections to ensure this happens.

16.6 Chapter Highlights and Comments

Although it is often assumed that religious individuals (particularly Christians) should have less fear of death, studies on the association between fear of death and religion have yielded some inconsistent results. Nevertheless, very consistent results have been found among Americans (a) who practice their faith as an end in itself (intrinsic religious motivation), and (b) who view their religious practices as a means to achieve their own social goals (extrinsic religious motivation). That is, individuals with intrinsic religious motivation are less afraid of death than individuals with extrinsic religious motivation. Related research suggests that the salubrious association between internal religiosity and fear of death is partially mediated by the fact that individuals who have internalized their religion are more likely than other individuals to believe in life-after-death. Overall, the findings of U.S. studies of primarily Christian samples indicate that belief in life-after-death is associated with less fear of death. However, people have many fears about death that do not appear to be affected by their belief in an afterlife. This is not surprising, since belief in an afterlife does not address the dying process or what happens in the material world after one's death. Nevertheless, some of these fears appear to be assuaged by other aspects of religion.

Obviously, one does not need ETAS Theory to explain why belief in life-after-death reduces a person's fear of death. One may ask, however, why the other religious beliefs that were discussed in the chapter affect fear of death or death anxiety. As "religious hope" is a measure of belief in a better future, and as the future includes life-after-death for many religious individuals, it is not surprising that "religious hope" is inversely associated with death anxiety. The explanation of why death anxiety is lower among Christians who believe they collaborate with God or have been forgiven by God is equally obvious. Since God decides whether someone gets into heaven or goes to hell, people who believe they work with God or have been forgiven by God probably expect they will to go to heaven when they die. On the other hand, doubting one's religious faith and beliefs undermines such certainty about going to heaven and increases death anxiety. Moreover, religious individuals who have doubts about their faith may be afraid that God will send them to hell to punish them for their lack of faith.

ETAS Theory was developed to explain how and why beliefs (including religious beliefs) affect mental health, particularly psychiatric symptoms. As explained in Chaps. 11 and 12, ETAS Theory proposes that the roots of psychiatric symptoms lie in proximate brain mechanisms that evolved over eons to protect us and our animal ancestors from harm. Although death anxiety has been widely discussed in the psychoanalytic literature, it is not a psychiatric disorder. Yet, some advocates of TM Theory have claimed that psychiatric disorders are the direct or indirect result of our fear of death [32]. This implies that the proximate mechanisms underlying anxiety and related psychiatric symptoms did not evolve until humans or our close human ancestors became consciously aware of their own mortality – a premise that I think is untenable.

References

1. Becker, E. (1973). *The denial of death*. New York: Free Press.
2. Heidegger, M. (1949). *Existence and being*. Chicago: Henry Regnery Co.
3. Stolorow, R. D. (1973). *Perspectives on death anxiety: A review*. Psychiatric Quarterly, 47(4), 473–486.

4. Malinowski, B. (1954). *Magic, science and religion*. New York: Doubleday.
5. Oates, W. E. (1973). *The psychology of religion*. Waco, TX: Word Books.
6. Jung, C. (1934/1969). The soul and death. In *The collected works of C. G. Jung* (Vol. 8). Princeton: Princeton University Press.
7. Rosenblatt, A., Greenberg, J., Solomon, S., Pyszczynski, T., & Lyon, D. (1989). Evidence for terror management theory: I. The effects of mortality salience on reactions to those who violate or uphold cultural values. *Journal of Personality and Social Psychology,* 57(4), 681–690.
8. Greenberg, J., Pyszczynski, T., Solomon, S., Rosenblatt, A., Veeder, M., Kirkland, S., et al. (1990). Evidence for terror management theory II: The effects of mortality salience on reactions to those who threaten or bolster the cultural worldview. *Journal of Personality and Social Psychology,* 58(2), 308–318.
9. Solomon, S., Greenberg, J., & Pyszczynski, T. (1991). A terror-management theory of self-esteem. In C. R. Snyder, & D. Forsyth (Eds.), *Handbook of social and clinical psychology: The health perspective* (pp. 21–40). New York: Pergamon Press.
10. Vail, K. E., 3rd, Rothschild, Z. K., Weise, D. R., Solomon, S., Pyszczynski, T., & Greenberg, J. (2010). A terror management analysis of the psychological functions of religion. *Personality and Social Psychology Review,* 14(1), 84–94.
11. Jonas, E., & Fischer, P. (2006). Terror management and religion: Evidence that intrinsic religiousness mitigates worldview defense following mortality salience. *Journal of Personality and Social Psychology,* 91(3), 553–567.
12. Templer, D. I., & Dotson, E. (1970). Religious correlates of death anxiety. *Psychological Reports,* 26, 895–897.
13. Neimeyer, R. A., Wittkowski, J., & Moser, R. P. (2004). Psychological research on death attitudes: An overview and evaluation. *Death Studies,* 28(4), 309–340.
14. Fortner, B. V., & Neimeyer, R. A. (1999). Death anxiety in older adults: A quantitative review. *Death Studies,* 23(5), 387–411.
15. Wink, P., & Scott, J. (2005). Does religiousness buffer against the fear of death and dying in late adulthood? Findings from a longitudinal study. *Journal of Gerontology: Psychological Sciences,* 60B(4), P207-P214.
16. Koenig, H. G. (1988). Religious behaviors and death anxiety in later life. *Hospice Journal,* 4(1), 3–24.
17. Ellis, L., & Wahab, E. (2013). Religiosity and fear of death: A theory-oriented review of the empirical literature. *Review of Religious Research,* 55(1), 149–189.
18. Allport, G. W. (1962). Prejudice: Is it societal or personal? *Journal of Social Issues,* 18(2), 120–134.
19. Allport, G. W. (1966). Religious context of prejudice. *Journal for the Scientific Study of Religion,* 5(3), 447–457.
20. Allport, G. W., & Ross, J. M. (1967). Personal religious orientation and prejudice. *Journal of Personality and Social Psychology,* 5(4), 432–443.
21. Feagin, J. R. (1964). Prejudice and religious types: A focused study of southern fundamentalists. *Journal for the Scientific Study of Religion,* 4(1), 3–13.
22. Falkenhain, M., & Handal, P. J. (2003). Religion, death attitudes, and belief in afterlife in the elderly: Untangling the relationships. *Journal of Religion and Health,* 42(1), 67–76.
23. Spilka, B., Stout, L., Minton, B., & Sizemore, D. (1977). Death and personal faith: A psychometric investigation. *Journal for the Scientific Study of Religion,* 16(2), 169–178.
24. Cohen, A. B., Pierce, J. D., Jr., Chambers, J., Meade, R., Gorvine, B. J., & Koenig, H. G. (2005). Intrinsic and extrinsic religiosity, belief in the afterlife, death anxiety, and life satisfaction in young Catholics and Protestants. *Journal of Research in Personality,* 39(3), 307–324.
25. Krause, N. (2005). God-mediated control and psychological well-being in late life. *Research on Aging,* 27(2), 136–164.
26. Krause, N. (2015). Trust in God, forgiveness by God, and death anxiety. *Omega – Journal of Death and Dying,* 72(1), 20–41.
27. Krause, N., Pargament, K. I., & Ironson, G. (2016). In the shadow of death: Religious hope as a moderator of the effects of age on death anxiety. *Journals of Gerontology Series B:*

Psychological Sciences and Social Sciences, Retrieved from http://psychsocgerontology.oxfordjournals.org/content/early/2016/04/10/geronb.gbw039.long
28. Henrie, J., & Patrick, J. H. (2014). Religiousness, religious doubt, and death anxiety. *The International Journal of Aging and Human Development,* 78(3), 203–227.
29. Hoelter, J. W. (1979). Multidimensional treatment of fear of death. *Journal of Consulting and Clinical Psychology,* 47(5), 996–999.
30. Hoelter, J. W., & Epley, R. J. (1979). Religious correlates of fear of death. *Journal for the Scientific Study of Religion,* 18(4), 404–411.
31. Silton, N. R., Flannelly, K. J., Ellison, C. G., Galek, K., Jacobs, M. R., Marcum, J. P., et al. (2011). The association between religious beliefs and practices and end-of-life fears among members of the Presbyterian Church (U.S.A). *Review of Religious Research,* 53, 357–370.
32. Arndt, J., Routledge, C., Cox, C. R., & Goldenberg, J. L. (2005). The worm at the core: A terror management perspective on the roots of psychological dysfunction. *Applied and Preventive Psychology,* 11(3), 191.

Chapter 17
Belief in Life-After-Death and Mental Health

Abstract The chapter summarizes the results of four major national and regional studies in the U.S. on the association between belief in life-after-death and psychological well-being and distress. The results found that belief in life-after-death tends to have a salutary association with psychological well-being and psychological distress, including several classes of psychiatric symptoms. Moreover, the results indicate that belief in an afterlife buffers against the pernicious effects of the threats posed by adverse life events and the uncertainty they create. In keeping with ETAS Theory, the chapter suggests that a major reason why belief in an afterlife reduces anxiety is that it reduces uncertainty about the future, because the brain structure called the amygdala responds to uncertainty with fear. The chapter contrasts this interpretation of the results, based on by ETAS Theory, to Terror Management Theory, which proposes that fear of death is the fundamental fear of humans. The chapter also discusses findings that social support is associated with lower levels of psychiatric symptoms in terms of ETAS Theory, which proposes that social support can provide a sense of security that reduces anxiety about one's current and future circumstances.

Keywords Afterlife • ETAS Theory • Life-after-death • Social support • Safety • Terror Management Theory • Psychological distress • Psychological well-being • Threat

17.1 Background

Despite the high prevalence of belief in life-after-death among Americans, very little research has explored whether belief in an afterlife contributes to mental health, aside from death anxiety. The influence of belief in an afterlife on psychological well-being has mainly been studied in relation to bereavement. Yet, even the research literature on bereavement is relatively sparse. Generally, belief in life-after-death tends to help people deal with the loss of a loved one and it can be a buffer against depression [1–3], whereas uncertainty about the existence of an afterlife may cause psychological distress among recently widowed individuals [4]. This chapter

K.J. Flannelly, *Religious Beliefs, Evolutionary Psychiatry, and Mental Health in America*, Religion, Spirituality and Health: A Social Scientific Approach 1,
DOI 10.1007/978-3-319-52488-7_17

summarizes findings on the relationship between belief in life-after death and mental health from four large-scale studies of U.S. adults.

17.2 Belief in Life-After-Death and Psychological Well-Being

Three studies by Chris Ellison of The University of Texas at San Antonio and his colleagues have examined the association between belief in an afterlife and psychological distress and well-being in the U.S. general public.[1] The first study [5], published in 2001, used data from the "Detroit Area Study" [6], and the second study, published in 2009, used data from the General Social Survey (GSS) [7]. The two studies were based on random samples, which were predominantly Catholic (22–24%) and Protestant (53–61%). Both studies used two dependent variables: one to assess psychological well-being (life satisfaction in 2001 and tranquility in 2009) and one to assess psychological distress (anxiety and depression in 2001 and anxiety in 2009).[2] The data were analyzed with ordinary least squares (OLS) regression,[3] controlling for age, gender, race, education, income, frequency of private prayer, frequency of church attendance, and other variables, including adverse life events.

Despite differences in their measures, samples, and other aspects of their methodology, belief in life-after-death had salubrious associations with psychological well-being and psychological distress in both studies (see Fig. 17.1). However, the strength of the associations (β's) were much larger in the 2009 study than in the 2001 study, and the net effects of belief in life-after death were statistically significant only for the measures of psychological well-being in the two studies: life satisfaction in 2001 and tranquility in 2009.

Two other sets of findings from these studies are important. First, the studies found that adverse life events (i.e., poor health and financial problems) had significant pernicious associations with both psychological well-being and psychological distress. Second, the studies found that belief in life-after-death buffered against the pernicious effects of poor health and financial problems on well-being and distress. This means that belief in life-after-death was particularly beneficial for individuals dealing with these adverse life effects.

From the perspective of ETAS Theory, poor health may pose a threat to one's life, and poor health and financial problems each pose a threat to one's way of life.

[1] The sample sizes in the three studies were, respectively: N = 921, N = 1139, and N = 1140/.

[2] The 2001 study measured belief in life-after-death on a 4-point scale, on which participants rated their agreement or disagreement with the statement, "I believe in eternal life." Belief in life-after-death was measured in the 2009 by responses to the question: "Do you believe there is life after death?" The measure of psychological distress in the 2001 study was the Kessler K6, which measures a combination of anxiety and depressive symptoms experienced during the past 30 days.

[3] The strength of association measured by OLS regression is typically reported as a standardized beta (β). When an OLS regression analysis involves only two variables, β is equivalent to Pearson's *r*.

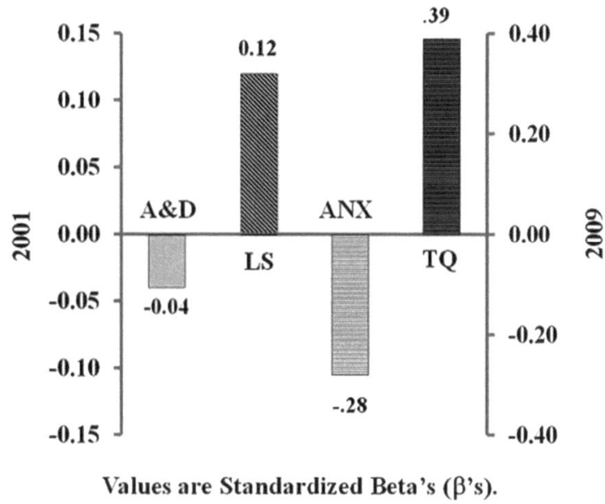

Fig. 17.1 Associations between belief in life-after-death and psychological distress and psychological well-being in studies by Ellison et al. in 2001 (A&D = Anxiety and Depression; LS = Life Satisfaction) and 2009 (ANX = Anxiety; TQ = Tranquility)

They also create uncertainty about the future, and uncertainty is known to produce anxiety [8, 9]. Hence, it is not surprising that these adverse life events were associated with higher levels of psychological distress in these studies, both of which measured anxiety. The results of the studies suggest that belief in life-after-death quells the anxiety posed by these threats and/or the uncertainty they create. I will demonstrate in later chapters how anxiety can affect psychological well-being.

The third study, which was conducted by Bradshaw and Ellison, also examined the degree to which belief in life-after-death buffers against the psychological distress produced by adversity in life (in this case, financial hardship) using data from the 1998 GSS [10]. The measure of psychological distress was the same one employed in the first study (Kessler's K6) [11], and the measure of belief in an afterlife was the same as the one used in the second study. Financial hardship was measured by participants' subjective impression of whether their income was about average or far below average.

Although belief in an afterlife had no main effect on psychological distress, survey participants experiencing financial hardship who believed in life-after-death reported significantly lower levels of psychological distress than those who did not believe in life-after-death, as the authors predicted. As seen in Fig. 17.2, psychological distress was nearly identical for study participants without financial hardship (Income Above Average), whether or not they believed in an afterlife. Among participants experiencing financial hardship (Income Far Below Average), however, psychological distress was significantly higher among those who said they do not believe in an afterlife.

Ellison and his colleagues interpreted the salubrious association of belief in an afterlife with psychological distress and well-being to be the product of a worldview within which individuals interpret their personal circumstances in a larger context. As people who believe in life-after-death view their earthly existence as temporary, they view their earthly problems as temporary, which provides a sense of calm, and reduces worry, fear, and other negative feelings [7]. The weaker associations of

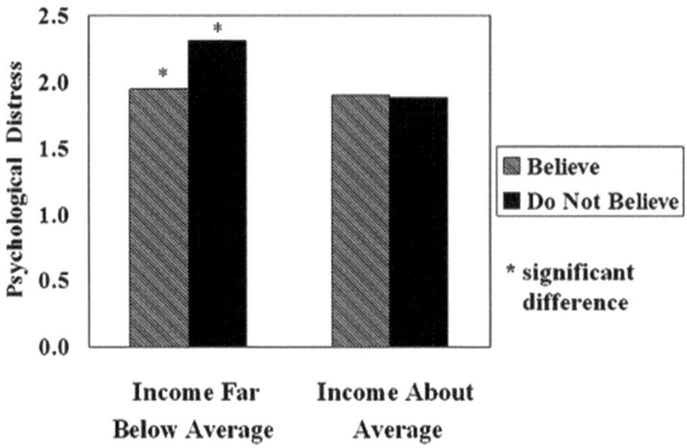

Fig. 17.2 Interaction of belief in an afterlife and financial hardship on psychological distress (Bradshaw & Ellison, 2010)

belief in life-after-death with psychological distress in the 2001 and 2010 studies may be due, in part, to the fact the measure of psychological distress they bout used combined symptoms of depression and anxiety, rather than using separate measures of depression and anxiety.

The relatively smaller association of belief in life-after-death with psychological well-being and distress observed in the 2001 study may be due to the fact that this study controlled for social support, which was found to have significant net effects on both psychological well-being and distress. Thus, the sense of personal safety provided by social support – according to ETAS Theory – may have reduced the effect size of belief in life-after-death on well-being and distress, which is consistent with the theory. Although belief in life-after-death provides a sense of safety or security by reducing uncertainty about the future, social support provides an immediate sense of security regarding one's current circumstances.

17.3 Belief in an Afterlife and Psychiatric Symptoms

A study by me, Chris Ellison, and our colleagues [12] used data from the 2004 "National Study of Religion and Health" (NSRH)[4] to examine the association between belief in life-after-death and six classes of psychiatric symptoms. The inde-

[4] The NSRH was an online survey, sponsored by *Spirituality and Health* magazine, that was completed by more than 1600 individuals from all 50 states and Washington, D.C. The sample was recruited from a sampling frame of U.S. adults that closely reflected the U.S. Census by gender, race, age, income, and state of residence. The sample was approximately 22% Catholic, 53% Protestant, 5% Jewish, and 20% other religions or unaffiliated.

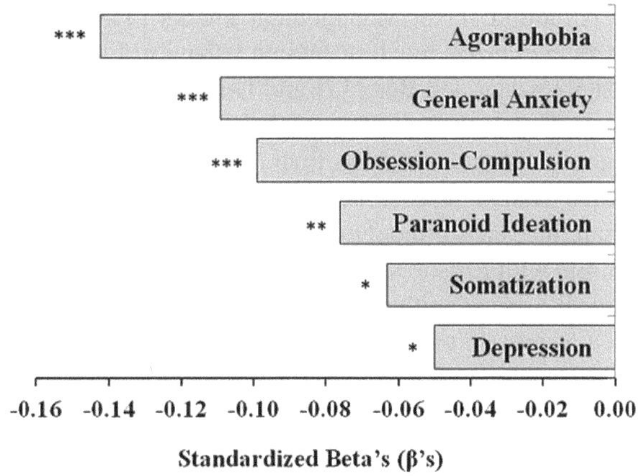

Fig. 17.3 Association between belief in life-after-death and six classes of psychiatric symptoms (Flannelly et al. 2006) [12]; * $p < .05$; ** $p < .01$; ***$p < .001$

pendent variable was based on responses to the question: "Do you believe in life after death?"[5] Six scales of the Symptom Assessment-45 (SA-45) Questionnaire [13, 14] were used as dependent variables.[6]

Belief in life-after-death had statistically significant inverse associations with all six classes of psychiatric symptoms (Fig. 17.3).[7] The association was strongest for agoraphobia, probably because many people with agoraphobia also suffer from panic attacks, which often include fear of imminent death. As seen in Fig. 17.3, the associations were successively weaker for general anxiety, obsession-compulsion, paranoid ideation, somatization, and depression.

The results suggest that part of the net effect of belief in life-after-death on psychiatric symptoms is that it provides a sense of certainty about the future. Behavioral studies have shown that uncertainty about life events are associated with anxiety [15, 16], and neuro-physiological studies have shown that the amygdala responds to uncertainty with fear, as if uncertainty poses a threat of harm [8, 9]. Hence, feeling secure about what will happen in the future should reduce anxiety and other psychiatric symptoms related to fears about the dangerousness of the world.

---

[5] The responses were coded as yes = +1, uncertain = 0, and no = −1.

[6] The paranoid ideation scale ($\alpha = .80$) contained items about blaming others for one's troubles and stealing credit for one's accomplishments, and being talked about and watched by others. The agoraphobia scale ($\alpha = .85$) measured fear of leaving home, crowded, open, or specific places, or public transportation. The anxiety scale ($\alpha = .84$) measured fearfulness, tension, and restlessness. The depression scale ($\alpha = .88$) measured loneliness, hopelessness, worthlessness and loss of interest in things. The obsessive-compulsive scale ($\alpha = .83$) measured problems with concentration and making decisions, excessive checking of things, and problems with one's mind "going blank." The somatization scale ($\alpha = .81$) measured vague physical symptoms, such as hot or cold spells, numbness, soreness, tingling, and heaviness in the limbs. Each scale included five items.

[7] The data were analyzed by ordinary least squares (OLS) regression, controlling for frequency of prayer and attending religious services, life stressors, social support, and socio-demographic characteristics. A value of $p < .05$ means the probability the observed result occurred by chance is 5 out of 100; $p < .01$ means the probability the result occurred by chance is 1 out of 100; and $p < .001$ means the probability the result occurred by chance is 1 out of 1000.

Although Terror Management Theory (TM Theory) proposes that the "terror of death" underlies much of human behavior, I tend to side with the Dutch psychologist Kees van den Bos [17] and Uncertainty Management Theory, that uncertainty about the future, including such things as health and financial well-being, are more common human concerns than death. I readily concede, however, that death is the major existential uncertainty of humans, which is why I think believing in eternal life reduces fears about present and future circumstances. I think this notion is compatible with Ellison's interpretation of the effects of belief in an afterlife on psychological distress in that belief in an afterlife provides certainty about a future life as well as putting one's present life in an eternal perspective.

17.4 Chapter Highlights and Comments

The research results presented in this chapter generally shows that belief in life-after-death has a salutary association with psychological well-being and psychological distress, including several classes of psychiatric symptoms. Moreover, they indicate that belief in life-after-death buffers against the pernicious effects of the threats posed by adverse life events and the uncertainty they create.

One reason why belief in an afterlife reduces anxiety and related fears and phobias may be that it reduces uncertainty about the future. This hypothesis, which follows from ETAS Theory, differs sharply from the basic proposition of TM Theory that the fundamental fear of humans is fear of death itself. Although my hypothesis has not been investigated, research indicates that uncertainty increases anxiety, and that the amygdala responds to uncertainty with fear, which is the biological basis of anxiety. This hypothesis differs from but is consistent with Ellison's explanation that belief in an afterlife may reduce anxiety by putting people's worldly problems in the broader perspective of an eternal life.

The findings mentioned above about social support are interesting for at least two reasons, from the perspective of ETAS Theory. First, they suggest that social support may provide a sense of safety, which reduces anxiety about one's current circumstances. Second, they call attention to the likelihood that the sense of immediate safety provided by social support may be equally or more important in reducing anxiety about one's current circumstances than the sense of security provided by the belief that things will be better in the next life.

References

1. Benore, E. R., & Park, C. L. (2004). Death-specific religious beliefs and bereavement: Belief in an afterlife and continued attachment. *International Journal for the Psychology of Religion, 14*(1), 1–22.

2. Smith, P. C., Range, L. M., & Ulmer, A. (1992). Belief in afterlife as a buffer in suicidal and other bereavement. *Omega: Journal of Death & Dying, 24*(3), 217–225.
3. Clarke, S. M., Hayslip Jr, B., Edmondson, R., & Guarnaccia, C. A. (2003). Religiosity, afterlife beliefs, and bereavement adjustment in adulthood. *Journal of Religious Gerontology, 14*(2–3), 207–224.
4. Carr, D., & Sharp, S. (2014). Do afterlife beliefs affect psychological adjustment to late-life spousal loss?. *Journals of Gerontology. Series B, Psychological Sciences and Social Sciences, 69*(1), 103–112.
5. Ellison, C. G., Boardman, J. D., Williams, D. R., & Jackson, J. S. (2001). Religious involvement, stress, and mental health: Findings from the 1995 Detroit area study. *Social Forces, 80*(1), 215–249.
6. Williams, D. R., Yu, Y., Jackson, J. S., & Anderson, N. B. (1997). Racial differences in physical and mental health socio-economic status, stress and discrimination. *Journal of Health Psychology, 2*(3), 335–351.
7. Ellison, C. G., Burdette, A. M., & Hill, T. D. (2009). Blessed assurance: Religion, anxiety, and tranquility among US adults. *Social Science Research, 38*(3), 656–667.
8. Grupe, D. W., & Nitschke, J. B. (2013). Uncertainty and anticipation in anxiety: An integrated neurobiological and psychological perspective. *Nature Reviews Neuroscience, 14*(7), 488–501.
9. Sarinopoulos, I., Grupe, D. W., Mackiewicz, K. L., Herrington, J. D., Lor, M., Steege, E. E., et al. (2010). Uncertainty during anticipation modulates neural responses to aversion in human insula and amygdala. *Cerebral Cortex, 20*(4), 929–940.
10. Bradshaw, M., & Ellison, C. G. (2010). Financial hardship and psychological distress: Exploring the buffering effects of religion. *Social Science & Medicine, 71*(1), 196–204.
11. Kessler, R. C., Andrews, G., Colpe, L. J., Hiripi, E., Mroczek, D. K., Normand, S.-L. T., et al. (2002). Short screening scales to monitor population prevalences and trends in non-specific psychological distress. *Psychological Medicine, 32*(6), 959–976.
12. Flannelly, K. J., Koenig, H. G., Ellison, C. G., Galek, K., & Krause, N. (2006). Belief in life after death and mental health: Findings from a national survey. *Journal of Nervous and Mental Disease, 194*(7), 524–529.
13. Sitarenios, G., Rayes, M., & Morrison, J. (2000). *SA-45: The symptom assessment-45 questionnaire*. North Tonawanda/New York: Multi-Health Systems Inc.
14. Davison, M. L., Bershadsky, B., Bieber, J., Silversmith, D., Maruish, M. E., & Kane, R. L. (1997). Development of a brief, multidimensional, self-report instrument for treatment outcomes assessment in psychiatric settings: Preliminary findings. *Assessment, 4*, 259–276.
15. Hirsh, J. B., Mar, R. A., & Peterson, J. B. (2012). Psychological entropy: A framework for understanding uncertainty-related anxiety. *Psychological Review, 119*(2), 304–320.
16. Sorrentino, R. M., Ye, Y., & Szeto, A. C. H. (2009). Uncertainty management: To fear of not to fear? *Psychological Inquiry, 20*(4), 240–244.
17. Van den Bos, K. (2009). Making sense of life: The existential self trying to deal with personal uncertainty. *Psychological Inquiry, 20*(4), 197–217.

Chapter 18
Beliefs About Life-After-Death and Psychiatric Symptoms

Abstract The chapter summarizes the findings of three national studies on the association between beliefs about life-after-death and psychiatric symptoms in the U.S. general population. The results of the first study found that pleasant beliefs about the nature of the afterlife had a salubrious association with psychiatric symptoms, whereas unpleasant beliefs about the afterlife had a pernicious association with psychiatric symptoms. The second study found that pleasant beliefs about the afterlife appeared to alter one's beliefs about the world, in that belief in a pleasant afterlife was positively associated with the belief that the world is equitable and negatively associated with the belief that the world is cynical. Belief in an equitable world, in turn, was associated with lower levels of psychiatric symptoms, whereas belief in a cynical world was associated with higher levels of psychiatric symptoms. The third study described in this chapter tested the major premise of Terror Management (TM) Theory that being made aware of one's own mortality increases anxiety: the "morality salience hypothesis." Contrary to TM Theory, the study found that whether morality salience elevated symptoms of anxiety depended on one's beliefs about the afterlife; morality salience elevated symptoms of anxiety only among people who believed the afterlife would be unpleasant. The chapter also challenges the claim of advocates of TM Theory that fear of death underlies many psychiatric disorders, arguing that Chaps. 11 and 12 explains how each class of psychiatric symptom is the product of a proximate mechanism that evolved to address a specific threat of harm.

Keywords Afterlife • Agoraphobia • Anxiety • ETAS Theory • Mortality salience • OCD • Paranoia • Psychiatric symptoms • Terror Management Theory • Uncertainty

The results described in Chap. 17 indicate that belief in life-after-death is generally associated with a salubrious effect on psychological well-being and psychological distress, including specific psychiatric symptoms. However, these studies ignore the possible effect of different beliefs about the afterlife on psychological distress. Therefore, the present chapter looks at three studies that attempted to determine the association between different beliefs about the afterlife and psychiatric symptoms.

K.J. Flannelly, *Religious Beliefs, Evolutionary Psychiatry, and Mental Health in America*, Religion, Spirituality and Health: A Social Scientific Approach 1,
DOI 10.1007/978-3-319-52488-7_18

18.1 Different Afterlife Beliefs and Psychiatric Symptoms

A 2008 study by me, Chris Ellison, and our colleagues [1] used data from the National Study of Religion and Health to analyze the degree to which seven beliefs about life-after-death were associated with the psychiatric symptoms examined in the 2006 Flannelly et al. study [2]. The seven beliefs were: "Union with God," "Reunion with family and loved ones," "A life of peace and tranquility," "A paradise of pleasures and delights," "A life of eternal reward or punishment," "Reincarnation into another life form," and "A pale, shadowy form of life, hardly life at all."[1] Rather than rehash the detailed results of the 2008 study here, I decided to summarize them in terms of two independent variables: Pleasant and Unpleasant beliefs about the afterlife.[2]

The association of pleasant beliefs about life-after-death with psychiatric symptoms (see Fig. 18.1) was generally similar to the association between belief in life-after-death and psychiatric symptoms that was observed in the 2006 Flannelly et al. study [2], which only examined belief in life-after-death, per se. The strongest association was found for agoraphobia, possibly because many people who suffer from agoraphobia also suffer from panic attacks, which entail intense fear of imminent death.[3] The associations were somewhat weaker for general anxiety paranoid ideation, and OCD, and no significant association was found between

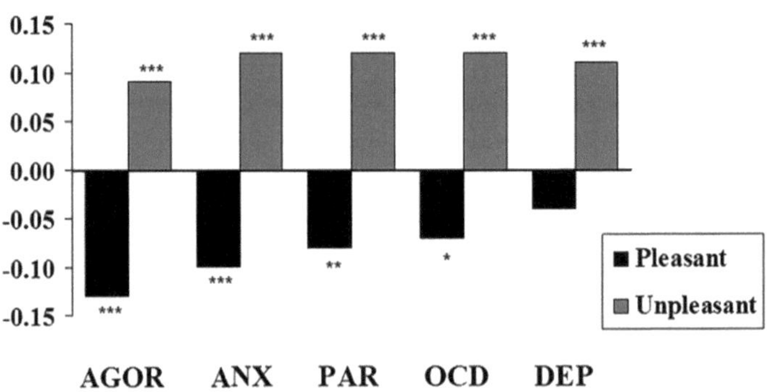

Fig. 18.1 Associations between pleasant and unpleasant beliefs about life-after-death and psychiatric symptoms (Flannelly et al. 2008); Values are standardized regression coefficients (β's); *AGOR* = Agoraphobia, *ANX* = General Anxiety, *PAR* = Paranoia, *OCD* = Obsessive-Compulsive Disorder, *DEP* = Depression; *** $p < .001$, ** $p < .01$, * $p < .05$

[1] The percentages of participants who expressed some degree of belief were: 96.7% for "Union with God"; 92.7% for "Reunion with family and loved ones"; 93.4% for "A life of peace and tranquility"; 85.5% for "A paradise of pleasures and delights"; 82.6% for "A life of eternal reward or punishment"; 61.7% for "Reincarnation into another life form"; and 45.5% for "A pale, shadowy form of life, hardly life at all."

[2] I excluded the belief "eternal reward or punishment" and somatization because only one significant association was found for each of them in the 2008 study. Since that study performed a total of 35 regression models, any single association that it found to be significant is likely to be due to chance.

[3] Agoraphobia was mislabeled social phobia in the 2008 article.

pleasant afterlife beliefs and depression. The latter finding is probably because the pleasant beliefs about the afterlife were more likely to tap into symptoms of anxiety than depression, and the presence of anxiety symptoms in depression (i.e., its comorbidity with depression) varies from 20 to 60% in Americans, depending on symptom severity [3, 4].

Unpleasant beliefs about life-after-death had a significant pernicious association with all five psychiatric symptoms in Fig. 18.1. Although far fewer participants believed in the unpleasant beliefs than the pleasant beliefs, such unpleasant beliefs apparently have a substantial pernicious affect on the mental health of those who do believe them. It is noteworthy that the two unpleasant beliefs we tested (the afterlife is "a pale shadowy place, hardy life at all" and "reincarnation into another life form") are very likely to raise uncertainty about what to expect after death, and uncertainty elicits fear from the amygdala.

18.2 Beliefs About the Afterlife, the World, and Psychiatric Symptoms

A later study by me and my colleagues, including Chris Ellison, provides evidence that belief in life-after-death may influence psychiatric symptoms by altering the way we think about the world [5]. The psychologist Jesse Bering [6] claimed that belief in an afterlife was part of a neuro-cognitive system that evolved to monitor social relations and human social exchanges. He proposed that this system underlies belief in life-after-death because it is predisposed to believe that people who are deceased are still alive. There are at least two reasons for this: (1) our inability to imagine our own non-existence [6, 7]; and (2) our experience that individuals and objects persist over time even when they are out of sight [8]. Because this system is intimately involved in social relations, beliefs about the afterlife may be intertwined with, and influence, beliefs about the nature of the social world [9–11].

Our study used data from the 2010 Baylor Religion Survey of American adults.[4] Five types of psychiatric symptoms served as the dependent variables (general anxiety, social anxiety, paranoia, obsession, and compulsion).[5] The data were analyzed

[4] Approximately 23% of survey respondents were Catholic, 55% were Protestant, 2% were Jewish, 4% were other religious faiths, and 11% had no religious affiliation.

[5] The root question was: "Over the past month, how often have you …" The response options were: Never =0; Rarely =1; Sometimes =2; Often =3; and Very Often =4. Three items measured each type of psychiatric symptomology. *Generalized Anxiety Disorder* ($\alpha = .84$) – Felt nervous; anxious or on edge; Unable to stop or control worrying; Worried too much about different things; *Social Anxiety* ($\alpha = .82$) – Feared that you might do something to embarrass yourself in a social situation; Became anxious doing things because people were watching; Endured intense anxiety in social or performance situations; *Paranoia* ($\alpha = .77$) – Felt like you were being watched or talked about by others; Felt that it is not safe to trust anyone; Felt that people were taking advantage of you; *Obsession* ($\alpha = .76$) – Been plagued by thoughts or images that you cannot get out of your mind; Thought too much about things that would not bother other people; Thought too much about

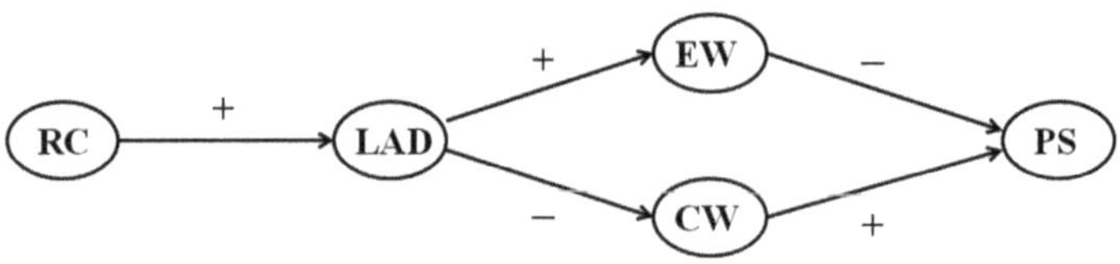

Fig. 18.2 Structural equation model of the direction of the hypothesized associations among religious commitment (*RC*), positive beliefs about life-after-death (*LAD*), belief in an equitable world (*EW*) and a cynical world (*CW*), and psychiatric symptoms (*PS*)

by structural equation modeling (SEM). Obsession and compulsion were analyzed separately because we thought they might be differentially affected by beliefs, in that obsessions, like beliefs, are forms of thought.

The first latent variable in the SEM was religious commitment (RC), which was measured by subjective religiosity and frequency of attending religious services. The second latent variable consisted of three pleasant beliefs about life-after-death (LAD) that were used in the 2008 study by Flannelly et al. Two types of beliefs about the world were tested simultaneously in the SEM: belief in a cynical world (CW) and belief in an equitable world (EW).[6] Separate SEM's were conducted for each of the five types of psychiatric symptoms (PS). Figure 18.2 illustrates the basic model, which hypothesized that: (1) religious commitment (RC) is positively associated with pleasant beliefs about life-after-death (LAD); that pleasant beliefs about life-after-death are (2) positively associated with the belief that the world is equitable (EW) and (3) negatively associated with the belief that the world is cynical (CW); and that (4) belief in an equitable world is negatively associated with psychiatric symptoms (PS), whereas (5) belief in a cynical world is positively associated with psychiatric symptoms.

As expected (see Fig. 18.3), religious commitment (RC) had a strong positive association ($\beta = +.74$) with pleasant beliefs about life-after-death (LAD), and pleasant beliefs about life-after-death (LAD) had a positive association with belief in an equitable world (EW, $\beta = +.36$)) and a negative association with belief in a cynical world (CW, $\beta = -.16$). Hence, as Fig. 18.3 shows, the association between belief in life-after-death and belief in an equitable world was more than twice as strong as the association between belief in life-after-death and belief in a cynical world. These findings are consistent with Bering's idea that belief in an afterlife is part of a neurocognitive system that monitors social exchanges and relationships, in that one might

---

pointless matters; *Compulsion* ($\alpha = .77$) – Felt compelled to perform certain actions for no justifiable reason; Repeated simple actions that realistically did not need to be repeated; Been afraid something terrible would happen if you did not perform certain rituals.

[6] Belief in an equitable world was measured by participant's agreement or disagreement with the statements, "Anything is possible if you work hard," and "Everyone starts out with the same chances in life." Belief in a Cynical World was measured by responses to the statements, "The world is controlled by a few powerful people," and "Finance is a field where people get rich without making a real contribution to society."

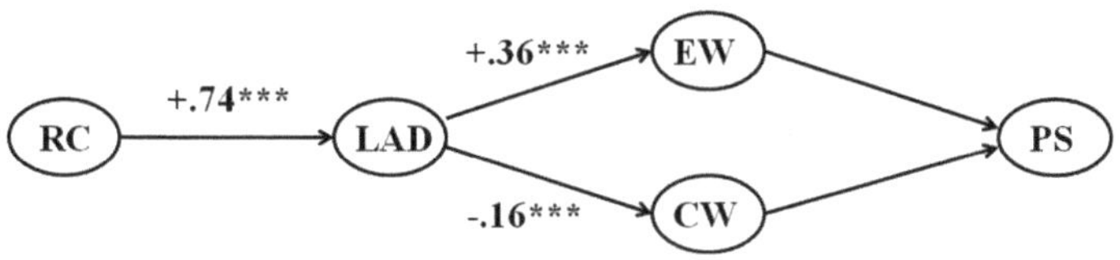

Fig. 18.3 The figure illustrates the results of structural equation models of the observed associations (β's) between religious commitment (*RC*) and positive beliefs about life-after-death (*LAD*), and between positive beliefs about LAD and belief in an equitable world (*EW*) and a cynical world (*CW*) (Flannelly et al. 2012); *** $p < .001$; the associations of equitable and cynical beliefs about the world with psychiatric symptoms (*PS*) are shown in Fig. 18.4

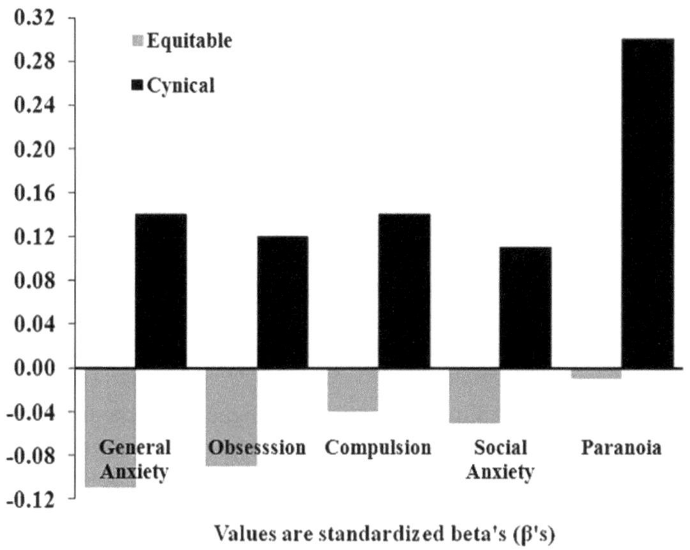

Fig. 18.4 Associations (β's) between five types of psychiatric symptoms and belief in an equitable world and belief in a cynical world (Flannelly et al. 2012)

expect people who believe in an afterlife would also believe such monitoring decreases cynical social behavior and increases social equity [6].

However, belief in an equitable world had significant salubrious associations with only two of the five types of psychiatric symptoms examined in the study: i.e., general anxiety and obsession (Fig. 18.4). Belief in a cynical world, on the other hand, had significant pernicious associations with all five types of psychiatric symptoms, probably because the items that comprised the latent variable "cynical world" implied that the world is dangerous. I have no doubt that the pronounced association of belief in a cynical world with paranoid ideation is because the two items that comprised the variable "cynical world" strongly implied that people cannot be trusted. In any case, I think these results provide support for Ellison's general premise that belief in life-after-death influences psychological distress by altering the way we think about the temporal world.

18.3 Terror Management Theory and Psychiatric Symptoms

Some advocates of Terror Management Theory (TM Theory) claim that the inability to manage the terror of death "leave[s] people vulnerable to anxiety and associated disorders" and that anxiety-related disorders are "attempts to compensate for compromised means of buffering existential anxiety" (p. 202) [12]. However, the proponents of this hypothesis do not even attempt to explain how fear of death could produce different psychiatric disorders [12], and there is no evidence that fear of death underlies any of the classes of psychiatrist disorders that exist. Moreover, TM Theory, unlike ETAS Theory, cannot explain why so many different classes of psychiatric symptoms exist – which is explained by their evolutionary functions, as discussed in Chaps. 11 and 12.

The "mortality salience" hypothesis, that a heighted awareness of one's own mortality increases anxiety, is a central element of TM Theory [13–15]. The results of the 2008 study by Flannelly et al. would seem to undermine this premise to some extent, as pleasant beliefs about the afterlife – which are reminders of death – were associated with lower psychiatric symptomology. Although the pleasant beliefs about death used in that study may not be sufficiently potent stimuli to create mortality salience, these results call attention to the need to reconsider TM Theory's notion that the function of religion is to reduce fear of death [16, 17], as some religious constructs (e.g., pleasant beliefs about the afterlife) may reduce anxiety, while other religious constructs (e.g., unpleasant beliefs about the afterlife) may increase anxiety.

A 2014 study by Chris Ellison, me, and a colleague used data from the National Study of Religion and Health to investigate the degree to which mortality salience moderates the association of beliefs about the afterlife with selected psychiatric symptoms [18]. I will briefly summarize the results for general anxiety and agoraphobia with respect to the pleasant belief that the afterlife is "a life of peace and tranquility" and the unpleasant belief that the afterlife is "a pale, shadowy form of life." The mortality salience variable was whether (1) or not (0) a person had experienced a serious illness of injury in the last 12 months. The regression analyses controlled for the same control variables used in the 2006 and 2008 Flannelly et al. studies on life-after-death [1, 2].

The belief that the afterlife was "a life of peace and tranquility" had a significant salutary association with agoraphobia ($\beta = -.133$), but not general anxiety ($\beta = -.026$). The belief that the afterlife was "a pale, shadowy form of life" had a significant pernicious association with both agoraphobia ($\beta = .128$) and general anxiety ($\beta = .091$). Mortality salience had significant interactions with both beliefs for agoraphobia and a significant interaction with a pale shadowy form of life for general anxiety.

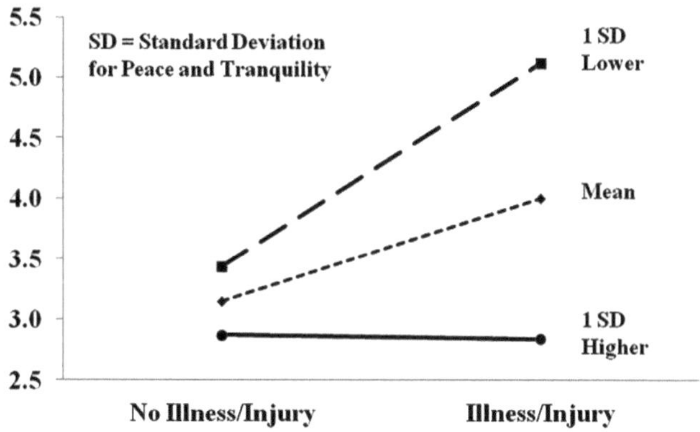

Fig. 18.5 Interaction of mortality salience with believing the afterlife is a life of peace and tranquility on agoraphobia (Ellison et al. 2014)

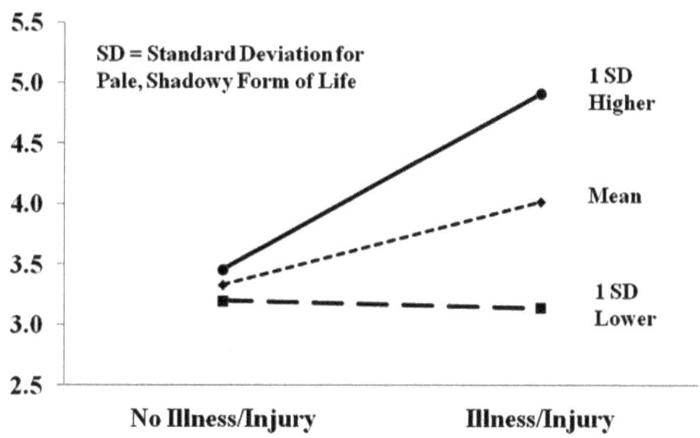

Fig. 18.6 Interaction of mortality salience with believing the afterlife is a pale, shadowy form of life on agoraphobia (Ellison et al. 2014)

Figures 18.5 and 18.6 show the interaction effects of mortality salience and the two beliefs about the afterlife on agoraphobia. Figure 18.5 shows that agoraphobia was highest among people who had a serious illness or injury during the past year (mortality salience) and only weakly believed the afterlife is a place of peace and tranquility (1 SD lower than the mean). Conversely (see Fig. 18.6), agoraphobia was highest among people who had a serious illness or injury during the past year (mortality salience) and strongly believed (1 SD higher than the mean) the afterlife is a pale, shadowy form of life. The interaction effect of mortality salience with belief in a pale shadowy life on general anxiety was nearly identical to the interaction effect of mortality salience with belief in a pale shadowy afterlife on agoraphobia.

Thus, the findings indicate that mortality salience does appear to have an effect on psychiatric symptoms, such as agoraphobia and general anxiety. However, the effect of mortality salience is influenced by one's beliefs about what the afterlife will be, not just the belief that there is an afterlife. It seems that for people who believe the afterlife will be pleasant (e.g., peace and tranquility), mortality salience decreases anxiety, whereas for people who believe the afterlife will be unpleasant (e.g., a palc, shadowy form of life), mortality salience increases anxiety. The findings are consistent with ETAS Theory, but not with TM Theory, which proposes that mortality salience increases anxiety and related psychiatric symptoms.

18.4 Chapter Highlights and Comments

Advocates of TM Theory claim that the terror of death can lead to anxiety and associated disorders, yet they do not provide a mechanism by which this can happen. Nor does TM Theory explain how fear of death could produce the variety of psychiatric symptoms that people commonly exhibit. ETAS Theory, in contrast, explains that a variety of psychiatric symptoms are linked to proximate mechanisms that evolved to promote survival, as described in Chaps. 11 and 12.

The results of the 2008 study by Flannelly et al. [1] indicate that pleasant beliefs about the afterlife tend to be associated with lower psychiatric symptomology, whereas unpleasant beliefs about the afterlife tend to be associated with higher psychiatric symptomology. These differential effects of beliefs about the afterlife on psychiatric symptoms generally undermine the simplistic premise of TM Theory that thoughts about death increase anxiety. According to ETAS Theory, pleasant beliefs about the afterlife decrease anxiety and related psychiatric symptoms because they reduce uncertainty and concerns about the future by offering assurance that the next life will be a pleasant one. On the other hand, unpleasant beliefs about the afterlife increase anxiety and related psychiatric symptoms by foretelling an unpleasant future life, possibly by enhancing amygdala activity via the "aversive amplification circuit" [19]. The two unpleasant beliefs we tested (the afterlife is "a pale shadowy place, hardy life at all" and "reincarnation into another life form") clearly forebode and unpleasant future and raise uncertainty about what the future holds. The latter point is important because uncertainty, itself, elicits fear from the amygdala.

The results of the 2014 study by Ellison et al. [18] on the association of mortality salience with agoraphobia and general anxiety further undermine the premise of TM Theory that reminders of one's mortality (mortality salience) necessarily increase anxiety. The findings of that study show that the association between mortality salience and psychiatric symptoms is mediated by beliefs about the afterlife. This is consistent with the more nuanced explanation of the relationship between beliefs and anxiety offered by ETAS Theory. Although mortality salience does appear to play a role in psychiatric symptomology, it seems to exacerbate symptoms in people who have unpleasant beliefs about the afterlife and to attenuate symptoms in people who have pleasant beliefs about the afterlife.

Finally, the results of the 2010 study on beliefs about the afterlife, beliefs about the world, and psychiatric symptoms are important because they suggest that afterlife beliefs may influence psychiatric symptoms by changing the way we think about the world [5]. These results provide support for Ellison's notion that belief an in life-after-death may reduce psychological distress, in part, by altering the way we think about our temporal problems in the context of an external life.

References

1. Flannelly, K. J., Ellison, C. G., Galek, K., & Koenig, H. G. (2008). Beliefs about life-after-death, psychiatric symptomology and cognitive theories of psychopathology. *Journal of Psychology & Theology,* 36, 94–103.
2. Flannelly, K. J., Koenig, H. G., Ellison, C. G., Galek, K., & Krause, N. (2006). Belief in life after death and mental health: Findings from a national survey. *Journal of Nervous and Mental Disease,* 194(7), 524–529.
3. Kessler, R. C., & DuPont, R. L. (1999). Impairment in pure and comorbid generalized anxiety disorder and major depression at 12 months. *American Journal of Psychiatry,* 156(12), 1915–1923.
4. Kessler, R. C., & Walters, E. E. (1998). Epidemiology of DSM-III-R major depression and minor depression among adolescents and young adults in the national comorbidity survey. *Depression and Anxiety,* 7(1), 3–14.
5. Flannelly, K. J., Galek, K., Ellison, C. G., & Silton, N. R. (2012). Belief in life-after-death, beliefs about the world, and psychiatric symptoms. *Journal of Religion and Health,* 51(3), 651–662.
6. Bering, J. M. (2006). The folk psychology of souls. *Behavioral and Brain Sciences,* 29, 453–498.
7. Pereira, V., Faísca, L., & de Sa-Saraiva, R. (2012). Immortality of the soul as an intuitive idea: Towards a psychological explanation of the origins of afterlife beliefs. *Journal of Cognition and Culture,* 12(1–2), 101–127.
8. Newman, G. E., Blok, S. V., & Rips, L. J. (2006). Belief in afterlife as a by-product of peristent judgments. *Behavioral and Brain Sciences,* 29(5), 480–481.
9. Gjersoe, N. L., & Hood, B. M. (2006). The supernatural guilt trip does not take us far enough. *Behavioral and Brain Sciences,* 29(5), 473–474.
10. Bering, J. M. (2006). The folk psychology of souls. *Behavioral and Brain Sciences,* 29(5), 453–462.
11. Bering, J. M. (2006). The cognitive science of souls: Clarifications and extensions of the evolutionary model. *Behavioral and Brain Sciences,* 29(5), 486–493.
12. Arndt, J., Routledge, C., Cox, C. R., & Goldenberg, J. L. (2005). The worm at the core: A terror management perspective on the roots of psychological dysfunction. *Applied and Preventive Psychology,* 11(3), 191.
13. Greenberg, J., Pyszczynski, T., Solomon, S., Rosenblatt, A., Veeder, M., Kirkland, S., et al. (1990). Evidence for terror management theory II: The effects of mortality salience on reactions to those who threaten or bolster the cultural worldview. *Journal of Personality and Social Psychology,* 58(2), 308–318.
14. Rosenblatt, A., Greenberg, J., Solomon, S., Pyszczynski, T., & Lyon, D. (1989). Evidence for terror management theory: I. The effects of mortality salience on reactions to those who violate or uphold cultural values. *Journal of Personality and Social Psychology,* 57(4), 681–690.
15. Pyszczynski, T., Greenberg, J., & Solomon, S. (1999). A dual-process model of defense against conscious and unconscious death-related thoughts: An extension of terror management theory. *Psychological Review,* 106(4), 835–845.

16. Vail, K. E., 3rd, Rothschild, Z. K., Weise, D. R., Solomon, S., Pyszczynski, T., & Greenberg, J. (2010). A terror management analysis of the psychological functions of religion. *Personality and Social Psychology Review,* 14(1), 84–94.
17. Jonas, E., & Fischer, P. (2006). Terror management and religion: Evidence that intrinsic religiousness mitigates worldview defense following mortality salience. *Journal of Personality and Social Psychology,* 91(3), 553–567.
18. Ellison, C. G., Flannelly, K. J., & Barrie, C. K. (2014). *Do afterlife beliefs moderate the association between recent serious illness and symptoms of anxiety-related disorders?*. Paper presented at the National Meeting of the Society for the Scientific Study of Religion, Indianapolis, IN, November 1.
19. Robinson, O. J., Krimsky, M., Lieberman, L., Allen, P., Vytal, K., & Grillon, C. (2014). Towards a mechanistic understanding of pathological anxiety: The dorsal medial prefrontal-amygdala "aversive amplification" circuit in unmedicated generalized and social anxiety disorders. *The Lancet. Psychiatry, 1*(4), 294.

Chapter 19
Beliefs About the Nature of God and Mental Health

Abstract The chapter reviews the results of several studies of convenience samples of students in the U.S. and U.K. and two large national studies of American adults that examined the association between beliefs about God and mental health. These studies indicate that belief in a benevolent God has a salubrious association with mental health, whereas belief in a malevolent God has a pernicious association with mental health. Based on ETAS Theory, the salubrious effects are interpreted to mean that belief in a benevolent God and the sense of safety that this belief provides increases the threshold of what constitutes a threat, thereby lowering anxiety and related psychiatric symptoms. Belief in a malevolent God, on the other hand, acts to lower the threshold of what constitutes a threat because God not only fails to provide protection from harm, but poses a direct threat of harm. Results related to belief in God and self-esteem are also presented and discussed in light of ETAS Theory. The chapter explains that self-esteem and self-efficacy reduce anxiety because belief in oneself and one's ability to address difficult situations and threats reduce the perception of the danger they pose. The chapter challenges the premise of Terror Management Theory that self-esteem evolved in humans as a buffer against fear of death, arguing instead, that both self-esteem and self-efficacy evolved long before our ancestors became aware or their own mortality. Finally, the chapter demonstrates that anxiety mediates the relationship between positive and negative beliefs about God and positive emotions (specifically, happiness).

Keywords Anxiety • Happiness • ETAS Theory • God • Nature of God • Psychiatric symptoms • Psychological well-being • Safety • Self-esteem • Threat

There is very little evidence that belief in God, in and of itself, is related to mental health, and there is some evidence that it is not related to mental health [1–3]. However, Chap. 15 demonstrated that Americans have many different beliefs about God, and different beliefs about the nature of God have been found to have either salubrious or pernicious associations with mental health. The present chapter summarizes that research on the relationship between specific beliefs about the nature of God and mental health among Americans.

K.J. Flannelly, *Religious Beliefs, Evolutionary Psychiatry, and Mental Health in America*, Religion, Spirituality and Health: A Social Scientific Approach 1,
DOI 10.1007/978-3-319-52488-7_19

19.1 Beliefs About the Nature of God and Psychological Well-Being

Bernard Spilka [4] and Richard Gorsuch [5] conducted studies in the 1960's on high school and college students' beliefs about God using lists of adjectives describing God. The student's ratings of the adjectives were then analyzed by factor analysis to create factors or clusters of beliefs about God. Subsequent studies by Benson and Spilka [6] and Schaefer and Gorsuch [7] examined the association of these clusters of beliefs with self-esteem and trait anxiety, respectively. This section presents results from these two studies, as well as the results of related studies.

Benson and Spilka studied a small convenience sample of male students attending a Catholic high school and Schaefer and Gorsuch studied a small convenience sample of undergraduate students at four Protestant colleges. Benson and Spilka measured self-esteem, which refers to the way a person feels about, or evaluates oneself [8], as their dependent or outcome variable [9], and Schaefer and Gorsuch used two measures of trait anxiety as their dependent variables [10, 11]. I used the average of the correlations of the two trait anxiety scales in my summary of the findings.

The clusters of beliefs about God that Spilka and Gorsuch found overlap with one another, but they differ in many respects, hence Spilka and Gorsuch gave them different names. I grouped the factors by the most prominent adjectives that they have in common and I combined the results of some factors that partially overlap. This produced four belief clusters that seem to be comparable to me. I used the most important common adjectives contained within each factor to name the variables in Fig. 19.1.

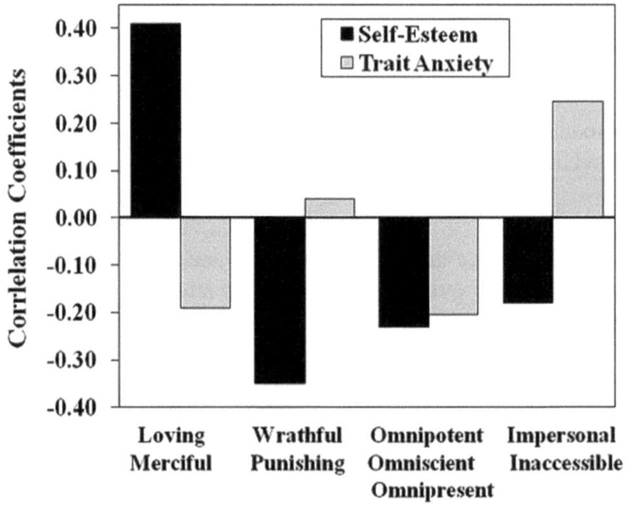

Fig. 19.1 Correlations of beliefs about God with self-esteem (Benson and Spilka, 1973) [6] and trait anxiety (Schaefer and Gorsuch, 1991) [7]

As seen in the Fig. 19.1, a loving and merciful God had a strong salubrious association with self- esteem and trait anxiety. The former association presumably reflects the fact that individuals who believe God is loving believe God loves them; the latter association probably reflects the fact that belief in a loving and merciful God provides a sense of personal security. In contrast, the belief that God is punishing and wrathful may be correlated with lower self-esteem because people who have this belief may feel that God is punishing them. Schaefer and Gorsuch did not find a significant correlation between belief in a wrathful and punishing God and anxiety, which is surprising, at first glance. However, the obvious explanation for this finding is that very few of the students at the four Protestant colleges believed that God is wrathful or punishing, which is in keeping with the Baylor Survey's results that relatively few American adults believe God is punishing or wrathful (see Chap. 15).

Although the Protestant college students in the Schaefer and Gorsuch study probably found a sense of safety or security in their belief that God is omnipotent, omniscient, and omnipresent, since these beliefs were correlated with lower anxiety in that sample, the Catholic high school students in the Benson and Spilka study apparently found these beliefs disturbing, since they were correlated with lower self-esteem in that sample. Benson and Spilka, themselves, thought these beliefs implied that God was detached from the world, which might have been disturbing to religious high school students, since devote Christians typically believe that God is active in their lives [12–14]. Hence, the belief that God is distant may have made the high school students feel unwanted, thereby, lowering their self-esteem [15]. The more explicit beliefs that God is impersonal and inaccessible had pernicious effects in both student samples: lower self-esteem among the high school students and higher anxiety among the college students.

The conclusions one can draw from these studies are limited by their small sample sizes, the fact that they used convenience samples, and the nature of the samples themselves. Nevertheless, the results indicate that beliefs about God may differentially affect self-esteem and anxiety. This is an important point from the perspective of ETAS Theory because some studies indicate that self-esteem buffers against the pernicious effect of the threat of physical harm on anxiety [16–18]. However, other studies indicate that threats to self-esteem increase anxiety [19–22], which also has implications for ETAS Theory, as I will examine in later chapters.

I know of only three other studies on beliefs about God and self-esteem. One was a 2012 online survey of over 400 college students – mostly from the U.S. and U.K. – who belonged to Christian fellowship organizations [23]. The other two were studies, which were conducted by Leslie Francis and his colleagues, used large convenience samples of secondary students in the U.K. The students in the 2001 study were not particularly religious [24][1]; the 2005 study was conducted with Catholic school students [25]. Figure 19.2 shows the adjectives used in the three studies to describe God and their correlations with self-esteem.

[1] Fifty-eight percent said they did not belong to any religion and 49% said they never attended church.

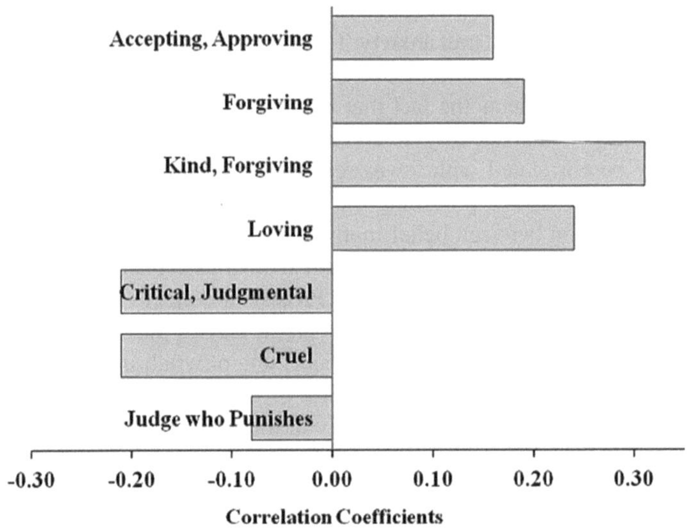

Fig. 19.2 Correlation of beliefs about God with self-esteem in three convenience samples

Overall, these three studies show that belief in a benevolent God (e.g., accepting, loving, forgiving) is associated with higher self-esteem, whereas belief in a punitive God (e.g., critical, cruel, judgmental) is associated with lower self-esteem. Since the studies used different measures of beliefs about God, different measures of self-esteem, and different kinds of samples it is difficult to compare their results directly. Nevertheless, belief in a benevolent God had a strong positive correlation with self-esteem among all three Christian groups. Although the direction of causality cannot be inferred from correlations, there is good evidence that religious beliefs and belonging to a faith tradition are positively associated higher self-esteem, and those findings suggest that religious involvement bolsters self-esteem [26, 27].

There appear to be only a few quantitative studies that have examined the relationship between beliefs about the nature of God and other measures of psychological well-being. Two studies I know of analyzed the association between beliefs about God and life-satisfaction. One is the online survey of Christian college students I mentioned above, [23]. It found a significant positive correlation ($r = .36$) between belief in a kind, forgiving, and approachable God and life satisfaction (Deiner's Satisfaction with Life Scale [28]).

The second study [29], which was conducted with convenience sample of Christian college students in the Midwest, used the same scale to examine the relationship of life satisfaction with belief in a loving-protective God. The set of beliefs used in this study were that God is loving, merciful, and comforting, and protects us from harm. This set of beliefs had a relatively small but significant, positive association with life satisfaction ($r = .18$). The last section of this chapter illustrates how psychiatric symptoms can mediate the effects of beliefs about the nature of God on positive emotions.

19.2 Beliefs About the Nature of God and Psychiatric Symptoms

Although research on the association between beliefs about God and psychiatric symptoms among the general public is rather limited, a review of research conducted in the 1990's noted that two studies found a salubrious association between depressive symptoms and belief in a personal God [3]. This section describes the results of two more recent studies on the association between beliefs about the nature of God and psychiatric symptoms in the U.S. general population [2, 30]. Both studies used data from large national surveys that were described in Chaps. 15 and 17: the 2004 National Study of Religion and Health and the 2010 Baylor Religion Survey.

The first study examined the associations between six classes of psychiatric symptoms (the dependent variables) and three sets of beliefs about God, each consisting of a pairs of adjectives (the independent variables) [30]. The independent variables were the mean ratings for each of a pair of adjectives describing God (close and loving, approving and forgiving, and creating and judging) in response to the question, "How much do you agree or disagree we each of these descriptions of God?" The six measures of psychiatric symptoms were the same as those used in the 2006 and 2008 studies by Flannelly et al. on belief in life-after death and psychiatric symptoms [31, 32]. Ordinary least square (OLS) regression was used to analyze the data.[2]

Based on ETAS Theory, we hypothesized that belief in a close and loving God would have a salubrious association with psychiatric symptomology because a close and loving God should provide a sense of security. Since we thought belief in a creating and judging God or an approving and forgiving God did not provide security, we hypothesized that these beliefs would not be related to psychiatric symptoms.[3] Finally, based on Dantz's theory that somatization does not involve cognitive input (see Chap. 12) [33], we hypothesized that somatization would not be affected by beliefs.[4]

The results are illustrated in Fig. 19.3; somatization is excluded from the figure because, as predicted, it did not have a significant association with any of the beliefs about God. As hypothesized, belief in a close and loving God (C&L: dark gray bars) had a significant salutary association with all the measures of psychiatric symptoms (except somatization), probably because a close and loving God provides a sense of

[2] The analyses controlled for demographic variables, social support, subjective religiousness, and the frequency of attending religious services. Survey respondents who were certain God *did not* exist were excluded from the analyses.

[3] This hypothesis, of course, is the same as the null hypothesis (i.e., there is no significant difference), which cannot be statistically tested. So, to test this prediction, we hypothesized that the association between overall psychiatric symptomology and a creating and judging God would be significantly lower than that for belief in a close and loving God, and, likewise, that belief in an approving and forgiving God would be significantly lower than that for belief in close and loving God.

[4] Since this prediction also is the same as the null hypothesis, to test it we hypothesized that the association between belief in a close and loving God would be significantly lower for somatic symptoms than for its association with all other symptoms.

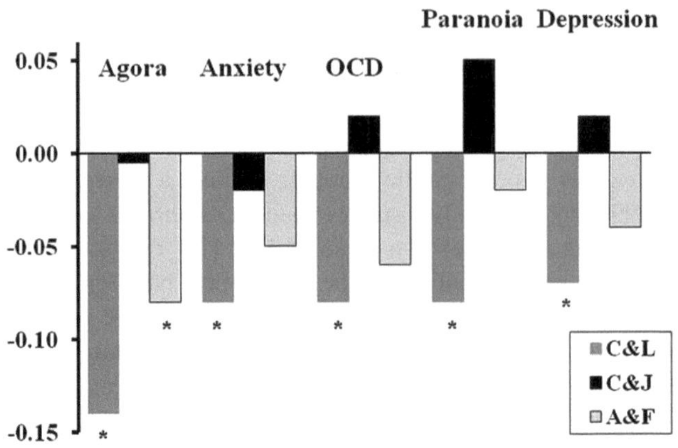

Fig. 19.3 Association of beliefs about God with psychiatric symptoms (Flannelly et al. 2010) [30]; *C&L* = Close & Loving, *C&J* = Creator & Judge, *A&F* = Approving & Forgiving, *Agora* = Agoraphobia, *OCD* = Obsessive-Compulsive Disorder. The values are standardized regression coefficients (β's); * statistically significant association between the belief and the class of psychiatric symptoms

safety in a dangerous world. On the other hand, belief in a creating and judging God (C&J: black bars) did not have a significant association with any symptom measures, probably because these beliefs about God do not offer security from harm. Belief in an approving and forgiving God (A&F: light gray bars) only had a significant salubrious association with agoraphobia, which suggests that an approving and forgiving God may provide a limited sense of security against some types of threats of harm.[5]

The study also found salubrious associations of social support with all of the measures of psychiatric symptoms (β's = −.14 to −.31), which were stronger than the net effects of belief in a close and loving God. This finding indicates that social support has a strong salutary association with psychiatric symptomology, which according to ETAS Theory, is due to the fact that close social relationships provide a strong sense of security. This finding also indicates that the net effects of belief in a close and loving God on psychiatric symptoms are above and beyond the effects of personal safety obtained from social support.

The second study, which was conducted by Silton et al. [2], analyzed data from the 2010 Baylor Religion Survey to examine the relationship between three beliefs about the nature of God and the five types of psychiatric symptoms. The independent variables were belief in a Deistic God (absolute and just), a Benevolent God (kind and accepting), and a Punitive God (wrathful and punishing). The OLS regression controlled for demographic variables, subjective religiousness, and belief in God, per se. We hypothesized that psychiatric symptomology would have no association with a Deistic God, a salubrious association with a Benevolent God, and a pernicious association with a Punitive God.

[5]Agoraphobia was mislabeled social anxiety in the 2010 article.

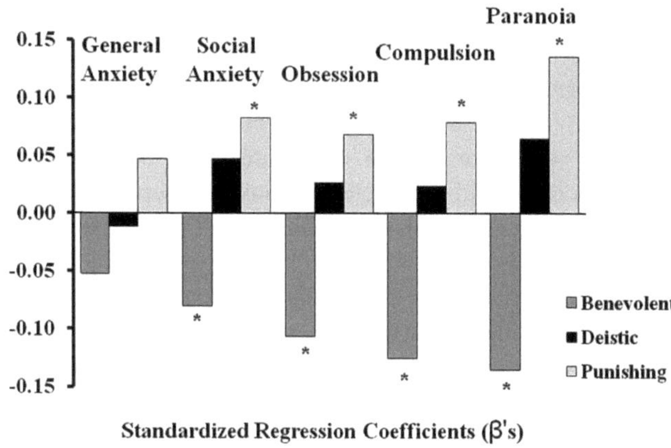

Fig. 19.4 Association of beliefs about God with psychiatric symptoms (Silton et al. 2014) [2]; * statistically significant association between the belief and the type of psychiatric symptoms

As expected, belief in a Deistic God was not significantly associated with psychiatric symptomology, as shown in black in Fig. 19.4. In contrast, belief in a Benevolent God had a salubrious association with all of the measures of psychiatric symptomology (dark gray bars), except general anxiety, whereas belief in a Punitive God had a pernicious association with all of the measures of psychiatric symptomology (light gray bars), except general anxiety. The results for a Deistic God and a Benevolent God are similar to the results of the 2010 Flannelly et al. study [30], presumably because belief in a Benevolent God provides a sense of safety and security and belief in a Deistic God does not, according to ETAS Theory. We hypothesized that belief in a Punitive God would have a pernicious association with psychiatric symptomology because a wrathful and punishing God poses a direct threat of harm.

19.3 Belief in a Harsh God, Psychiatric Symptoms, and Happiness

Although ETAS Theory does not explain positive emotions, themselves, it proposes that psychiatric symptoms influence positive emotions. Given this premise, I decided to examine if anxiety (in the broad sense of anxiety disorders) would mediate the association between beliefs about God and positive emotions. A mediation effect would mean that beliefs about God (the independent variable) affect positive emotions (the dependent variable) indirectly, through the effects of beliefs about God on anxiety (the mediator variable).

The only dataset available to me that measured psychiatric symptoms and positive emotions was the Baylor Religion Survey, and it only measured one positive emotion – happiness. However, I was fortunate to have happiness available to study because over a half-dozen studies of convenience samples in the U.K. have found that happiness is positively associated with religion [34, 35]. Happiness is also very important from the perspective of evolution. Charles Darwin described the expression of happiness (which he considered to be synonymous with joy), in apes, monkeys, canines, and horses, mainly in the context of social relationships [36]. Moreover, the psychologist and neuroscientist Jaak Panksepp considers "social joy" to be an ancient positive emotion that solidifies social relationships within species of mammals [37, 38].

I created a mediator variable that consisted of the combined symptoms of anxiety disorders in the Baylor Religion Survey (i.e., general anxiety, social anxiety, obsession, and compulsion). After creating the mediator variable (called AD symptoms, for short), I created two new sets of beliefs about God, rather than use the beliefs from the Silton et al. study, to analyze the mediating effects of AD symptoms on the association between happiness and positive and negative beliefs. The first set of beliefs, which I call a Harsh God, combined the adjectives severe and critical. The second set combined beliefs about God's Love ("God's love in eternal" and "God's love never fails"), which have not used in any other study of which I am aware.

The inter-correlations of the three key variables in each mediation analysis are shown in Table 19.1.[6] The analyses excluded self-proclaimed atheists in the Baylor Religion Survey.

Model 1 in Fig. 19.5 shows the results of a simple OLS model regressing Happiness on (a) belief in a Harsh God, and (b) belief in God's Love. The standardized regression coefficients (β's) between Happiness and belief in a Harsh God and belief in God's Love in Fig. 19.5 are the same as the correlation coefficients shown in Table 19.1 because there are no other variables in regression Model 1. However, when AD symptoms were added to Model 2, the β's for each belief were reduced in size, indicating that AD symptoms mediated the effects of belief in a Harsh God and belief in God's Love on Happiness.

The fact that the association between belief in a Harsh God and Happiness is not significant in Model 2 means that anxiety-disorder symptoms fully mediated this relationship. The fact that the association between belief in God's Love and Happiness remains significant in Model 2 means that anxiety-disorder symptoms only partially mediated this relationship.[7]

These findings indicate that positive emotions, such as happiness, are influenced by the negative affect linked to psychiatric symptoms, particularly anxiety, and that anxiety mediates the influences of religious beliefs on positive emotions. Hence, it appears that threat assessments and the beliefs that modulate them affect positive emotions. Therefore, the mediation results illustrate that ETAS Theory can help to explain the association of positive and negative beliefs about God with positive emotions.

---

[6]The three key variables in a mediation analysis (the independent variable, mediator, and dependent variable) have to be significantly correlated with each other in order to test mediation. Since belief in a Harsh God and belief in God's Love are used as mediators in separate analyses their inter-correlation is not relevant, so they are not shown below in Table 19.1.

[7]The Sobel-Goodman test confirmed that anxiety-disorder symptoms meditated the association between beliefs and Happiness.

Table 19.1 Correlations between the three key variables in the two mediation analyses

	AD symptoms	Harsh God	God's Love
Happiness	−.437***	−.057*	.128***
AD symptoms		−.073**	−.061**

**p* < .05; ***p* < .01; ****p* < .001

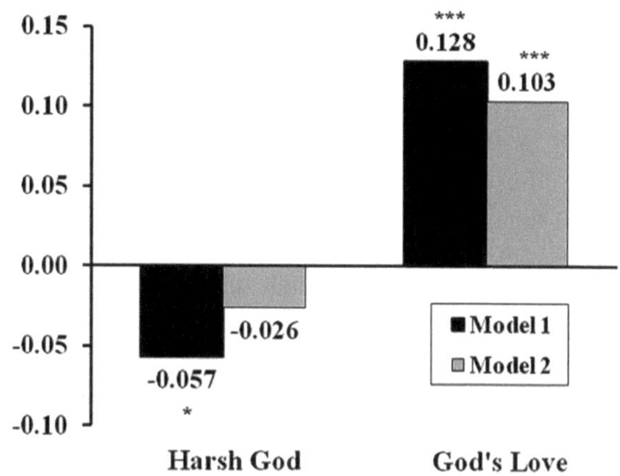

Fig. 19.5 Mediating effects of symptoms of anxiety disorders on the association of happiness with belief in a Harsh God and belief in God's Love; values are β's; **p* < .05; ****p* < .001

19.4 Chapter Highlights and Comments

The research described in this chapter demonstrates that belief in a benevolent God has a salubrious association with mental health, whereas belief in a malevolent God has a pernicious association with mental health. According to ETAS Theory, the salubrious effects of belief in a benevolent God on anxiety and other psychiatric symptoms results from the combined effects of the perception of threat and a sense of safety. Belief in a benevolent God causes the ventromedial PFC to raise the threshold of what constitutes a threat, thereby reducing amygdala activity and anxiety-related psychiatric symptoms. Belief in a malevolent God, on the other hand, acts to lower the threshold of what constitutes a threat because God not only fails to provide protection from harm but poses a direct threat of harm. The latter effect probably involves activation of the "aversive amplification circuit," which consists of the dorsomedial prefrontal cortex, the anterior cingulated cortex, and the amygdala, and enhances amygdala activity [39]. Belief in a deistic God generally had no association with symptomology because it does not provide imply protection from harm, according to ETAS Theory.

Terror Management Theory, which was mentioned in Chaps. 17 and 18, considers self-esteem to be an evolved mechanism that buffers against anxiety about death, and other forms of anxiety that the terror of death creates, because self-esteem provides a sense of security [40–42]. It seems more plausible to me, however, that self-esteem evolved in primates, long before our ancestors became aware of their own mortality, as a cognitive mechanism to assess one's relative status within a dominance hierarchy. It strikes me as equally plausible that self-efficacy evolved around the same time as a cognitive mechanism to assess ones' ability to succeed in moving up that dominance hierarchy or maintain one's position in that dominance hierarchy by defeating one's social rivals. This would account for the close relationship between the two concepts [43–45].

As noted above, the observed relationships between beliefs about God and self-esteem are important for at least two reasons. One is that threats to self-esteem can increase anxiety and other psychiatric symptoms, which will be discussed in later chapters. The other is that higher self-esteem is associated with lower anxiety [42, 46]. If, as I think, self-esteem arose as a mechanism to assess one's social status, then self-esteem should lower anxiety because it indicates a superior social status, which should reduce threats of harm from social rivals. Self- efficacy (one's belief in one's own abilities), on the other hand, should reduce anxiety because the belief that one has the ability to handle difficult situations reduces the threat posed by any situations [47], including threats from social rivals. A large 2001 study by Chris Ellison and his colleagues found that both self-esteem and self-efficacy had independent salutary effects on psychological distress [48], which is consistent with ETAS Theory.

The findings of the 2010 Flannelly et al. [30] study showed, consistent with past research, that social support had a significant salubrious association with mental health. Unlike prior interpretations of the effects of social support on mental health, however, ETAS Theory proposes that social support can have a direct effect on psychiatric symptoms by providing a sense of security that counters the effects of perceived threats on psychiatric symptomology.

The mediation results illustrate that ETAS Theory can help to explain the association of positive and negative beliefs about God with psychological well-being in addition to their association with psychiatric symptoms. This point will be explored further in Chap. 21 in which I analyze the association between happiness and other variables from the Baylor Religion Survey.

References

1. Cranney, S. (2013). Do people who believe in God report more meaning in their lives? The existential effects of belief *Journal for the Scientific Study of Religion, 52*(3), 638–646.
2. Silton, N. R., Flannelly, K. J., Galek, K., & Ellison, C. G. (2014). Beliefs about God and mental health among American adults. *Journal of Religion and Health, 53*(5), 1285–1296.
3. McCullough, M. E., & Larson, D. B. (1999). Religion and depression: A review of the literature. *Twin Research, 2*(2), 126-136.
4. Spilka, B., Armatas, P., & Nussbaum, J. (1964). The concept of God: A factor analytic approach. *Review of Religious Research, 6*(1), 28–36.
5. Gorsuch, R. L. (1968). The conceptualization of God as seen in adjective ratings. *Journal for the Scientific Study of Religion, 7*(1), 56–64.
6. Benson, P., & Spilka, B. (1973). God image as a function of self-esteem and locus of control. *Journal for the Scientific Study of Religion, 12*(3), 297–310.

7. Schaefer, C. A., & Gorsuch, R. L. (1991). Psychological adjustment and religiousness: The multivariate belief-motivation theory of religiousness. *Journal for the Scientific Study of Religion, 30*(4), 448–461.
8. Jonas, E., & Fischer, P. (2006). Terror management and religion: Evidence that intrinsic religiousness mitigates worldview defense following mortality salience. *Journal of Personality and Social Psychology, 91*(3), 553–567.
9. Coopersmith, S. (1967). *The antecedents of self-esteem*. San Francisco: Freeman.
10. Spielberger, C. R., Gorsuch, R. L., & Lushene, R. (1970). *Manual for the state-trait anxiety inventory*. Palo Alto: Consulting Press.
11. Krug, S. E., Scheirer, I. H., & Cattell, R. B. (1963). *Handbook for the IPAT anxiety scale*. Champaign: Institute for Personality and Ability Testing, Inc.
12. Hammersla, J. F., Andrews-Qualls, L. C., & Frease, L. G. (1986). God concepts and religious committment among Christian university students. *Journal for the Scientific Study of Religion, 25*(4), 424–435.
13. Froese, P., & Bader, C. D. (2010). *America's four Gods*. New York: Oxford University Press.
14. Noffke, J. L. M. S. H. (2001). Denominational and age comparisons of god concepts. *Journal for the Scientific Study of Religion, 40*(4), 747–756.
15. Schieman, S., Pudrovska, T., & Milkie, M. (2005). The sense of divine control and the self-concept: A study of race differences in later-life. *Research on Aging, 27*, 165–196.
16. Martens, A., Greenberg, J., & Allen, J. J. B. (2008). Self-esteem and autonomic physiology: Parallels between self-esteem and cardiac vagal tone as buffers of threat. *Personality and Social Psychology Review, 12*(4), 370–389.
17. Baldwin, M. W., & Wesley, R. (1996). Effects of existential anxiety and self-esteem on the perception of others. *Basic and Applied Social Psychology, 18*(1), 75–94.
18. Karademas, E. C., Kafetsios, K., & Sideridis, G. D. (2007). Optimism, self-efficacy and information processing of threat- and well-being-related stimuli. *Stress and Health, 23*(5), 285–294.
19. Gruenewald, T. L., Aziz, N., Fahey, J. L., & Kemeny, M. E. (2004). Acute threat to the social self: Shame, social self-esteem, and cortisol activity. *Psychosomatic Medicine, 66*(6), 915–924.
20. Leary, M. R., Barnes, B. D., & Griebel, C. (1986). Cognitive, affective, and attributional effects of potential threats to self-esteem. *Journal of Social and Clinical Psychology, 4*(4), 461.
21. Houston, B. K., Olson, M., & Botkin, A. (1972). Trait anxiety and beliefs regarding danger and threat to self-esteem. *Journal of Consulting and Clinical Psychology, 38*(1), 152.
22. van Dellen, M. R., Campbell, W. K., Hoyle, R. H., & Bradfield, E. K. (2001). Compensating, resisting, and breaking: A meta-analytic examination of reactions to self-esteem threat. *Personality and Social Psychology Review, 15*(1), 51–74.
23. Zahl, B. P., & Gibson, N. J. S. (2012). God representations, attachment to God, and satisfaction with life: A comparison of doctrinal and experiential representations of God in Christian young adults. *The International Journal for the Psychology of Religion, 22*(3), 216–230.
24. Francis, L. J., Gibson, H. M., & Robbins, M. (2001). God images and self-worth among adolescents in Scotland. *Mental Health, Religion and Culture, 4*(2), 103–108.
25. Francis, L. J. (2005). God images and self-esteem: A study among 11–18 year olds. *Research in the Social Scientific Study of Religion,* 18(1), 105–121.
26. Ellison, C. G., & Levin, J. S. (1998). The religion-health connection: Evidence, theory and future directions. *Health Education & Behavior, 2516*(700–720).
27. Thompson, M. S., Thomas, M. E., & Head, R. N. (2012). Race, socioeconomic status, and self-esteem: The impact of religiosity. *Sociological Spectrum, 32*(5), 385–405.
28. Diener, E. D., Emmons, R. A., & Larsen, R. J. G. S., (1985). The satisfaction with life scale *Journal of Personality Assessment, 49*(1), 71–75.
29. Steenwyk, S. A. M., Atkins, D. C., Bedics, J. D., & Whitley, B. E., Jr. (2010). Images of God as they relate to life satisfaction and hopelessness. *The International Journal for the Psychology of Religion, 20*(2), 85–96.

30. Flannelly, K. J., Koenig, H., Galek, K., & Ellison, C. G. (2010). Beliefs about God, psychiatric symptoms and evolutionary psychiatry. *Journal of Religion and Health, 49*(2), 246–261.
31. Flannelly, K. J., Koenig, H. G., Ellison, C. G., Galek, K., & Krause, N. (2006). Belief in life after death and mental health: Findings from a national survey. *Journal of Nervous and Mental Disease, 194*(7), 524–529.
32. Flannelly, K. J., Ellison, C. G., Galek, K., & Koenig, H. G. (2008). Beliefs about life-after-death, psychiatric symptomology and cognitive theories of psychopathology. *Journal of Psychology & Theology, 36,* 94–103.
33. Dantzer, R. (2005). Somatization: A psychoneuroimmune perspective. *Psychoneuroendocrinology, 30*(10), 947–952.
34. Lewis, C. A., & Cruise, S. M. (2006). Religion and happiness: Consensus, contradictions, comments and concerns. *Mental Health, Religion and Culture, 9*(3), 213–225.
35. Francis, L. (2010). Religion and happiness. J. Atherton, E. Graham, & I. Steedman (Eds.), *The practices of happiness, political economy, religion and well-being* (pp. 114–124). London: Routledge.
36. Darwin, C. (1872). *The expression of emotions in man and animals*. London: John Murray.
37. Burgdorf, J., & Panksepp, J. (2006). The neurobiology of positive emotions. *Neuroscience and Biobehavioral Reviews, 30*(2), 173–187.
38. Panksepp, J. (2000). The riddle of laughter neural and psychoevolutionary underpinnings of joy. *Current Directions in Psychological Science, 9*(6), 183–186.
39. Robinson, O. J., Krimsky, M., Lieberman, L., Allen, P., Vytal, K., & Grillon, C. (2014). Towards a mechanistic understanding of pathological anxiety: The dorsal medial prefrontal-amygdala "aversive amplification" circuit in unmedicated generalized and social anxiety disorders. *The Lancet Psychiatry, 1*(4), 294.
40. Arndt, J., Routledge, C., Cox, C. R., & Goldenberg, J. L. (2005). The worm at the core: A terror management perspective on the roots of psychological dysfunction. *Applied and Preventive Psychology, 11*(3), 191.
41. Dechesne, M., Arndt, J., Ransom, S., Sheldon, K. M., Pyszczynski, T., Van Knippenberg, A., et al. (2003). Literal and symbolic immortality: The effect of evidence of literal immortality on self-esteem striving in response to mortality salience. *Journal of Personality and Social Psychology, 84*(4), 722–737.
42. Pyszczynsi, T., Greenberg, J., Solomon, S., Arndt, J., & Schimel, J. (2004). *Why do people need self-esteem? A theoretical and empirical review. Psychological Bulletin, 130*(3), 435–468.
43. Welch, D. C., & West, R. L. (1995). Self-efficacy and mastery: Its application to issues of environmental control, cognition, and aging. *Developmental Review, 15*(2), 150–171.
44. Chen, G., Gully, S. M., & Dov, E. (2004). General self-efficacy and self-esteem: Toward theoretical and empirical distinction between correlated self-evaluations. *Journal of Organizational Behavior, 25*(3), 375–395.
45. Lightsey, O. R., Burke, M., Ervin, A., Henderson, D., & Yee, C. (2006). Generalized self-efficacy, self-esteem, and negative affect. *Canadian Journal of Behavioural Science, 38*(1), 72–80.
46. Rosenberg, M. (1962). The association between self-esteem and anxiety. *Journal of Psychiatric Research,* 1(2), 135–152.
47. Thompson, S. C. (1981). Will it hurt less if I can control it? A complex answer to a simple question. *Psychological Bulletin, 90*(1), 89–101.
48. Ellison, C. G., Boardman, J. D., Williams, D. R., & Jackson, J. S. (2001). Religious involvement, stress, and mental health: Findings from the 1995 Detroit area study. *Social Forces, 80*(1), 215–249.

Chapter 20
Beliefs About One's Relationship with God and Mental Health

Abstract The chapter summarizes the results of research indicating that believing one has a relationship with God is associated with mental health. For example, a 1991 study of a large national sample of American adults found that believing one has a close relationship with God was related to psychological well-being. The chapter describes several subsequent avenues of research into the ways in which Americans say they rely on God to help them cope with life stressors. At least three separate but similar lines of research have demonstrated that believing one collaborates with God in some way has a salutary association with many measures of mental health. The chapter also presents the results of related research that demonstrate that believing one has a poor relationship with God has a pernicious association with many measures of mental health, including psychiatric symptoms. According to ETAS Theory, the salubrious association between believing one has a good relationship with God and mental health reflects the fact this belief provides a sense of safety, which causes ETAS to raise the threshold of what constitutes a threat, thereby lowering anxiety and other forms of psychological distress. Since Chap. 19 showed that anxiety mediates the association between religious beliefs and psychological well-being, believing one has a good relationship with God increases psychological well-being. On the other hand, believing one has a poor relationship with God reduces the sense of safety that belief in God would otherwise provide, thereby lowering the threshold of what is a threat and increasing psychiatric symptoms and other forms of psychological distress.

Keywords Collaboration with God • ETAS Theory • God • God-mediated control • Psychiatric symptoms • Relationship with God • Safety • Psychological distress • Psychological well-being • Religious coping • RCOPE • Spiritual struggles

20.1 Believing One Has a Relationship with God

Neal Krause, a Professor of Public Health at the University of Michigan who has done extensive research on religion and health, has said that "having a close personal relationship with God is the hallmark of leading a religious life" (p. 17) [1]. One's relationship with God is a vital element of the Christian experience, and some

K.J. Flannelly, *Religious Beliefs, Evolutionary Psychiatry, and Mental Health in America*, Religion, Spirituality and Health: A Social Scientific Approach 1,
DOI 10.1007/978-3-319-52488-7_20

authors consider it to be the core of Christian spirituality [2, 3]. Williams James recognized the psychological importance of believing one has a personal relationship with God in his 1902 book *The Varieties of Religious Experience* [4]. However, this concept apparently was considered to lie outside the scope of scientific investigation until the 1970s. The studies I discuss in this chapter are different from the research I discussed in Chap. 19 because they explicitly examine how people's beliefs about their relationship with God (not just their beliefs about God) are related to mental health.

A 1978 article by the anthropologist John L. Caughey argued that the social science definition of social relations was far too narrow, noting that people in some non-Western societies believe that nonhuman entities, such as gods, mythical monsters, and deceased ancestors directly interact with humans [5]. Although such interactions, by Western standards, would not be defined as social relations, Caughey recognized that they can be an important part of a person's subjective social experience.

As Caughey saw it, the "real social world" of most Americans consists of only a few people with whom we "actually interact," yet there are many more people in our "artificial social world" with whom we never interact face-to-face. This artificial social world "includes all those beings that are known to the individual via television, radio, movies, books, magazines, and newspapers" (p. 71) [5], to which we would now add the internet. Even though people do not have actual interactions with media figures, they may have artificial interactions with them, in a sense, when they see or hear them or read about them. Moreover, many people may even see such figures as sources of guidance for dealing with problems in their personal lives [5].

20.2 Early Research on Mental Health and Believing One Has a Relationship with God

A 1989 article by the sociologist Melvin Pollner drew upon Caughey's ideas and the writings of Swedish psychologist Hjalmar Sunden in the 1970s [6] to make the case that one's relationship with God is a form of social relationship, and therefore, open to scientific inquiry [7]. Pollner believed that God "was one of the most prominent … imagined significant others of Americans" (p. 92) [7]. He thought that individuals interacted with God symbolically and that the main mechanism of this symbolic interaction was prayer. He also thought that interaction with God probably had a salutary effect on psychological well-being by providing individuals with a sense of safety and security.

Chris Ellison, who was then at Duke University, tested Pollner's idea that interacting with God has a salutary association with psychological well-being in a 1991 study that used data from the 1988 General Social Survey [8]. The dependent variables were personal happiness and life satisfaction. The independent variable, which Ellison called Divine Interaction, was measured by averaging the answers to two

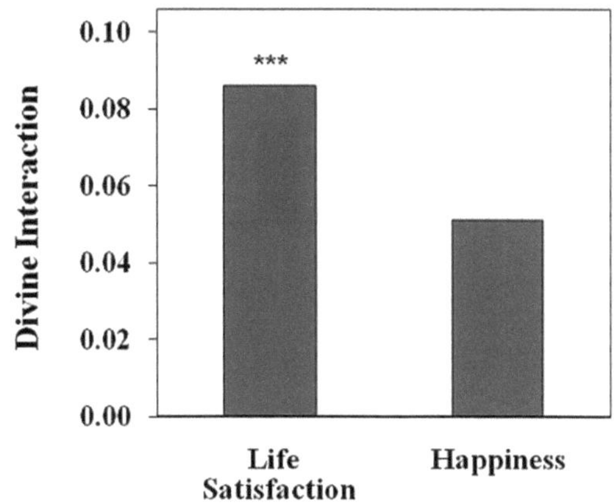

Fig. 20.1 The association of Divine Interaction with life satisfaction and happiness (Ellison 1991); $^{***}p < .001$

questions: "How close do you feel to God most of the time?" and "How often do you pray?" Research by Neal Krause suggests that prayer, for many Christians, is the overt expression of their belief that God will do what is best for them [8, 9].

Figure 20.1 shows the results of Ellison's study, controlling for socio-demographic variables, religious denomination, church attendance, and other variables. As seen in the figure, people who believed they had a closer relationship with God and prayed more frequently (i.e., Divine Interaction) reported significantly greater life satisfaction and somewhat greater happiness than other people did.

The results indicate that believing one has a positive relationship with God has a salubrious association with psychological well-being. Since Ellison's measure of Divine Interaction included the beliefs that one has a close relationship with God and that one interacts with God through prayer, it captures the notion of a close and caring God that the studies in Chap. 19 found to have a salubrious association with psychiatric symptoms. Although the research in Chap. 19 examined people's beliefs about God, not their belief that they interact with God, the mechanisms underlying the association of psychological well-being with both types of beliefs are probably the same: i.e., both types of beliefs affect anxiety.

20.3 Three Beliefs About One's Relationships with God and Mental Health

Many Americans turn to their religion and God in times of stress [1, 10, 11], particularly when situations pose a threat to life or serious physical harm [10, 12–14], and they often to seek support [15] and protection from God [16] when difficult situations are beyond their control [17]. A 1988 study by Ken Pargament and his colleagues at Bowling Green State University identified three types of religious problem-solving used by people when confronted with stressful situations [18]. The first two, which they called collaborative and deferring styles, involve reliance on

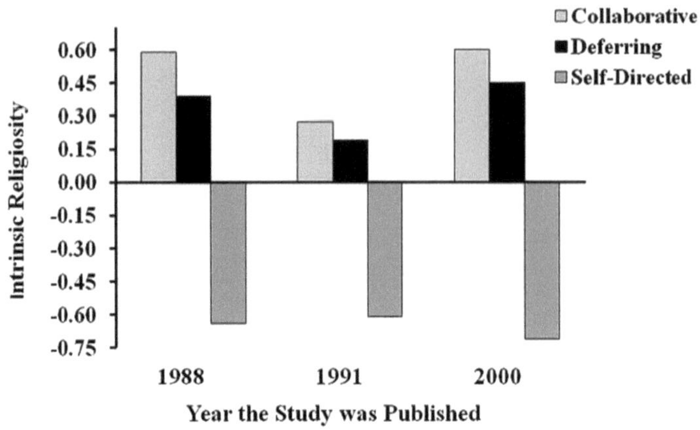

Fig. 20.2 Association between intrinsic religiosity and three styles of religious problem-solving reported in three studies; Values are standardized regression coefficients (β's); All the associations are statistically significant

God. Pargament et al. linked the collaborative style to Judeo-Christian traditions and the belief that one can "partner with God" to receive support and guidance from God in order to cope with worldly problems. The deferring style entails turning a difficult situation completely over to an omnipotent God to determine its ultimate outcome.

Of course, not everyone turns to God in times of stress, and this fact is reflected in the third problem-solving style that Pargament et al. identified [18]. This third style, called self-directed problem-solving, neither embraces nor dismisses God's role in the world, but assumes that individuals are responsible for resolving their own problems, and "stresses the power of the person rather than the power of God" (p. 91) [18]. The 1988 study, which developed a 36-item scale to measure these three styles, tested the scale with convenience samples of congregants of two Protestant churches in the Midwestern U.S. A subsequent study with Protestant clergy and their spouses confirmed the three-factor structure of the original scale [19]: that is, collaborative, deferring, and self-directed problem-solving styles.

As one would expect (see Fig. 20.2), the 1988 study found that people who were more intrinsically religious (i.e., had a stronger intrinsic religious orientation) were more likely to say they collaborated or deferred to God to address their problems, and they were less likely to exclude God from their efforts to solve problems (the self-directed style) [18]. Two studies of undergraduate students at U.S. Christian colleges, published by Gorsuch and his colleagues in 1991 and 2000, confirmed the general pattern of correlations between intrinsic religiosity and collaborative, deferring, and self-directed problem-solving [20, 21] (see Fig. 20.2). The 1988 study by Pargament and his colleagues also reported the pattern of correlations between extrinsic religiosity and the three problem-solving styles, but this pattern was not confirmed by Gorsuch and his colleagues.

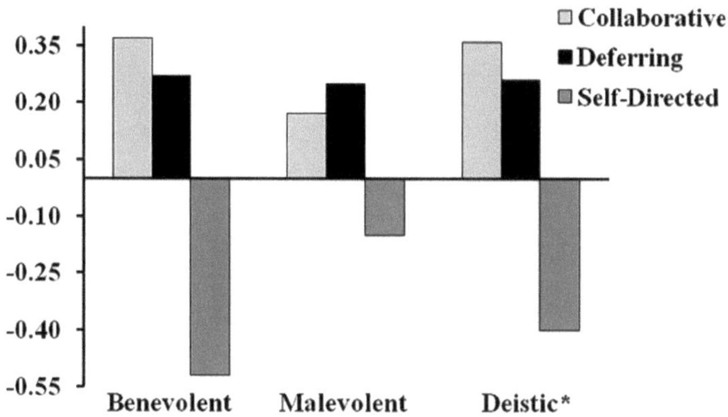

Fig. 20.3 Associations between beliefs about God and three styles of religious problem-solving. Values are standardized regression coefficients (β's); All values are statistically significant; * Omnipotent, Omnipresent, and Omniscient

The 1991 study, which was conducted by Schaefer and Gorsuch, also correlated the three problem-solving styles with beliefs about God. The correlations, which are shown in Fig. 20.3, indicate that the Christian college students with a self-directed style took an independent approach to solving problems, regardless of their beliefs about God. My own analysis of the correlations for collaborative and deferring problem-solving indicates that students were equally likely to defer to all three kinds of God, but they were significantly less likely to collaborate with a malevolent God than with a benevolent God or a deistic God (i.e., an omnipotent, omnipresent, and omniscient God). Since there is no way of knowing if people actually interact with God, I consider statements about one's interactions with God (e.g., collaboration) to be expressions of a person's belief that s/he interacts with God.

In addition, the 1991 Schaefer and Gorsuch study investigated the association between each of the three problem-solving styles and anxiety [21], as measured by the Institute for Personality and Ability Testing's (IPAT) anxiety scale [22] and the trait anxiety subscale of the State-Trait Anxiety Inventory (STAI) [23]. Their findings are shown in Fig. 20.4. The belief that one collaborates with or defers to God was significantly associated with lower anxiety, whereas self-directed problem-solving, which does not involve God, was significantly associated with higher anxiety.

Another study of undergraduate students at a religiously affiliated university in the Midwest found that both collaborative and deferring religious coping styles had significant salubrious associations with psychological well-being and psychological distress [24]. In addition, the belief that one is collaborating with God [25, 26] or deferring to God have been found to have salubrious association with depression [25], anxiety about health [27], and psychological adjustment to a health crisis [28]. Some of the same research has found that that self-directed coping has a pernicious association with depression and quality of life in hospital patients, and other U.S. research has reported that it is associated with trait anxiety [29] and depression [30]

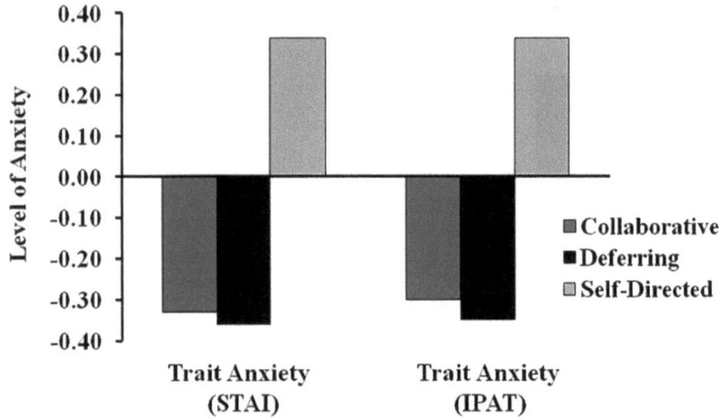

Fig. 20.4 Association of two measures of trait anxiety with three styles of religious problem-solving; The values are standardized regression coefficients (β's); All the associations are statistically significant

among Protestants church members. However, the results about self-directed coping have been mixed in other U.S. samples [25, 31, 32].

20.4 Collaboration with God and Mental Health

Neal Krause explored the concept of collaboration with God (which he calls God-mediated control) in a series of national surveys of U.S. adults [33–38]. The results of two surveys are of special interest because they investigated the relationship between believing that one collaborates with God and psychological well-being. The two studies, published in 2005 and 2010, used the following items to measure collaboration with God: "I rely on God to help me control my life." "I can succeed with God's help." and "All things are possible when I work together with God" (p. 148) [35].

The Americans in these and other studies by Krause who embraced the concept of God-mediated control clearly believed that God controlled their lives, but because they believed they had a close relationship with God, they trusted God, and they believed God would do what was best for them [34, 35, 39]. Their own role in this relationship, therefore, may be seen as following God's guidance about what they should do for themselves. Krause's research also indicates that African-Americans are significantly more likely than White Americans to believe they have a close relationship with God [1], even after statistically controlling for the fact that African-Americans, in general, are more religious than Whites [40, 41].

Figure 20.5 shows the results of two large-scale studies by Neal Krause, the first of which interviewed over 1200 older Americans in 2005, and the second of which interviewed many of the same people in 2010. The survey participants were asked

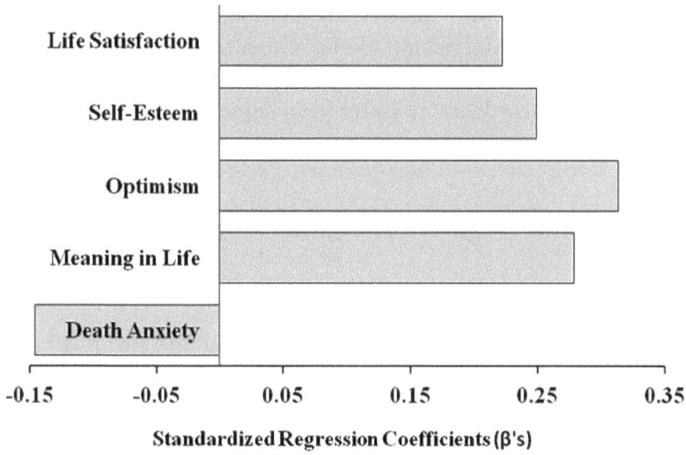

Fig. 20.5 Association between measures of psychological well-being and believing that one collaborates with God (Krause, 2005, 2010) [35, 37]; Values are standardized regression coefficients (β's)

about their collaboration with God (God-mediated control) and optimism, life satisfaction, self-esteem, optimism, and death anxiety [35], and the belief that life has meaning [37].[1]

Overall, believing that one collaborates with God had significant positive associations with life-satisfaction, self-esteem, and optimism, and the belief that there is meaning in life (see Fig. 20.5). The belief that one collaborates with God had a significant negative association with death anxiety. The 2005 study also found that the salubrious associations between believing one collaborates with God and life satisfaction, self-esteem, and optimism were more pronounced in African-Americans than in White Americans.

The results of a series of studies by Scott Schieman – a sociologist at the University of Toronto – and his colleagues complement Krause's research. One study, for example, asked a national sample of 1800 older Americans to rate the extent to which they thought God controlled ("divine control") and they controlled ("personal control") their own lives [42]. Naturally, there was an inverse relationship between belief in divine control and belief in personal control for the entire sample, but this inverse relationship was most pronounced among people who were not religious. Very religious Americans, on the other hand, were more likely to give equal weight to God's control and their own control over their lives. Studies of older adults in the Washington, D.C. area found that belief in divine control was greater in African Americans than White Americans [43], and they suggest that this difference may be related to the fact that African Americans tend to pray and attend church more often than Whites do [43]. Divine control, which included relying on God, being part of God's plan, and seeking guidance from God, was found to have

[1] Figure 20.5 shows the mean results for optimism, which was measured in both studies.

a salubrious association with anxiety, depression, and self-esteem in African Americans but not White Americans [44–46]. Other research on African-Americans has found that those who believe their religion provides "a great deal of guidance in day-to-day living" are less likely to suffer from depression [47].

20.5 Positive and Negative Religious Coping and Mental Health

Research by Pargament and his colleagues during the 1990s identified many different methods of religious coping and how they were related mental health [11, 48, 49]. The different methods of religious coping, most of which are related to one's relationship with God [50], were broadly classified as positive and negative religious coping. Key examples of the different positive methods of religious coping included: viewing things as part of God's plan, seeking a closer connection to God, seeking God's intercession, seeking God's forgiveness, seeking comfort from God, working together with God, and deferring or surrendering to God's will. Negative methods of coping included: doubting God's power and feeling punished or abandoned by God.

A 1998 paper by Pargament et al. called attention to the negative consequences of having a poor relationship with God, particularly, the belief that God has abandoned you or is punishing you. That paper and subsequent studies found that believing you are being punished by God has a pernicious association with anxiety in convenience samples of U.S. college students (r's = .15 to .32) [51], Catholic church parishioners ($r = .33$) [51], and lung transplant patients ($r = .55$) [32], as well as depression in college students [31] and transplant patients [32]. Similarly, the belief that one has been abandoned by God was found to have a significant pernicious associations with anxiety ($r = .15$), depression ($r = .15$), and life satisfaction ($r = -.21$) in a convenience sample of U.S. college students [31].

The pernicious association between believing one has been punished or abandoned by God with psychological well-being and distress has been partially confirmed in two large studies by Harold Koenig et al. [25] and Ellison and Lee [52] (see Fig. 20.6).[2] The Koenig study found that hospital patients who believed they had been abandoned and/or punished by God reported a significantly lower quality of life and a significantly higher level of depressed mood than other patients did, controlling for socio-demographic variables and social support [25]. The Ellison and Lee study found American adults who believed God had abandoned and/or punished them had significantly higher psychological distress [53] than other adults had, controlling socio-demographic variables and frequency of prayer and church attendance.

[2] The Koenig study used a convenience sample of nearly 600 older hospitalized patients in North Carolina. The Ellison study used a representative sample of U.S. adults.

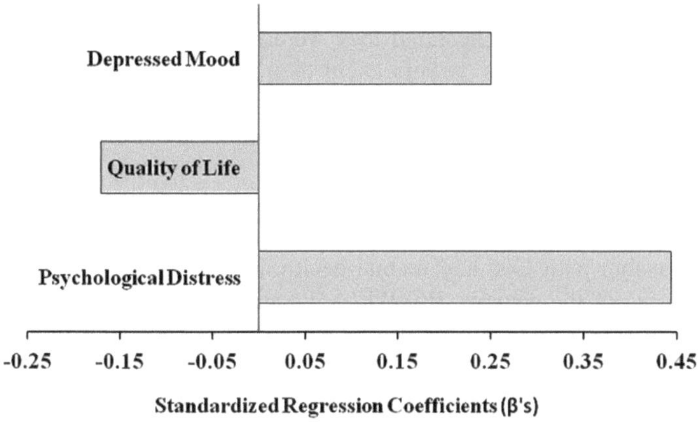

Fig. 20.6 Association between psychological well-being and believing that you have been abandoned or punished by God (Koenig et al. 1998; Ellison and Lee, 2010) [25, 52]; Values are standardized regression coefficients (β's); All associations are statistically significant

20.6 The RCOPE

Research by Pargament and his colleagues led to the development of the Brief RCOPE, which consists of 14 items: 7 measuring positive religious coping and 7 measuring negative religious coping.[3] The authors involved in the development of the RCOPE specifically assumed that individuals who exhibited positive patterns of religious coping shared a specific set of religious beliefs: (1) the belief that one has "a secure relationship with God" (p. 712), (2) the "belief that there is meaning to be found in life" (p. 712), and (3) the belief that individuals have "spiritual connectedness with others" (p. 712) [48]. Research by Neal Krause and his colleagues provides some support for these assumptions [33, 37, 54, 55]. However, the seven items of the positive RCOPE items do not specifically measure beliefs about one's relationship with God, but thoughts that religious persons might have, or the activities in which they might engage, if they believed they have a good relationship with God.

In contrast, Pargament and his colleagues "believed that the negative religious coping pattern is an expression of a less secure relationship with God, a tenuous and ominous view of the world, and a religious struggle in search of significance" (p. 712) [48]. Most of the negative coping items of the Brief RCOPE can be interpreted as expressions of belief about one's relationship with God. Despite this fact, I think

[3] The seven positive items are: Looked for a stronger connection with God; Sought God's love and care; Sought help from God in letting go of my anger; Tried to put my plans into action together with God; I tried to see how God might be trying to strengthen me in this situation; Asked God's forgiveness for my sins; and Focused on religion to stop worrying about my problems. The seven negative items are: Wondered whether God had abandoned me; Felt punished by God for my lack of devotion; Wondered what I did for God to punish me; Question God's love for me; Wondered whether my church had abandoned me; Decided the devil made this happen; and Questioned the power of God.

the negative RCOPE items would be more useful for studying the association between beliefs and mental health if they were rephrased to make them explicit statements about individuals' beliefs about their relationship with God. I do not think this is a mere matter of semantics because I think beliefs are stored in the brain and that beliefs are actively involved in the threat assessment that underlie psychiatric symptoms.

A study by my colleagues Holly Gaudette and Kathy Jankowski [56] used a scale that contained the kind of items I think are more useful for studying beliefs about one's relationship with God and mental health. The scale's six items, which are similar to some of the negative RCOPE items are: (1) I believe God protects me from harm; (2) I believe God is punishing me; (3) I believe God is involved in my life; (4) I believe God has abandoned me; (5) I believe God loves and care for me; and (6) I believe my life and death follow a plan from God. The study reported that the scale had a significant inverse correlation with general anxiety in a small sample of hospitalized palliative care patients ($r = -.42$).

20.7 The RCOPE and Mental Health

A 2005 meta-analysis by American psychologists Gene G. Ano and ErinB. Vasconcelles found that positive religious coping tends to be associated with positive psychological outcomes (psychological well-being) and negative religious coping tends to be associated with negative psychological outcomes (psychological distress) [57]. However, very few of the studies in their meta-analysis used the RCOPE; so I did a literature search on Medline and PsycNet of studies that used the RCOPE. Although numerous have used items from the Brief RCOPE, relatively few have used all seven items from either subscale, and many of studies that have used all the items of either subscale fail to report any useable statistical results about their association with a specific psychological outcomes.

Nevertheless, I was able to find and analyze the correlations of the positive RCOPE subscale (P-RCOPE: n = 14) and the negative RCOPE subscale (N-RCOPE: n = 16) with 30 mental-health outcomes (i.e., dependent variables) that I broadly categorized as being either measures of psychological well-being (n = 16) or psychological distress (n = 14). The measures of psychological well-being included life satisfaction, optimism, positive affect, and quality of life; the measures of psychological distress included trait and generalized anxiety, depressive mood, clinical depression, and combined measures of anxiety and depressive symptoms.

The results of my analysis revealed significant main effects of RCOPE subscales (P-RCOPE vs. N-RCOPE) and psychological outcomes (Well-Being vs. Distress) and a significant interaction between the subscales and the type of psychological

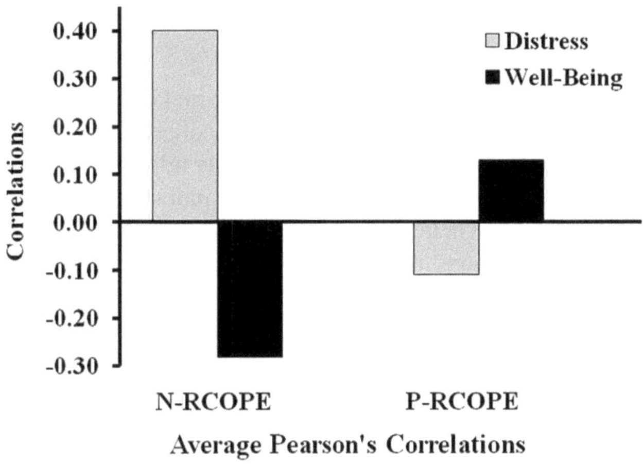

Fig. 20.7 Average correlations of the N-RCOPE and the P-RCOPE with psychological well-being and psychological distress in various studies

outcomes (see Fig. 20.7).[4] Contrary to the findings of Ano and Vasconcelles' meta-analysis [57], negative religious coping was significantly associated with both positive (psychological well-being) and negative psychological outcomes (psychological distress), though the direction of the associations differed, as one would expect. As shown in Fig. 20.7, the N-RCOPE had a significant positive association with psychological distress and a significant negative association with psychological well-being. On the other hand, positive religious coping (the P-RCOPE) only had minor association with either positive or negative psychological outcomes.

The N-RCOPE has come to be known as a measure of "spiritual struggles." Although a number of small-scale studies, which are included in my above analysis of the N-RCOPE, have examined the relationship between spiritual struggles and mental health, only a few national studies have done so [58–60]. The first of these is a study by McConnell et al. that examined the association between the spiritual struggles and six classes of psychiatric symptoms, using data from the 2004 National Study of Religion and Health [60]. The study found that believing one has a poor relationship with God (spiritual struggles) had a significant positive association with six classes of symptoms: agoraphobia, depression, general anxiety, obsessive-compulsive disorder, paranoid ideation, and somatization. A later national study found that believing one has a poor relationship with God was, as one might expect, particularly distressing for clergy [58].

[4] The analysis was a 2 × 2 analysis of variance with the RCOPE subscales (P-RCOPE vs. N-RCOPE) and psychological outcomes (well-being vs. distress) as between factors.

20.8 Chapter Highlights and Comments

Many Americans believe they have a relationship with God. For some, this entails deferring to God's will and for others this entails collaborating with God to deal with everyday problems. People who are intrinsically religious tend to do both, but they are more likely to collaborate with God. Some individuals defer to God's will, regardless of whether they believe God is benevolent, malevolent, or deistic, but religious individuals are more inclined to collaborate with a benevolent or deistic God than with a malevolent God. Thus, people's beliefs about the nature of God and their beliefs about their relationship with God appear to interact with each other.

Three of the most important findings from the studies reviewed in this chapter are that individuals who believe they collaborate with God have better mental-health outcomes than other individuals, that individuals who have a poor relationship with God have poorer mental health outcomes, and that African Americans are more likely to benefit from the belief that God controls their lives. Most of the association observed between a poor relationship with God and poor mental health are based on small studies that used convenience samples. However, the results of the national study by McConnell et al. confirm that believing one has a poor relationship with God has a pernicious association with poor mental health, specifically, psychiatric symptoms.

According to ETAS Theory, the salubrious association of mental health with the belief that one has a good relationship with God reflects the fact that God provides a sense of safety, which causes ETAS to raise the threshold of what constitutes a threat, thereby lowering anxiety and other forms of psychological distress. The belief that one has a poor relationship with God undermines this sense of safety. The belief that one has been abandoned by God presumably eliminates whatever sense of safety that even a poor relationship with God may provide, whereas believing God is punishing you makes God a direct threat of harm, which may activate the "aversive amplification circuit." To the degree that anxiety mediates the relationship between beliefs and psychological well-being, the effects of religious and other beliefs on anxiety indirectly affect positive measures of psychological well-being, such as happiness.

References

1. Krause, N. (2007). Stressors arising in highly valued roles and change in feeling close to God over time. *The International Journal for the Psychology of Religion, 17*(1), 17–36.
2. Proctor, M. T., Miner, M., McLean, L. D. S, & Bonab, B. G. (2009). Exploring Christians' explicit attachment to God representations: The development of a template for assessing attachment to God experiences. *Journal of Psychology and Theology, 37*(4), 245–264.
3. Miner, M. H. (2007). Back to the basics in attachment to God: revisiting theory in light of theology. *Journal of Psychology & Theology, 35*(2), 112–122.
4. James, W. (1902). *The varieties of religious experience: A study of human nature*. London: Longmans, Green, and Company.

5. Caughey, J. L. (1978). Artificial social relations in modern America. *American Quarterly, 30*(1), 70–89.
6. Wikstrom, O. (1987). Attribution, roles and religion: A theoretical analysis of Sunden's role theory of religion and the attribution approach to religious experience. *Journal for the Scientific Study of Religion, 26*(3), 390–400.
7. Pollner, M. (1989). Divine relations, social relations and well-being. *Journal of Health and Social Behavior, 30*(March), 92–104.
8. Ellison, C.G. (1991). Religious involvement and subjective well-being. *Journal of Health and Social Behavior, 32*(1), 80–99
9. Krause, N. (2004). Assessing the relationships among prayer expectancies, race, and self-esteem in late life. *Journal for the Scientific Study of Religion, 43*(3), 395–408.
10. Kirkpatrick, L. A. (2005). *Attachment, evolution, and the psychology of religion.* Guilford Press: New York.
11. Pargament, K. I. (1997). *The psychology of religion and coping: Theory, research, practice.* New York: Guilford Press.
12. Chen, Y. Y., & Koenig, H. G. (2006). Do people turn to religion in times of stress?: An examination of change in religiousness among elderly, medically ill patients. *Journal of Nervous and Mental Disease, 194*(2), 114–120.
13. Pargament, K. I., & Hahn, J. (1986). God and the just world: Causal and coping attributions to God in health situations. *Journal for the Scientific Study of Religion, 25*(2), 193–207.
14. Schuster, M. A., Stein, B. D., Jaycox, L. H., Collins, R. L., Marshall, G. N., Elliott, M. N., et al. (2001). A national survey of stress reactions after the September 11, 2001, terrorist attacks. *New England Journal of Medicine, 345*(20), 1507–1512.
15. Lynn Gall, T., & Cornblat, M. W. (2002). Breast cancer survivors give voice: A qualitative analysis of spiritual factors in long-term adjustment. *Psycho-Oncology, 11*(6), 524–535.
16. Jenkins, R. A., & Pargament, K. I. (1988). Cognitive appraisals in cancer patients. *Social Science & Medicine, 26*(6), 625–633.
17. Pargament, K. I. (1990). God help me: Toward a theoretical framework of coping for the psychology of religion. *Journal for the Scientific Study of Religion, 29*, 195–224.
18. Pargament, K. I., Kennell, J., Hathaway, W., Grevengoed, N., Newman, J., & Jones, W. (1988). Religion and the problem-solving process: Three styles of coping. *Journal for the Scientific Study of Religion, 27*(1), 90–104.
19. Fox, C. A., Blanton, P. W., & Morris, M. L. (1998). Religious problem-solving styles: Three styles revisited. *Journal for the Scientific Study of Religion, 37*(4), 673–677.
20. Wong-McDonald, A., & Gorsuch, R. L. (2000). Surrender to God: An additional coping style? *Journal of Psychology & Theology, 28*(2), 149–161.
21. Schaefer, C. A., & Gorsuch, R. L. (1991). Psychological adjustment and religiousness: The multivariate belief-motivation theory of religiousness. *Journal for the Scientific Study of Religion, 30*(4), 448–461.
22. Wittchen, H. U., & Boyer, P. (1998). Screening for anxiety disorders: Sensitivity and specificity of the Anxiety Screening Questionnaire (ASQ-15). *British Journal of Psychiatry, 34*, 10–17.
23. Spielberger, C. R., Gorsuch, R. L., & Lushene, R. (1970). *Manual for the state-trait anxiety inventory*. Palo Alto: Consulting Press.
24. Fabricatore, A. N., Handal, P. J., Rubio, D. M., & Gilner, F. H. (2004). Stress, religion, and mental health: Religious coping in mediating and moderating roles. *The International Journal for the Psychology of Religion, 14*(2), 91–108.
25. Koenig, H. G., Pargament, K. I., & Nielsen, J. (1998). Religious coping and health status in medically ill hospitalized older adults. *Journal of Nervous and Mental Disease, 186*(9), 513–521.
26. Bosworth, H. D., Park, K.-S., & McQuoid, D. R. (2003). The impact of religious practice and religious coping on geriatric depression. *International Journal of Geriatric Psychiatry, 18*(10), 905–914.

27. Bowie, J., Curbow, B., Laveist, T., Fitzgerald, S., & Pargament, K. (2001). The relationship between religious coping style and anxiety over breast cancer in African American women. *Journal of Religion and Health, 40*(4), 411–422.
28. Pargament, K. I., Cole, B., Vandecreck, L., Belavich, T., Brant, C., & Perez, L. (1999). The vigil: Religion and the search for control in the hospital waiting room. *Journal of Health Psychology, 4*(3), 327–341.
29. Schaefer, C. A., & Gorsuch, R. L. (1993). Situational and personal variations in religious coping. *Journal for the Scientific Study of Religion, 32*(2), 136–147.
30. Bickel, C. O., Ciarrocchi, J. W., Sheers, N. J., Estadt, B. K., Powell, D. A., & Pargament, K. I. (1998). Perceived stress, religious coping styles, and depressive affect. *Journal of Psychology and Christianity, 17*(1), 33–42.
31. Phillips, R. E., Pargament, K. I., Lynn, Q. K., & Crossley, C. D. (2004). Self-directing religious coping: A deistic God, abandoning God, or no God at all? *Journal for the Scientific Study of Religion, 43*(3), 409–418.
32. Burker, E. J., Evon, D. M., Sedway, J. A., & Egan, T. (2005). Religious and non-religious coping in lung transplant candidates: Does adding God to the picture tell us more? *Journal of Behavioral Medicine, 28*(6), 513–526.
33. Krause, N. (2010). The social milieu of the church and religious coping responses: A longitudinal investigation of older Whites and older Blacks. *The International Journal for the Psychology of Religion, 20*(2), 109–129.
34. Krause, N., & Hayward, D. (2013). Older Mexican Americans and God-mediated control: Exploring the influence of Pentecostal/Evangelical affiliation. *Mental Health, Religion and Culture, 16*(3), 319–333.
35. Krause, N. (2005). God-mediated control and psychological well-being in late life. *Research on Aging, 27*(2), 136–164.
36. Krause, N. M. (2007). Social involvement in religious institutions and God-mediated control beliefs: A longitudinal investigation. *Journal for the Scientific Study of Religion, 46*(4), 519–537.
37. Krause, N. (2010). God-mediated control and change in self-rated health. *The International Journal for the Psychology of Religion, 20*(4), 267–287.
38. Hayward, R. D., & Krause, N. (2013). Trajectories of late-life change in God-mediated control. *The Journals of Gerontology. Series B, Psychological Sciences and Social Sciences, 68*(1), 49–58.
39. Krause, N. (2002). Church-based social support and health in old age: Exploring variations by race. *Journal of Gerontology, 57B*(6), S332–S347.
40. Taylor, R. J., Chatters, L. M., Jayakody, R., & Levin, J. S. (1996). Black and White differences in religious participation: A multisample comparison. *Journal for the Scientific Study of Religion, 35*(4), 403–410.
41. Taylor, R. J., Mattis, J., & Chatters, L. M. (1999). Subjective religiosity among African Americans: A synthesis of findings from five national samples. *Journal of Black Psychology, 25*(4), 524–543.
42. Schieman, S. (2008). The religious role and the sense of personal control. *Sociology of Religion, 69*(3), 273–296.
43. Schieman, S., & Bierman, A. (2007). Religious activities and change in the sense of divine control: Dimensions of social stratification as contingencies. *Sociology of Religion, 68*(4), 361–381.
44. Schieman, S., Pudrovska, T., & Milkie, M. (2005). The sense of divine control and the self-concept: A study of race differences in later-life. *Research on Aging, 27*, 165–196.
45. Schieman, S., Pudrovska, T., Pearlin, L. I., & Ellison, C. G. (2006). The sense of divine control and psychological distress: Variations across race and socioeconomic status. *Journal for the Scientific Study of Religion, 45*(4), 529–549.

46. Schieman, S., Bierman, A., & Ellison, C. G. (2010). Religious involvement, beliefs about God, and the sense of mattering among older adults. *Journal for the Scientific Study of Religion, 49*(3), 517–535.
47. Ellison, C. G., & Flannelly, K. J. (2009). Religious involvement and risk of major depression in a prospective nationwide study of African American adults. *Journal of Nervous and Mental Disease, 197*(8), 568–573.
48. Pargament, K. I., Smith, B. W., Koenig, H. G., & Perez, L. (1998). Patterns of positive and negative religious coping with major life stressors. *Journal for the Scientific Study of Religion, 37*(4), 710–724.
49. Harrison, M. O., Koenig, H. G., Hays, J. C., Eme-Akwari, A. G., & Pargament, K. I. (2001). The epidemiology of religious coping: A review of recent literature. *International Review of Psychiatry, 13*(2), 86–93.
50. Pargament, K. I., Koenig, H. G., & Perez, L. M. (2000). The many methods of religious coping: Development and Initial Validation of the RCOPE. *Journal of Clinical Psychology, 56*(4), 519–543.
51. Pargament, K. I., Zinnbauer, B. J., Scott, A. B., Butter, E. M., Zerowin, J., & Stanik, P. (1998). Red flags and religious coping: Identifying some religious warning signs among people in crisis. *Journal of Clinical Psychology, 54*(1), 77–89.
52. Ellison, C. G., & Lee, J. (2010). Spiritual struggles and psychological distress: Is there a dark side of religion? *Social Indicators Research, 98*(3), 501–517.
53. Kessler, R. C., Andrews, G., Colpe, L. J., Hiripi, E., Mroczek, D. K., Normand, S.-L. T., et al. (2002). Short screening scales to monitor population prevalences and trends in non-specific psychological distress. *Psychological Medicine, 32*(6), 959–976.
54. Krause, N., & Hayward, R. (2012). Social factors in the church and positive religious coping responses: Assessing differences smong older Whites, older Blacks, and older Mexican Americans. *Review of Religious Research, 54*(4), 519–541.
55. Krause, N., Ellison, C. G., Shaw, B. A., Marcum, J. R., & Boardman, J. D. (2001). Church-based social support and religious coping. *Journal for the Scientific Study of Religion, 40*(4), 637–656.
56. Gaudette, H., & Jankowski, K. R. (2013). Spiritual coping and anxiety in palliative care patients: A pilot study. *Journal of Health Care Chaplaincy, 19*(4), 131–139.
57. Ano, G. G., & Vasconcelles, E. B. (2005). Religious coping and psychological adjustment to stress: A meta-analysis. *Journal of Clinical Psychology, 61*(4), 461–480.
58. Ellison, C. G., Roalson, L. A., Guillory, J. M., Flannelly, K. J., & Marcum, J. P. (2010). Religious resources, spiritual struggles, and mental health in a nationwide sample of PCUSA clergy. *Pastoral Psychology, 59*(3), 287–304.
59. Ellison, C. G., Fang, Q., Flannelly, K. J., & Steckler, R. A. (2013). Spiritual struggles and mental health: Exploring the moderating effects of religious identity. *The International Journal for the Psychology of Religion, 23*, 214–229.
60. McConnell, K. M., Pargament, K. I., Ellison, C. G., & Flannelly, K. J. (2006). Examining the links between spiritual struggles and symptoms of psychopathology in a national sample. *Journal of Clinical Psychology, 62*(12), 1469–1484.

Chapter 21
Belief in God as an Attachment Figure and Mental Health

Abstract The first section of the chapter explains Attachment Theory, what an attachment figure is, and attachment styles (avoidant, anxious, and secure attachment). The second section covers the application of Attachment Theory to religion, including the concept that God can be an attachment figure because God provides a sense of security and safety to individuals (a "safe base" in Attachment Theory terms) and a "safe haven" when facing threats of potential harm. As these are two essential characteristics of secure attachment in mother-infant relationships, believing one has a secure attachment to God is a special case of believing one has a positive relationship with God, which is supported by a large nationwide survey of American Protestants. The next sections summarize the results of studies of convenience samples of primarily U.S. college students and three large national studies of American adults, which found: (a) that believing one has a secure attachment to God has a salubrious association with mental health, including psychiatric symptoms, and (b) believing one has an anxious or avoidant attachment to God has a pernicious association with mental health, including psychiatric symptoms. The final section of the chapter demonstrates that anxiety symptoms mediate the relationship between perceived attachment to God and happiness. The main results of all the research are interpreted within ETAS Theory to mean that believing one has a secure attachment to God provides a sense of safety, which reduces the brain's assessment that the world is dangerous, whereas believing one has an anxious or avoidant attachment to God does not provide this sense of safety.

Keywords Attachment to God • Attachment Theory • God • Happiness • ETAS Theory • Psychiatric symptoms • Psychological distress psychological well-being • Safety • Threat • Uncertainty

The present chapter briefly traces the history of Attachment Theory, and summarizes research on its application to various religious phenomena, including research on the premise that people can have an attachment to God. Then, it summarizes research on the relationship between mental health and the belief that God is an attachment figure. I consider beliefs about one's attachment to God to be a special case of beliefs about one's relationship with God in that the former beliefs are linked to a well-established theory of psychological development that leads to specific

K.J. Flannelly, *Religious Beliefs, Evolutionary Psychiatry, and Mental Health in America*, Religion, Spirituality and Health: A Social Scientific Approach 1,
DOI 10.1007/978-3-319-52488-7_21

predictions about mental health. Paul Gilbert has implied that the "attachment system" is the "safety system" of the brain, which may be partially true, although I think there are other proximate mechanisms that provide a sense of safety.

21.1 Attachment Theory

The British psychologist John Bowlby developed Attachment Theory based on his research into the mother-infant bond [1–3], which he began in the 1940s as a complement to his work as a child psychiatrist [4]. Bowlby wanted to introduce an evolutionary perspective to psychoanalytical thought about human development by applying ethological concepts and analyses [5, 6] to personality development [4, 7]. Bowlby was especially interested in Konrad Lorenz's concept of imprinting, which describes how young birds bond with their parents. Imprinting had been shown to have profound effects on adult relationships, and Bowlby [1] recognized that imprinting had implications for human development. Whereas psychoanalytic theory presumed that the mother-infant bond was a by-product of oral gratification related to hunger and feeding [8], Bowlby proposed that the mother-infant bond was a primary motivational system that evolved to ensure the survival of offspring. This perspective was supported, in part, by research conducted by American psychologist Harry Harlow [9], whose findings showed that infant monkeys formed attachments to their mothers through bodily contact ("contact comfort" as Harlow called it) rather than through food reinforcement.

Bowlby said the fundamental tenets of Attachment Theory "are that the human infant comes into the world genetically biased to develop a set of behavioral patterns that, given an appropriate environment, will result in his keeping more or less close proximity to whomever cares for him, and that this tendency to maintain proximity serves the function of protecting the mobile infant and growing child from a number of dangers, amongst which in man's environment of evolutionary [history] the danger of predation [was] likely to have been paramount" (p. 9) [7] . The basic repertoire of behaviors the child exhibits to facilitate attachment are innate, species-typical, fixed-action patterns [1, 5]. They are what I have referred to elsewhere in this book as proximate mechanisms, some of which maintain contact (e.g., sucking, clinging, following) and some of which signal the child's interest in keeping close to its mother (e.g., smiling and gurgling) [1]. Since the major purpose of the human attachment system is to protect young children from physical harm, it interacts with the child's brain systems involved in fear and defense. Bowlby proposed that the attachment system responds not only to immediate threats of harm, but also to potential threats of harm, saying: "man, like other animals, responds with fear to certain situations, not because they carry a *high* risk of pain or danger, but because they signal an *increase* of risk" (p. 9) [7].

Bowlby thought children form an "internal working model" of their own self-worth (or self-esteem) and an "internal working model" of their "attachment figure" (typically, their mother) around 1 year of age [10]. Both of these internal models are strongly influenced by the ability of the attachment figure to provide attention and care. The American psychologist Lee Kirkpatrick described children's "internal working model" of their attachment figure as "a set of expectations and beliefs – a *schema* in cognitive terms – about the availability and responsiveness of their primary caregivers" (p. 38). Such working models of ourselves and others are thought to affect the quality of our relationships throughout life [11–13] – especially, romantic relationships [14–16].

The American psychologist Mary Ainsworth, who worked with Bowlby in the early 1950s [4] , later conducted two classic studies that confirmed and extended Attachment Theory. A major finding of her research was the observation that there were substantial differences in the quality of mother-infant interactions [17], which she classified into three basic styles of attachment based on the patterns of behavior exhibited by the child: secure, anxious-avoidant, anxious-ambivalent attachment [17, 18]. Anxious-avoidant and anxious-ambivalent attachment came to be known simply as avoidant attachment and anxious attachment, respectively. The most obvious differences between children with different attachment styles was the behavior of children with secure attachment: (1) they used their mother as a "safe base" from which to interact with strangers and explore strange places, (2) they became upset when separated from their mother, and (3) they quickly sought proximity to their mother when their mother returned after being out of sight [4, 18, 19].

Ainsworth's observations about the behavior of children with secure attachment were consistent with Bowlby's [1, 3] prototypical or ideal infant-mother attachment relationship, in which proximity to the attachment figure provides a sense of the security and safety (a "safe base") that encourages play, exploration, and affiliative relationships. The ideal attachment figure should also provide a "safe haven" when the child is threatened with harm or frightened for whatever reason, according to Attachment Theory. Some theorists and researchers have characterized Ainsworth's three attachment styles as answers to a child's question: Can I rely on this person to be available and responsive when I need him/her? The answers to the question are: "yes" (secure), "no" (avoidant), and "maybe" (anxious) [20, 21]. Bowlby considered the "safe haven" and "secure base" roles of the attachment figure to be closely related in that both roles provide a sense of protection, such that individuals who are confident they can rely on their attachment figure will be "much less prone to either intense or chronic fear than will an individual who … has no such confidence" (p. 202) [3].

Several criteria have been proposed to define attachment relationships [11, 22], including the following: (1) that the individual believes the attachment figure provides (a) care and protection and a safe haven from harm, and (b) a sense of security in the absence of a threat of harm – a secure base from which to explore the word; and (2) that the individual (a) seeks proximity to the attachment figure – especially when alarmed or afraid, and (b) becomes anxious when separated from the attachment figure [11, 20, 23]. Attachment relationships are thought to differ from other types of social relationships and other familial or kinship relationships that lack these characteristics [11, 24] in that attachment relationships tend to be more inherently stable and more enduring than other social relationships [11, 20, 23].

Research on adult attachment styles began in the 1970s [21, 24] and interest in adult attachment has increased over the years. American psychologists Cindy Hazan and Phillip Shaver [25] developed a self-report questionnaire modeled on Ainsworth's attachment styles. Their work and subsequent research has found that the proportions of the three attachment styles in adults [15, 25] are generally comparable to those found in Ainsworth's experimental studies of infants: 55% secure attachment, 25% avoidant attachment, and 20% anxious attachment [26]. Other studies of adult attachment have recognized up to three styles other than secure attachment in adults [27, 28], but many studies have only distinguished between two broad categories of attachment styles: "secure" and "insecure" [16, 20, 28]. It is important to note that even though attachment reflects the relationship between two individuals, it is usually measured in adults only from the perspective of the attached person.

Although most research on the neural foundations of Attachment Theory has focused on neurochemistry [29–31], neuro-anatomical studies have implicated areas of the limbic system (i.e., the amygdala, anterior cingulate cortex, hippocampus, and insula) [30, 32–37] and the prefrontal cortex (i.e., the dorsolateral PFC, orbitofrontal PFC, and ventromedial PFC (vmPFC) in attachment) [30, 32–38]. The role of the vmPFC appears to be particularly important because it is specifically attuned to safety cues [33] and it inhibits the amygdala's ability to generate fear [39, 40].

21.2 Attachment Theory Applied to Religion

Lee Kirkpatrick and Philip Shaver [41] contended that the application of Attachment Theory to religion follows logically from the notion that religion provides security in a world of uncertainty [42, 43]. Since their early research, Attachment Theory has been applied to explain various religious phenomena [44–50], including "new age" spiritual attitudes [22], religious coping styles [51], religious doubts [47], religious conversion [44, 46], and other changes in religious beliefs and behavior [48].

Three articles by Kirkpatrick and his colleagues in the early 1990s proposed that a person's relationship with God should be considered to be an attachment relationship [23, 41, 52]. Kirkpatrick based this proposal, in part, on the writings of the Christian theologian Gordon D. Kaufman [53] and the sociologist Bruce D. Reed [54]. In Kirkpatrick and Shaver's words: "Much like an infant's primary caregiver, God may serve as a secure base and as a safe haven of safety and comfort for believers" (p. 267) [52].

While all three articles by Kirkpatrick proposed that God serves the functions of an attachment figure in being a safe haven and a secure base, the evidence that these articles provided to support this proposition was limited. A 1992 article by Kirkpatrick probably made the best case that God is a safe haven for religious persons [23], citing studies that show Americans are more likely to turn to religion and God when confronted by a crisis. This point is supported by other studies, as well [55, 56]. However, one study cited by Kirkpatrick [23] is especially relevant because it indicated that people are more likely to look to God when faced with a threat of severe illness or physical injury than they are to look to God when faced with moral issues [57]; this may be taken to imply that some people are more inclined to view God as a source of comfort and protection from harm than they are to view God as a source of moral guidance.

Kirkpatrick proposed that attachment to God meets another criterion of an attachment relationship in that praying to God is equivalent, in some sense, to seeking proximity with an attachment figure. The Anglican theologian Bruce Reed, for instance, drew a parallel between a child's crying to attract the attention of its attachment figure and petitionary prayer (i.e., asking God for something) [54], and a study by the German theologian Friedrich Heiler reported that religious persons believe they are in a close personal relationship with God and are speaking directly to God when they pray [58].

Many studies on attachment to God have examined the nature and plausibility of the concept, and how one's attachment to one's parents is related to one's attachment to God, e.g., [49, 59–61]. The findings of that research generally indicate that the attachment style individuals report to have had with their parents is the same as the attachment style they reportedly have with God. Nevertheless, it is still an open question whether individuals' attachment relationship with their parents is associated with their beliefs about their current attachment to God [62–64].

Several American studies have reported that adult attachment is related to one's beliefs about God [41, 65]. For instance, a study of more than 200 American adults found that believing one has a secure attachment to God had a significant positive correlation ($r = .25$) with their belief in a loving God, whereas believing that one has as an avoidant attachment to God had a significant negative correlation with belief in a personal God ($r = -.52$) [41]. Similarly a large nationwide survey of members of the Presbyterian Church (USA) found that believing one has a secure attachment to God is associated with the belief that God is loving ($r = .39$), whereas believing one has an anxious attachment to God is associated with the belief that God is remote ($r = .30$) [66].

21.3 Beliefs About One's Attachment to God and Mental Health

21.3.1 Attachment to God and Psychological Well-Being

Two small studies of college students by Lee Kirkpatrick and his colleagues in the 1990s found that individuals who believed they had a secure attachment to God were more satisfied with their lives, and less anxious, lonely, and depressed than those who believed they had an avoidant or anxious attachment to God [52, 67]. Subsequent research primarily has used sophisticated scales to measure attachment to God that were published by Wade Rowatt and Lee Kirpatrick in 2002 [68] and Richard Beck and Angie McDonald in 2004 [69]. Both scales measure the same two styles of attachment – avoidant and anxious attachment – with secure attachment being the opposite of avoidant attachment on the Rowatt and Kirpatrick scale.

Four studies have reported that avoidant and anxious attachment are negatively related to self-esteem, life satisfaction, and positive affect [70–73], as measured, respectively, by the Roesenberg [74], the Diener [75], and Watson [76] scales. Figure 21.1 shows the results from the two studies that analyzed the association

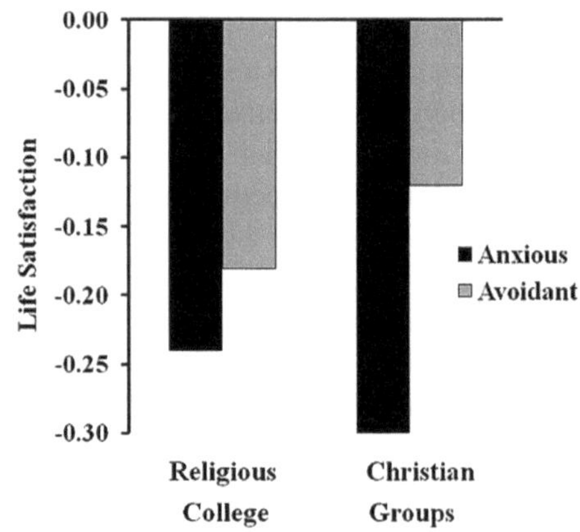

Fig. 21.1 Association between life satisfaction and anxious and avoidant attachment in two studies; All associations are statistically significant

between life satisfaction and believing that one has an avoidant and anxious attachment with God. One studied a sample of undergraduates at a religious college in the U.S. (labeled Religious College), and the other studied students who belonged to university-based Christian organizations (labeled Christian Groups) in the U.S. and U.K. The studies found that believing that one has either of these two types of poor attachment to God had pernicious associations with life satisfaction. However, believing that one has an anxious attachment to God had a larger pernicious association with life satisfaction than believing one has an avoidant attachment to God in both samples (see Fig. 21.1).

A Canadian study of Christian church congregants found an even larger inverse association between anxious attachment and life satisfaction ($\beta = -.41$), after controlling for age and life stressors. The results of all five studies indicate that believing that one has a poor relationship with God (avoidant attachment) or that one has an ambivalent or inconsistent relationship with God (anxious attachment) undermines psychological well-being among Christians. Conversely, the studies conducted by Kirkpatrick and his colleges in the 1990s indicated that believing one has a secure relationship with God enhances psychological well-being.

21.3.2 *Attachment to God and Psychological Distress*

Two studies by Chris Ellison and his colleagues examined the degree to which secure attachment and anxious attachment to God were associated with psychological distress [66, 77], (measured by the K6 [78]),[1] controlling for demographic, religious, and other variables. The first study surveyed over 1000 members of the Presbyterian Church (USA), and the second study surveyed the same sample 1 year later. The first study (Study 1 in Fig. 21.2) found that church members who believed they had a secure attachment to God had a significant salubrious association with psychological

[1] The K6 consists of six items that measure symptoms of anxiety and depression.

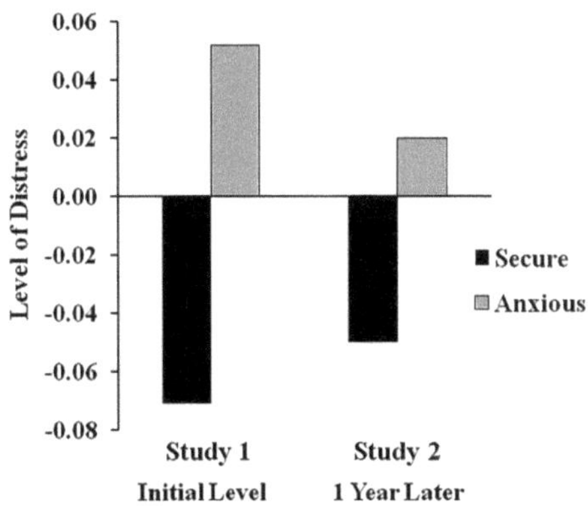

Fig. 21.2 Association between psychological distress and secure and anxious attachment in two studies; Study 1 measured the participants' "initial" level of distress and Study 2 measured their level of distress 1 year later; Values are standardized regression coefficients (β's)

distress whereas church members who believed they had an anxious attachment to God had a significant pernicious association with psychological distress. The second study (Study 2) found that psychological distress decreased during the intervening year among the church members who believed they had a secure relationship with God. Because the second study compared changes in the net effects of attachment styles over 1 year, it provides evidence that believing one has a secure attachment with God is causally related to lower levels of psychological distress.

21.3.3 Attachment to God and Psychiatric Symptoms

A more recent study by Ellison and his colleagues examined attachment to God and psychiatric symptoms using data from the 2010 Baylor Religion Survey. The study analyzed the association between the four classes of anxiety disorders and beliefs about one's attachment to God: i.e., secure attachment and anxious attachment.

As shown in Fig. 21.3, bivariate correlations (Pearson's r) showed that the symptoms of all four of classes of anxiety disorders had significant salubrious associations with secure attachment to God and significant pernicious associations with anxious attachment to God (black bars). Subsequent multivariate regression analyses controlled for demographic, religious, and other variables.

The results of the multivariate analyses (gray bars in Fig. 21.3, β's) found a pernicious association between anxious attachment to God and all four classes of symptoms. However, no significant association was found for secure attachment.[2] Nevertheless,

[2] As mentioned earlier in the book, the correlation coefficient (r) is a measure of the strength of association between two numerical variables in correlational analysis and beta (β) is a measure of the strength of association between one numerical variable and one or more other numerical variables in regression analysis. If the regression model only involves two variables, β is identical to r, but β usually decreases when the association between one variable and another variable (such as secure attachment with GA, SA, Obs, or Comp in Fig 21.3) when control variables are included in the regression model. However, the inclusion of secure attachment and anxious attachment (which had a strong negative correlation with each other) in the same regression model accentuated the effect of the anxious attachment while reducing the effect of secure attachment.

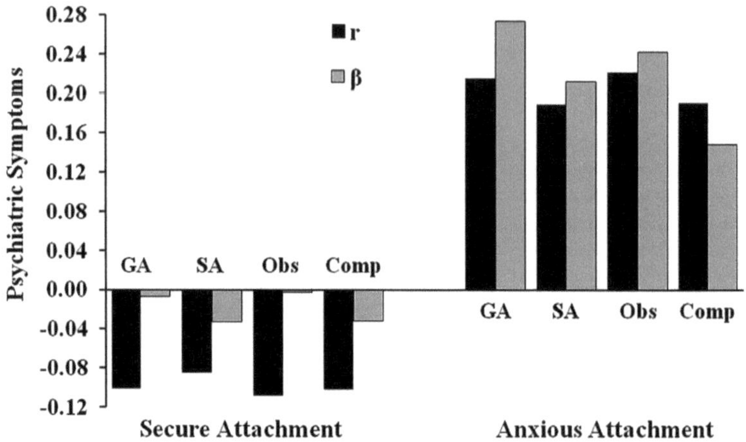

Fig. 21.3 Associations between symptoms of anxiety disorders and beliefs about one's attachment to God in bivariate and multivariate analyses (Ellison et al. [81]); *GA* General Anxiety, *SA* Social Anxiety, *Obs* Obsession, *Comp* Compulsion; All Pearson *r*'s are significant; All β's are significant for anxious attachment

the effect of secure attachment emerged again in moderation analyses that examined the interaction of secure attachment and prayer. The analyses showed that people who believed they had a secure attachment to God and prayed frequently had less severe symptoms than those who prayed less frequently. Thus, prayer appears to have reduced psychiatric symptoms among people who believed they had a secure attachment to God. No interaction effect was found between prayer and anxious attachment.

21.3.4 Mediating Effect of Anxiety on the Association Between Attachment to God and Happiness

Once again, I used the Baylor Religious Survey's measure of happiness as a dependent variable to analyze the potential mediating effect of anxiety-disorder symptoms on the association between beliefs and psychological well-being. In this case, I used the three items measuring anxious attachment to God and the first three of the items measuring secure attachment to God as the independent variables. Anxiety-disorder symptoms were significantly correlated with anxious attachment ($r = .246$, $p < .001$) and secure attachment ($r = -.086$, $p < .001$), and happiness was significantly correlated with anxious attachment ($r = -.241$, $p < .001$) and secure attachment ($r = .188$, $p < .001$).

Figure 21.4 shows that believing one has an anxious attachment to God had a significant pernicious association with happiness and believing one has a secure attachment to God had a significant salubrious association with happiness in regression Model 1. Both associations were reduced in magnitude but remained statistically significant in regression Model 2, which included anxiety-disorder symptoms.

Fig. 21.4 Mediation effects of symptoms of anxiety-disorders on the association of happiness with beliefs about having an anxious attachment or a secure attachment with God; Values are standardized regression coefficients; ***$p < .001$

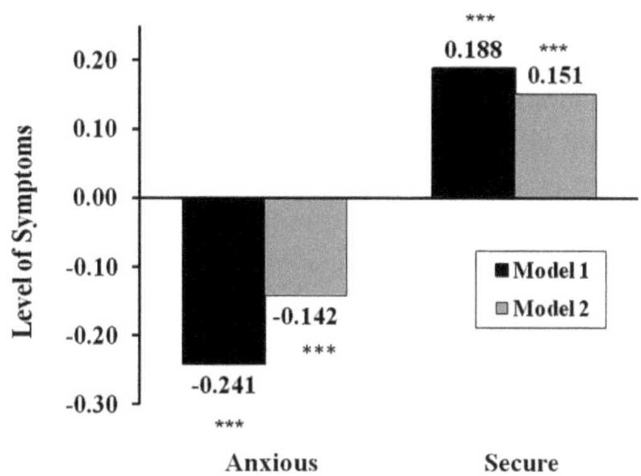

These results indicate that anxiety-disorder symptoms partially mediated the association between happiness and both beliefs about attachment to God.[3]

21.4 Chapter Highlights and Comments

Attachment Theory has been applied to several aspects of religious experience, including one's attachment to God. Overall, the belief that one has a secure attachment to God has a salubrious association with psychological well-being, psychological distress, and psychiatric symptoms. Despite the obvious fact that believing one has a secure attachment to God is not the same as having a secure attachment to another person, such a belief may activate the same neural systems involved in being attached to a person. Based on the ETAS Theory, the salubrious effect of believing one has a secure attachment to God results from the fact that this belief provides a sense of safety, which makes the vmPFC increase the threshold of what constitutes a threat; thus, it inhibits amygdala activity, which decreases anxiety-related psychiatric symptoms.

The belief that one has an anxious or avoidant attachment to God, on the other hand, has a pernicious association with psychological well-being, psychological distress, and psychiatric symptoms. As avoidant attachment entails the belief that God is cold, unsupportive, and unconcerned about one's life, this belief does not provide a sense of security; hence, psychological distress among people who have these beliefs is elevated relative to persons who believe they have a secure attachment with God. Belief that one has an anxious attachment to God may have a more pernicious effect on mental health because it involves uncertainty about God's caring and responsiveness, and research related to ETAS Theory demonstrates that uncertainty directly elicits anxiety.

It is possible that some of the observed effects of beliefs about God on mental health, which were described in the preceding chapters, may be attributable to the fact that these beliefs tap into the attachment system, which Paul Gilbert claims is the

[3] The mediation effect which was confirmed by the Sobel-Goodman test.

safety system of the brain. Although the existence of a safety system is not directly relevant to ETAS Theory, the attachment system is thought to be involved in the development of self-esteem, which is directly relevant to ETAS Theory. Therefore, it would be worthwhile to be able to differentiate between (a) the direct effects of a sense of safety on anxiety that are attributable to believing one has a secure attachment to God and (b) the indirect effects of a sense of safety attributable to the elevated self-esteem that results from believing one has a secure attachment to God.

Kirkpatrick considered praying to God to be the equivalent of seeking proximity with an attachment figure in Attachment Theory. Prayer can also be regarded as an expression of belief, in the context of ETAS Theory, based on the findings of Neal Krause [79, 80]. Thus, the interaction effect of prayer and secure attachment on the symptoms of anxiety disorders observed by Ellison et al. [81] presumably reflects the interaction of beliefs, as proposed by ETAS Theory.

The findings reported in this chapter confirm the findings from Chap. 19 that happiness is influenced by anxiety, which is consistent with the ETAS Theory notion that anxiety mediates the influences of religious beliefs on positive emotions. Thus, the mediation effects reported in this and Chap. 19 support the idea that the threat assessments and the beliefs that modulate them appear to affect positive emotions.

References

1. Bowlby, J. (1969). *Attachment and loss: Volume 1: Attachment.* New York: Basic Books.
2. Bowlby, J. (1980). *Attachment and Loss: Volume 3: Loss.* New York: Basic Books.
3. Bowlby, J. (1973). *Attachment and loss: Volume 2. Separation: Anxiety, and anger.* New York: Basic Books.
4. Bretherton, I. (1992). The origins of attachment theory: John Bowlby and Mary Ainsworth. *Developmental Psychology, 28*(5), 759–775.
5. Tinbergen, N. (1972). *The animal in its world: Explorations of an ethologist, 1932–1972.* Cambridge, MA: Harvard University Press.
6. Lorenz, K. Z. (1981). *The foundations of ethology* (R. W. Kickert, Trans.). New York: Springer.
7. Bowlby, J. (1984). Psychoanalysis as a natural science. *Psychoanalytic Psychology, 1*(1), 7–21.
8. Bowlby, J. (1958). The nature of the child's tie to his mother. *The International Journal of Psycho-Analysis, 39*, 350–373.
9. Harlow, H. F. (1958). The nature of love. *American Psychologist, 13*(12), 673–685.
10. Bowlby, J. (1988). *A secure base.* New York: Basic Books.
11. Ainsworth, M. D. S. (1985). Attachments across the life span. *Bulletin of the New York Academy of Medicine, 61*(9), 792–812.
12. Ainsworth, M. S. (1989). Attachments beyond infancy. *American Psychologist, 44*(4), 709–716.
13. Ainsworth, M.D.S. (1991). Attachments and other affectional bonds across the life span. In C. M. Parkes, J. Stevenson-Hinde, & P. Marris (Eds.), *Attachment across the life cycle* (pp. 33–51). London: Routledge.
14. Collins, N. L., & Read, S. J. (1990). Adult attachment, working models, and relationship quality in dating couples. *Journal of Personality and Social Psychology, 58*(4), 644–663.
15. Feeney, J. A., & Noller, P. (1990). Attachment style as a predictor of adult romantic relationships. *Journal of Personality and Social Psychology, 58*(2), 281–291.
16. Brennan, K. A., Clark, C. L., & Shaver, P. R. (1998). Self-report measurement of adult romantic attachment: An integrative overview. In J. A. Simpson, & W. S. Rholes (Eds.), *Attachment theory and close relationships* (pp. 46–76). New York: Guilford Press.

17. Ainsworth, M. S. (1979). Infant–mother attachment. *American Psychologist, 34*(10), 932–937.
18. Ainsworth, M. D. S. (1985). Patterns of infant-mother attachments: Antecedents and effects on development. *Bulletin of the New York Academy of Medicine, 61*(9), 771–791.
19. Ainsworth, M. S., & Bowlby, J. (1991). An ethological approach to personality development. *American Psychologist, 46*(4), 333–341.
20. Kirkpatrick, L. A. (2005). *Attachment, evolution, and the psychology of religion*. New York: Guilford Press.
21. Hazan, C., & Shaver, P. R. (1994). Attachment as an organizational framework for research on close relationships. *Psychological Inquiry, 5*(1), 1–22.
22. Granqvist, P., & Hagekull, B. (2001). Seeking security in the new age: On attachment and emotional compensation. *Journal for the Scientific Study of Religion, 40*(3), 527–545.
23. Kirkpatrick, L. A. (1992). An attachment-theory approach to the psychology of religion. *The International Journal for the Psychology of Religion, 2*(1), 3–28.
24. Weiss, R. S. (1982). Attachment in adults. In C. M. Parkes, & J. Stevenson-Hinde (Eds.), *The place of attachment in human behavior* (pp. 171–184). New York: Basic Books.
25. Hazan, C., & Shaver, P. (1987). Romantic love conceptualized as an attachment process. *Journal of Personality and Social Psychology, 52*(3), 511–524.
26. Campos, J. J., Barrett, K., Lamb, M. E., Goldsmith, H. H., & Stenberg, C. (1983). Socioemotional development. In P. H. Mussen (Ed.), *Handbook of child psychology: Vol. 2, Infancy and developmental psychobiology* (pp. 783–915). New York: Wiley.
27. Bartholomew, K., & Horowitz, L. M. (1991). Attachment styles among young adults: A test of a four-category model. *Journal of Personality and Social Psychology, 61*(2), 226–244
28. Bartholomew, K., & Shaver, P. R. (1998). Methods of assessing adult attachment: Do they converge? In J. A. Simpson, & W. S. Rhodes (Eds.), *Attachment theory and close relationships* (pp. 25–45). New York: Guilford Press.
29. Hruby, R., Hasto, J., & Minarik, P. (2011). Attachment in integrative neuroscientific perspective. *Neuroendocrinology Letters, 32*(2), 111–120.
30. Vrticka, P., & Vuilleumier, P. (2012). Neuroscience of human social interactions and adult attachment style. *Frontiers in Human Neuroscience, 6,* 212.
31. Young, K. A., Liu, Y., & Wang, Z. (2008). The neurobiology of social attachment: A comparative approach to behavioral, neuroanatomical, and neurochemical studies. *Comparative Biochemistry and Physiology; Part C: Toxicology & Pharmacology, 148*(4), 401–410.
32. Coria-Avila, G. A., Manzo, J., Garcia, L. I., Carrillo, P., Miguel, M., & Pfaus, J. G. (2008). Neurobiology of social attachments. *Comparative Biochemistry and Physiology. Toxicology & Pharmacology, 148*(4), 401–410.
33. Eisenberger, N. I., Master, S. L., Inagaki, T. K., Taylor, S. E., Shirinyan, D., Lieberman, M. D., et al. (2011). Attachment figures activate a safety signal-related neural region and reduce pain experience. *Proceedings of the National Academy of Sciences, 108*(28), 11721–11726.
34. Moutsiana, C., Fearon, P., Murray, L., Cooper, P., Goodyer, I., Johnstone, T., et al. (2014). Making an effort to feel positive: Insecure attachment in infancy predicts the neural underpinnings of emotion regulation in adulthood. *Journal of Child Psychology & Psychiatry, 55*(9), 999–1008.
35. Noriuchi, M., Kikuchi, Y., & Senoo, A. (2008). The functional neuroanatomy of maternal love: Mother's response to infant's attachment behaviors. *Biological Psychiatry, 63*(4), 415–423.
36. Vrticka, P., Sander, D., Vuilleumier, P., & Bondolfi, G. (2012). The neural substrates of social emotion perception and regulation are modulated by adult attachment style. *Social Neuroscience, 7*(5), 473–493.
37. Coan, J. A. (2010). Adult attachment and the brain. *Journal of Social and Personal Relationships, 27*(2), 210–217.
38. Minagawa-Kawai, Y., Matsuoka, S. D. I, Naoi, N., Nakamura, K., & Kojima, S. (2009). Prefrontal activation associated with social attachment: Facial-emotion recognition in mothers and infants. *Cerebral Cortex, 19*(2), 284–292.

39. Motzkin, J. C., Philippi, C. L., Wolf, R. C., Koenigs, M., & Baskaya, M. K. (2015). Ventromedial prefrontal cortex is critical for the regulation of amygdala activity in humans. *Biological Psychiatry, 77*(3), 276–284.
40. Greenberg, T., Carlson, J. M., Cha, J., Hajcak, G., & Mujica-Parodi, L. R. (2013). Ventromedial prefrontal cortex reactivity is altered in generalized anxiety disorder during fear generalization. *Depression and Anxiety, 30*(3), 242–250.
41. Kirkpatrick, L. A., & Shaver, P. R. (1990). Attachment theory and religion: Childhood attachments, religious beliefs, and conversations. *Journal for the Scientific Study of Religion, 29*(3), 315–334.
42. Radin, P. (1957). *Primitive religion: Its nature and origin*. New York: Dover Press.
43. Thouless, R. (1971). An introduction to the psychology of religion (3rd ed.). Cambridge: *Cambridge University Press*.
44. Granqvist, P. (2003). Attachment theory and religious conversions: A review and a resolution of the classic and contemporary paradigm chasm. *Review of Religious Research, 45*(2), 172–187.
45. Granqvist, P., & Hagekull, B. (2003). Longitudinal predictions of religious change in adolescence: Contributions from the interaction of attachment and relationship status. *Journal of Social and Personal Relationships, 20*(6), 793–817.
46. Granqvist, P., & Kirkpatrick, L. A. (2004). Religious conversion and perceived childhood attachment: A meta-analysis. *The International Journal for the Psychology of Religion, 14*(4), 223–250.
47. Urbán, S., Kézdy, A., & Martos, T. (2011). The relationship between adult attachment and religious doubts. *Studia Universitatis Babes-Bolyai, Theologia Catholica Latina, 56*(2), 95–118.
48. Kirkpatrick, L. A. (1997). A longitudinal study of changes in religious belief and behavior as a function of individual differences in adult attachment style. *Journal for the Scientific Study of Religion, 36*(2), 207–217.
49. Granqvist, P., & Hagekull, B. (1999). Religiousness and perceived childhood attachment: Profiling socialized correspondence and emotional compensation. *Journal for the Scientific Study of Religion, 38*(2), 254–273.
50. Granqvist, P., & Hagekull, B. (2000). Religiosity, adult attachment, and why " singles" are more religious. *The International Journal for the Psychology of Religion, 10*(2), 111–123.
51. Granqvist, P. (2005). Building a bridge between attachment and religious coping: Tests of moderators and mediators. *Mental Health, Religion and Culture, 8(1)*, 35–47.
52. Kirkpatrick, L. A., & Shaver, P. R. (1992). An attachment-theoretical approach to romantic love and religious belief. *Personality and Social Psychology Bulletin, 18*(3), 266–275.
53. Kaufman, G. D. (1981). *The theological imagination: Constructing the concept of God*. Philadelphia: Westminister.
54. Reed, B. (1978). *The dynamics of religion: Process and movement and Christian churches*. London: Darton, Longman and Todd.
55. Argyle, M., & Beit-Hallahmi, B. (1975). *The social psychology of religion*. Boston: Routledge.
56. Pargament, K. I., Kennell, J., Hathaway, W., Grevengoed, N., Newman, J., & Jones, W. (1988). Religion and the problem-solving process: Three styles of coping. *Journal for the Scientific Study of Religion,* 27(1), 90–104.
57. Pargament, K. I., & Hahn, J. (1986). God and the just world: Causal and coping attributions to God in health situations. *Journal for the Scientific Study of Religion, 25*(2), 193–207.
58. Heiler, F. (1932). *Prayer: A study in the history and psychology of religion*. New York: Oxford University Press.
59. Biregard, A., & Granqvist, P. (2004). The correspondence between attachment to parents and God: Three experiments using subiminal separation cues. *Personality and Social Psychology Bulletin, 30*(9), 1122–1135.
60. Granqvist, P. (1998). Religiousness and perceived childhood attachment: On the question of compensation or correspondence. *Journal for the Scientific Study of Religion,* 37(2), 350–367.

61. Granqvist, P. (2002). Attachment and religiosity in adolescence: Cross-sectional and longitudinal evaluations. *Personality and Social Psychology Bulletin, 28*(2), 260–270.
62. Hall, T. W., Fujikawa, A., Halcrow, S. R., Hill, P. C., & Delaney, H. (2009). Attachment to God and implicit spirituality: Clarifying correspondence and compensation models. *Journal of Psychology and Theology, 37*(4), 227–242.
63. Miner, M. (2009). The impact of child-parent attachment, attachment to God and religious orientation on psychological adjustment. *Journal of Psychology and Theology, 37(2)*, 114–124.
64. Sim, T. N., & Loh, B. S. M. (2003). Attachment to God: Measurement and dynamics. *Journal of Social and Personal Relationships, 20*(3), 373–389.
65. Kirkpatrick, L. A. (1998). God as a subsitute attachment figure: A longitudinal study of adult attachment style and religious change in college students. *Personality and Social Psychology Bulletin, 24*(9), 961–973.
66. Bradshaw, M., Ellison, C. G., & Marcum, J. P. (2010). Attachment to God, images of God, and psychological distress in a nationwide sample of Presbyterians. *The International Journal for the Psychology of Religion, 20*(2), 130–147.
67. Kirkpatrick, L. A., Shillto, D. J., & Kellas, S. L. (1999). Loneliness, social support, and perceived relationships with God. *Journal of Social and Personal Relationships, 16*(4), 513–522.
68. Rowatt, W. C., & Kirkpatrick, L. A. (2002). Two dimensions of attachment to God and their relation to affect, religiosity, and personality constructs. *Journal for the Scientific Study of Religion, 41*(4), 637–651.
69. Beck, R., & McDonald, A. (2004). Attachment to God: The attachment to God inventory, tests of working model, correspondence, and an exploration of faith group differences. *Journal of Psychology and Theology, 32(*2), 92–103.
70. Wei, M., Ku, T. Y., Chen, H. J., Wade, N., Liao, K. Y. H., & Guo, G. J. (2012). Chinese Christians in America: Attachment to God, stress, and well-being. *Counseling and Values, 57*(2), 162–180.
71. Freeze, T. A., & Di Tommaso, E. (2015). Attachment to God and church family: Predictors of spiritual and psychological well-being. *Journal of Psychology and Christianity, 34*(1), 60–72.
72. Homan, K. J. (2014). A mediation model linking attachment to God, self-compassion, and mental health. *Mental Health, Religion and Culture, 17*(10), 977–989.
73. Zahl, B. P., & Gibson, N. J. S. (2012). God representations, attachment to God, and satisfaction with life: A comparison of doctrinal and experiential representations of God in Christian young adults. *The International Journal for the Psychology of Religion, 22*(3), 216–230.
74. Rosenberg, M. (1962). The association between self-esteem and anxiety. *Journal of Psychiatric Research, 1*(2), 135–152.
75. Diener, E. D., Emmons, R. A., & Larsen, R. J. G.S (1985). The satisfaction with life scale *Journal of Personality Assessment, 49*(1), 71–75.
76. Watson, D., Clark, L. A. T., & Tellegen, A. (1988). Development and validation of brief measures of positive and negative affect: The PANAS scales. *Journal of Personality and Social Psychology,* 54(6), 1063–1070.
77. Ellison, C., Bradshaw, M., Kuyel, N., & Marcum, J. (2012). Attachment to God, stressful life events, and changes in psychological distress. *Review of Religious Research, 53*(4), 493–511.
78. Kessler, R. C., Andrews, G., Colpe, L. J., Hiripi, E., Mroczek, D. K., Normand, S.-L. T., et al. (2002). Short screening scales to monitor population prevalences and trends in non-specific psychological distress. *Psychological Medicine,* 32(6), 959–976.
79. Krause, N., & Hayward, R. D. (2013). Prayer beliefs and change in life satisfaction over time. *Journal of Religion and Health, 52*, 674–694.
80. Krause, N. (2004). Assessing the relationships among prayer expectancies, race, and self-esteem in late life. *Journal for the Scientific Study of Religion, 43*(3), 395–408.
81. Ellison, C. G., Bradshaw, M., Flannelly, K. J., & Galek, K. C. (2014). Prayer, attachment to God, and symptoms of anxiety-related disorders among US adults. *Sociology of Religion, 75*(2), 208–233.

Chapter 22
Belief in Meaning in Life and Mental Health

Abstract The chapter presents evidence from convenience samples of mainly Christian students in the U.S. and U.K. that various facets of religion have a positive association with believing that life has meaning and purpose, and in turn, that believing life has meaning is associated with psychological well-being. A large national study of U.S. Christians supports these findings. Some psychologists have suggested that the need to believe one's life has meaning and purpose is so universal that it must be an evolutionary adaptation. ETAS Theory proposes that believing life has meaning and purpose may partly bolster mental health by fostering the belief, especially among religious people, that one's life is part of a plan, which reduces concerns about life's vicissitudes and uncertainties, particularly uncertainty, which elicits fear from the amygdala. Belief in meaning and purpose in life is also theoretically and empirically linked to the beliefs that one is a worthy (vis-a-vis self-esteem) and capable (vis-a-vis self-efficacy) person, which provides a sense of safety. According to ETAS Theory, the sense of safety provided by self-esteem and self-efficacy counter the ability of threats of harm to produce psychiatric symptoms.

Keywords ETAS Theory • Meaning in life • Purpose • Psychiatric symptoms • Psychological well-being • Threat

22.1 Background

Many psychologists and sociologists believe that one of the major psychological benefits of religion is that it provides a sense of meaning and purpose in life [1–4]. The Austrian psychiatrist and Holocaust survivor Victor Frankl made a compelling case for the importance of meaning in the life to people under ordinary and extraordinary circumstances in his 1946 book *Man's Search for Meaning* [5]. Frankl believed the things that provide meaning in life to a person may change over time but the need for meaning exists throughout life. The American social psychologist Roy Baumeister classified the need to believe life has meaning into four categories: (1) to believe that one's life has purpose; (2) to believe that one is able to meet challenges and achieve goals; (3) to believe that one is a worthy person with desirable characteristics; and (4) to believe that one's actions are good and justified [6].

K.J. Flannelly, *Religious Beliefs, Evolutionary Psychiatry, and Mental Health in America*, Religion, Spirituality and Health: A Social Scientific Approach 1,
DOI 10.1007/978-3-319-52488-7_22

Though individuals find meaning in life many ways [7, 8], religion is unique in providing answers to existential questions that we all have [2, 7, 9]. Besides addressing issues that are commonly recognized as being religious, such as death and suffering, religion addresses issues about other aspects of the world, such as fairness and equity, and one's vulnerability to the vagaries of life [2, 9, 10]. The Canadian psychologist Paul T.P. Wong, who has done extensive research on meaning, says that existential questions about meaning and purpose in life fall into seven areas of personal concern: "Who am I? What should I do with my life to make it worthwhile? What can I do to find happiness and life satisfaction? How can I make the right choices in an age of moral ambiguity and conflicting values? Where do I belong and where can I call home? What is the point of living in the face of suffering and death? What happens after death?" (p. xxx) [4]. For many people, religion provides answers to all or most of these questions.

Some psychologists have suggested that the need to believe one's life has meaning and purpose is so universal that it must be an evolutionary adaptation [11–13]. Eric Klinger [12], for example, suggested that the need for ultimate purposes and goals, which are embodied in the search for meaning, arose from proximate mechanisms that evolved in animals to seek food and other resources that are necessary for survival. Similarly, my colleagues Nava Silton, Laura Flannelly, Kathleen Galek and I specifically proposed that the need for meaning and other higher needs discussed by the American psychologist Abraham H. Maslow [14] are rooted in the mammalian goal-seeking system identified by the neuroscientist Jaak Panksepp [15, 16].

Other psychologists, such as Dov Shmotkin and Amit Shrira, who have studied meaning and psychological well-being, think the nearly universal tendency to believe that life has meaning can be maladaptive. They think there is a cognitive mechanism that they call the "hostile world scenario" [17, 18], which they say "functions as a system of appraisal that scans for any potential negative condition" in the surrounding world (p. 146) [18]. Although they think the system is adaptive in keeping individual's vigilant about potential danger, they also think it can be maladaptive because it generates "a continuous sense of survivorship in a disastrous world" (p. 146), which makes the world seem less dangerous than it actually is [18]. This is possible, they claim, because the brain mechanism underlying the "hostile world scenario" interacts with a hypothetical meaning system in the brain, such that the positive bias of the meaning system counteracts the negative perspective of the hostile world scenario by offering a favorable, and sometimes unreasonable, interpretations of adverse life events [17, 18]. Shmotkin and Shrira believe this can have adverse consequences [18].

22.2 Religion and Meaning

Although a substantial body of research in the U.K. has demonstrated there is a significant positive relationship between religion (e.g., prayer, church attendance, Bible reading, belief in God, and intrinsic religiosity) and the belief that life has meaning [19–24], this topic has received little attention in the U.S. until recently. A few U.S. studies, which were conducted in the 1970s with convenience samples of church congregants and primarily Christian college students, found the belief that life has meaning was significantly related to intrinsic religiosity, religious commitment, and belief in an afterlife [25–27].

I conducted electronic literature searches that failed to identify any other U.S. studies that explicitly explored this topic for nearly three decades. However, I found four U.S. studies published since 2005 that were specifically designed to analyze the relationship between religion and meaning in life. Two of them, which were studies of college students, reported that belief in meaning in life was positively correlated with a combined measure of religiosity (i.e., church attendance, private prayer, and religious commitment) [28], and believing that one has a close relationship with God [29]. The other two studies used national representative samples of U.S. adults. The first national study found that individuals who believed in God were more likely to believe that life has a purpose [30], whereas the second study found that individuals who believed God is loving were twice as likely to believe that their life had purpose than did individuals who did not believe God was loving [31].[1]

22.3 Meaning and Mental Health

A literature review by psychologist Michael Steger [32] of research in the U.S. and elsewhere showed that there is a consistent positive association between belief in meaning in life and mental-health outcomes. Cross-sectional studies, mainly of U.S. college students, have shown (see Fig. 22.1) that belief in meaning and purpose in life is positively correlated with hope [33, 34], personal growth [35], and positive affect [36–38], and negatively correlated with negative affect [37, 38] and depressive symptoms [33, 34].

The research reviewed by Steger also indicates that believing life has meaning has a salubrious relationship with psychiatric symptoms, as demonstrated in studies on meaning in life and anxiety in college students, patients, and community-dwelling adults [32]. Moreover, studies of U.S. college students have helped to establish a causal connection between belief in meaning and purpose in life and psychiatric symptoms by demonstrating that belief in meaning at a given point in time predicts depressive symptoms at a later point in time [33, 34]. In addition, a large national study by Neal Krause of over 1000 older Americans revealed that believing life has meaning predicts lowers levels of affective and somatic symptoms of depression [39].

[1] The first national study used data from the General Social Survey; the second used data from the Baylor Religion Survey.

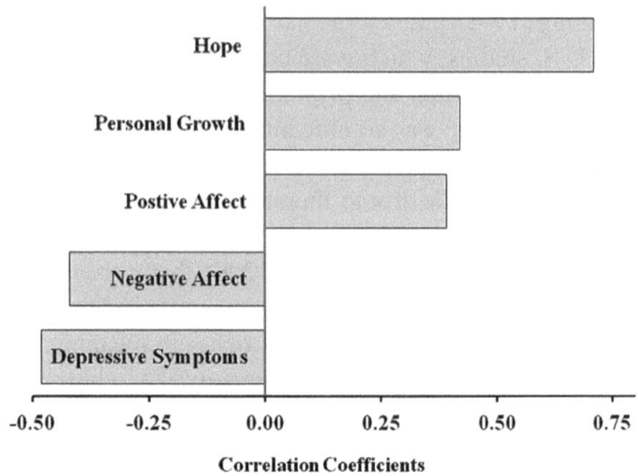

Fig. 22.1 Average correlations between mental-health outcomes and believing that there is meaning and purpose in life

22.4 Religious Meaning and Mental Health

A 2003 study of the relationship between meaning in life and psychological well-being in a large sample of older Christian Americans is particularly interesting for several reasons. First, the study, which was conducted by Neal Krause, specifically linked meaning in life to religion [40]. Krause's 6-item measure of religious meaning, including the items: "God put me in this life for a purpose"; "God has a specific plan for my life" and "My faith gives me a sense of direction in my life."

Second, some studies suggest that belief in meaning in life underlies the salubrious connection between religion and psychological well-being [28, 40], and Krause's 2003 study provides further evidence that this is so. Specifically, Krause's study examined the degree to which belief in meaning accounted for the apparent salutary association between church attendance and psychological well-being. Third, Krause's study compared differences in religious meaning and the differential effects of meaning on psychological well-being in Black and White Americans, which revealed that Black Americans had a stronger sense of religious meaning than White Americans.

Krause's analysis of psychological well-being began by examining the net effects of church attendance on optimism, self-esteem, and life-satisfaction, controlling for age, gender, marital status, race, and prayer. Before religious meaning was added to the regression model, church attendance had a positive association with all three measures of psychological well-being, particularly optimism and self-esteem (see Fig. 22.2).

However, when religious meaning was added to the models, the associations were substantially reduced, indicating that the associations between church attendance and the three measures were partially mediated by religious meaning. This indicates that what appeared to be an association between church attendance and psychological well-being included an association between belief in religious meaning and the three measures of psychological well-being.

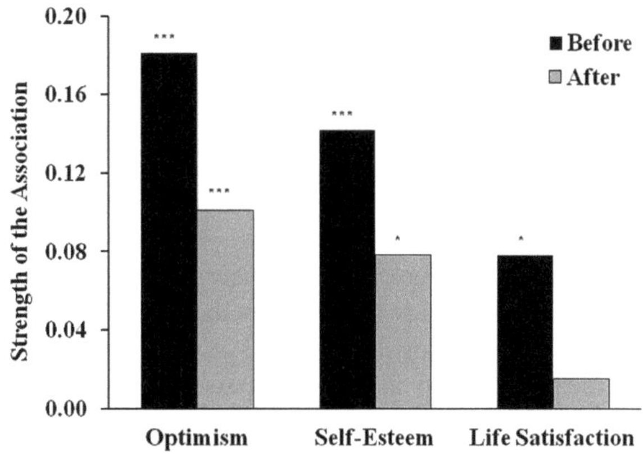

Fig. 22.2 Association between church attendance and measures of psychological well-being before and after belief in religious meaning was added to the regression models [40]; Values are standardized regression coefficients (β's); * $p < .01$; *** $p < .001$

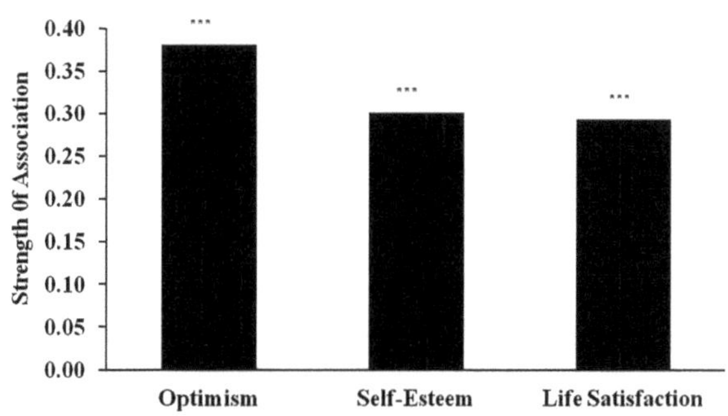

Fig. 22.3 Association between belief in religious meaning and measures of psychological well-being [40]; Values are standardized regression coefficients (β's); *** $p < .001$

Figure 22.3 shows the association between religious meaning, itself, and optimism, self-esteem, and life-satisfaction, controlling for other variables. If one compares the strength of the association of religious meaning with these three measures of psychological well-being in Fig. 22.3 to the strength of the association of church attendance with the same three measures of well-being in Fig. 22.2 ("Before"), it is obvious that the association of religious meaning is substantially higher. Further analyses of the data revealed that Black Americans benefited more from religious meaning than did White Americans on all three outcome measures.

22.5 Chapter Highlights and Comments

There is reasonable evidence to conclude that religion has a positive association with believing that life has meaning and purpose, at least among Christians in the U.S. and U.K. In turn, the belief that life has meaning is associated with psychological well-being among American Christians. There also is sufficient evidence to support the notion that the salubrious association of religion with mental health is partially attributable to the belief that life has meaning and purpose. Meaning and purpose in life may partly bolster mental health by instilling the belief, especially among religious people, that one's life is part of a plan, which reduces concerns about life's uncertainties and vicissitudes. Uncertainty elicits fear from the amygdala and reducing uncertainty reduces anxiety, according to ETAS Theory, so the belief that there is meaning and purpose in life reduces anxiety, related psychiatric symptoms, and other forms of psychological distress. From Roy Baumeister's perspective, meaning and purpose also entail the beliefs that one is a worthy (vis-a-vis self-esteem) and capable (vis-a-vis self-efficacy) person. ETAS Theory claims that self-esteem and self-efficacy provide a sense of safety that counters the ability of threats of harm to elicit psychiatric symptoms by raising the threshold of what constitutes a threat.

Ideas similar to those encompassed in ETAS Theory have been proposed by researchers investigating meaning and purpose in life, but those ideas have not been fully developed. Shmotkin and Shrira's concept of a "hostile world scenario" [17, 18], for example, is similar to ETAS theory in that the scenario proposes a vigilance system that scans for potential threats of harm in the environment, However, only ETAS Theory provides a biologically plausible explanation of such a system and its scope. While Shmotkin and Shrira hypothesize that positive beliefs about the meaning of adverse life events can undermine more realistic interpretations of the danger they pose, I think this possibility is less likely than they think it is. Even though ETAS Theory explains how cognitive assessments of safety can over-ride subcortical assessments of danger, cognitive control over subcortical areas evolved, in part, to balance the strong bias of subcortical areas to perceive threats when none exists. Nevertheless, any brain system that consistently denied the harm posed by adverse life events could not have evolved. I think a brain system that finds meaning in adversity (if such a system exists) is more likely to be a mechanism to deal retroactively with the psychological consequences of personal harm, rather than a proactive process that discounts the possibility of potential harm posed by current or future adverse events.

References

1. Clark, W. H. (1958). *The psychology of religion*. New York: McMillan.
2. Pargament, K. I. (1997). *The psychology of religion and coping: Theory, research, practice*. New York: Guilford Press.
3. Park, C. L., & Edmondson, D. (2012). Religion as a source of meaning. In P. R. Shaver, & M. Mikulincer (Eds.), *Meaning, mortality, and choice: The social psychology of existential concerns* (pp. 145–162). Washington, DC: American Psychological Association.
4. Wong, P. T. P. (Ed.). (2012). *The human quest for meaning: Theories, research, and application* (2nd ed.). New York: Routledge/Taylor & Francis.
5. Frankl, V. E. (1946/1992). *Man's search for meaning*. Boston: Beacon Press.
6. Baumeister, R. F. (1991). *Meaning of life*. New York: Guilford Press.
7. Wong, P. T. P. (1998). Spirituality, meaning, and successful aging. In: Wong, PTP (Ed.), *The human quest for meaning: A handbook of psychological research and clinical applications*. (2nd ed., 359–394). Mahwah: Erlbaum.
8. Wong, P. T. P. (2012). From logotherapy to meaning-centered counseling. In: P. T. P. Wong (Ed.), *The human quest for meaning: Theories, research, and application* (2nd ed., pp. 619–647). New York: Routledge/Taylor & Francis.

9. Park, C. L. (2005). Religion as a meaning-making framework in coping with life stress. *Journal of Social Issues, 61*(4), 707–729.
10. Flannelly, K. J., Galek, K., Ellison, C. G., & Silton, N. R. (2012). Belief in life-after-death, beliefs about the world, and psychiatric symptoms. *Journal of Religion and Health, 51*(3), 651–662.
11. King, L. A., & Hicks, J. A. (2012). Positive affect and meaning in life. The intersection of hedonism and eudiamonia. In P. T. P. Wong (Ed.), *The human quest for meaning: Theories, research, and application* (2nd ed., pp. 125–142). New York: Routledge/Taylor & Francis.
12. Klinger, E. (2012). The search for meaning in evolutionary goal-theory perspective and its clinical implications. In P. T. P. Wong (Ed.), *The human quest for meaning: Theories, research, and application* (2nd ed., pp. 23–56). New York: Routledge/Taylor & Francis.
13. Sommer, K. L., Baumeister, R. F., & Stillman, T. F. (2012). The construction of meaning from life events: Empirical studies of personal narratives. In P. T. P. Wong (Ed.), *The human quest for meaning: Theories, research, and application* (2nd ed., pp. 297–314) New York: Routledge/Taylor & Francis.
14. Silton, N. R., Flannelly, L. T., Flannelly, K. J., & Galek, K. (2011). Toward a theory of holistic needs and the brain. *Holistic Nursing Practice, 25*(5), 258–265.
15. Panksepp, J. (1998). *Affective neuroscience: The foundations of human and animal emotions.* New York: Oxford University Press.
16. Panksepp, J. (2005). Affective consciousness: Core emotional feelings in animals and humans. *Consciousness and Cognition, 14*(1), 30–80.
17. Shrira, A., Palgi, Y., Ben-Ezra, M., & Shmotkin, D. (2011). How subjective well-being and meaning in life interact in the hostile world? *The Journal of Positive Psychology, 6*(4), 273–285.
18. Shmotkin, D., & Shrira, A. (2012). On the distinction between subjective well-being and meaning in life. In P. T. P. Wong (Ed.), *The human quest for meaning: Theories, research, and application* (2nd ed., pp. 143–163). New York: Routledge/Taylor & Francis.
19. Robbins, M., & Francis, L. J. (2000). Religion, personality, and well-being: The relationship between church attendance and purpose in life. *Journal of Research on Christian Education, 9*(2), 223–238.
20. Francis, L. J. (2000). The relationship between bible reading and purpose in life among 13–15-year-olds. *Mental Health, Religion and Culture, 3*(1), 27–36.
21. Francis, L. J., & Burton, L. (1994). The influence of personal prayer on purpose in life among Catholic adolescents. *Journal of Beliefs & Values, 15*(2), 6–9.
22. Francis, L. J., & Evans, T. E. (1996). The relationship between personal prayer and purpose in life among churchgoing and non-churchgoing twelve-to-fifteen year-olds in the UK. *Religious Education, 91*(1), 9–18.
23. Francis, L. J., Jewell, A., & Robbins, M. (2010). The relationship between religious orientation, personality, and purpose in life among an older Methodist sample. *Mental Health, Religion and Culture, 13*(7–8), 777–791.
24. Francis, L. J., & Robbins, M. (2009). Prayer, purpose in life, and attitudes toward substances: A study among 13- to 15-year-olds in England and Wales. *Counselling and Spirituality/Counseling et Spiritualité, 28*(2), 83–104.
25. Crandall, J. E., & Rasmussen, R. D. (1975). Purpose in life as related to specific values. *Journal of Clinical Psychology, 31*(3), 483–485.
26. Soderstrom, D., & Wright, E. W. (1977). Religious orientation and meaning in life. *Journal of Clinical Psychology, 33*, 65–68.
27. Weinstein, L., & Cleanthous, C. C. (1996). A comparison of protestant ministers and parishioners on expressed purpose in life and intrinsic religious motivation. *Psychology: A Journal of Human Behavior, 33*(1), 26–29.
28. Steger, M. F., & Frazier, P. (2005). Meaning in life: one link in the chain from religiousness to well-being. *Journal of Counseling Psychology, 52*(4), 574–582.

29. Holmes, J. D., & Hardin, S. I. (2009). Religiosity, meaning in life, and clinical symptomology: A comparison of African-American and European-American college students. *Journal of College Student Psychotherapy, 23*(2), 103–117.
30. Cranney, S. (2013). Do people who believe in God report more meaning in their lives? The existential effects of belief *Journal for the Scientific Study of Religion, 52*(3), 638–646.
31. Stroope, S., Draper, S., & Whitehead, A. L. (2013). Images of a loving God and sense of meaning in life. *Social Indicators Research, 111*(1), 25–44.
32. Steger, M. F. (2012). Making meaning in life. *Psychological Inquiry, 23*(4), 381–385.
33. Mascaro, N., & Rosen, D. H. (2008). Assessment of existential meaning of and its longitudinal relations with depressive symptoms. *Journal of Social and Clinical Psychology, 27*(6), 576–599.
34. Mascaro, N. D. H. (2005). Existential meaning's role in the enhancement of hope and prevention of depressive symptoms. *Journal of Personality, 73*(4), 985–1014.
35. Ryff, C. D., & Keyes, C. L. M. (1995). The structure of psychological well-being revisited. *Journal of Personality and Social Psychology, 69*(4), 719–727.
36. Hicks, J. A., Cicero, D. C., Trent, J., Burton, C. M., & King, L. A. (2010). Positive affect, intuition, and feelings of meaning. *Journal of Personality and Social Psychology, 98*(6), 967–979.
37. King, L. A., Hicks, J. A., Krull, J. L., & Del Gaiso, A. K. (2006). Positive affect and the experience of meaning in life. *Journal of Personality and Social Psychology, 90*(1), 179–196.
38. Hicks, J. A., Trent, J., Davis, W. E., & King, L. A. (2012). Positive affect, meaning in life, and future time perspective: An application of socioemotional selectivity theory. *Psychology and Aging, 27*(1), 181–189.
39. Krause, N. (2007). Evaluating the stress-buffering function of meaning in life among older people. *Journal of Aging and Health, 19*(5), 792–812.
40. Krause, N. (2003). Religious meaning and subjective well-being in late life. Journals of Gerontology. *Series B, Psychological Sciences and Social Sciences, 58*(3), S160–S170.
41. Krok, D. (2014). The religious meaning system and subjective well-being. *Archive for the Psychology of Religion, 36*(2), 253–273.

Chapter 23
Religious Doubt and Mental Health

Abstract The first section of the chapter briefly presents historical (Augustine of Hippo and Thomas Aquinas) and modern (James H. Snowden and Paul Tillich) theological perspectives about religious doubt, as well as psychological perspectives about religious doubt, including Gordon Allport's ideas about the causes of religious doubt. The rest of the chapter summarizes the research findings from convenience samples of religious Americans and several large studies of random samples of Americans (including a random sample of Christian Americans), all of which demonstrate that religious doubt has a pernicious association with psychological well-being. The chapter also presents the results of several large national and regional U.S. studies that indicate religious doubt has a pernicious association with psychiatric symptoms. Based on ETAS Theory, the pernicious effects of religious doubt at least partly reflect the fact (a) that doubts undermine the sense of meaning and security provided by religious faith, and (b) that uncertainty about one's beliefs increases anxiety, just as uncertainty about the future increases anxiety. Some of the large studies also found that the adverse effects of religious doubt on mental health were more pronounced in persons who had a strong religious commitment or religious identity. This finding is important because it suggests that religious doubt threatens the social role (and therefore, the self-esteem) of religious people within their religious community, which is consistent with Identity Theory and ETAS Theory. According to ETAS Theory, this threat to self-esteem makes people more vulnerable to other forms of threats, which further exacerbates psychiatric symptoms.

Keywords Aquinas • Augustine • ETAS Theory • Identity Theory • Meaning • Psychiatric symptoms • Psychological distress • Psychological well-being • Religious doubt • Self-esteem • Threat • Uncertainty

K.J. Flannelly, *Religious Beliefs, Evolutionary Psychiatry, and Mental Health in America*, Religion, Spirituality and Health: A Social Scientific Approach 1,
DOI 10.1007/978-3-319-52488-7_23

23.1 Religious Doubt

Despite the fact that religious beliefs can provide meaning in life by helping people to make sense of the world, some people do not find the explanation of life events that religion provides to be satisfactory at an intellectual or emotional level, which may lead them to doubt their religious beliefs [1]. The anthropologist and psychiatrist Simon Dein [2] defined religious doubt as "a feeling of uncertainty toward, and the questioning of, religious teachings and beliefs." Other psychologists have offered similar definitions, and have distinguished doubts about one's religious beliefs from the lack of, or the rejection of religious beliefs, which some call "unbelief" [3–5].

The 5th Century Catholic theologian Augustine of Hippo recounted his religious doubts in his *Confessions* [6, 7], including his concern that a omnipotent and good God could allow the existence of evil in the world. In other writings, he repeatedly expressed his doubt that the *Book of Genesis* was literally true [8–10]. The 13th Century Catholic theologian Thomas Aquinas took a more circumspect stance about religious doubts. Aquinas realized that doubt was an aspect of both science and religious faith and he acknowledged that "the believer may sometimes suffer … doubt … about matters of faith" (p. 2684) [11]. He claimed, however, " …the fact that some happen to doubt … articles of faith is not due to the uncertain nature of the truths, but to the weakness of human intelligence" (p. 10) [11].

Several modern theologians have addressed the fact that religious doubts often arise among the faithful. The American Protestant theologian James H. Snowden published a paper in 1916 that shared Aquinas' opinion that doubt is an inherent part of both science and religion, but he did not think doubt reflected a failure of faith or intellect [12]. Snowden thought that doubts about religious beliefs could lead to stronger religious faith, and the contemporary Christian theologians Paul Tillich [13, 14] and James W. Fowler [15, 16] considered religious doubt to be a necessary element of religious faith. Yet, Tillich and other theologians have recognized that Christians and other people of faith feel guilt and anxiety about having religious doubts [14, 17, 18].

Although the American psychologist Gordon Allport thought beliefs about science, philosophy, and religion were all subject to doubt, he thought religious beliefs were particularly prone to doubt because of the unworldly nature of many religious beliefs [19]. He also thought some religious beliefs were subject to doubt because of disparities between what is practiced and what is preached by religious organizations, clergy, and congregants. Another major source of religious doubt is the conflict between the belief that God is good and omnipotent and the existence of evil in the world, which is called the problem of theodicy [20]. Finally, religious doubt may arise from the disparate explanations of nature offered by religion and science [19]. Though relatively few studies have explicitly explored the roots of religious doubt, their results are in agreement with the causes of doubt enumerated by Allport [21–23].

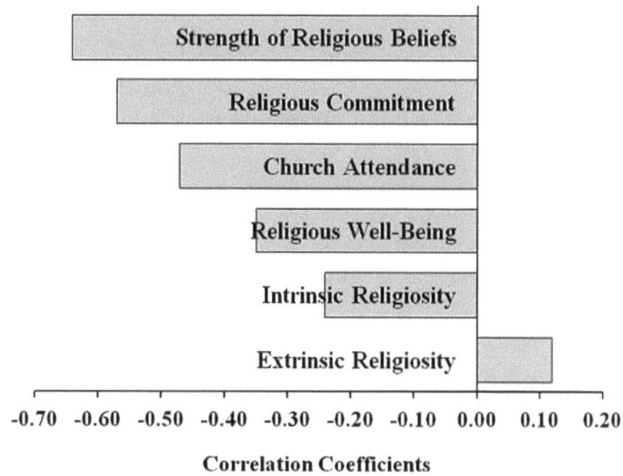

Fig. 23.1 Correlation of religious doubt with six measures of religion in three studies

Three studies of convenience samples of church members, Christian youth, and/or college students all support the idea that religious doubt undermines religious faith (see Fig. 23.1) [5, 24, 25]. All three studies found that religious doubt [26][1] had significant negative correlations with the religious variables they measured, except extrinsic religiosity (i.e. extrinsic religious orientation). Naturally, the largest negative correlation was between religious doubt and strength of religious beliefs. As seen in Fig. 23.1, religious doubt had smaller, but significant negative correlations, with religious commitment, church attendance, religious well-being, and intrinsic religiosity (i.e., intrinsic religious orientation).

23.2 Religious Doubt and Psychological Well-Being

Three other studies using convenience samples of religious Americans provide evidence for a pernicious association between religious doubt and psychological well-being (Fig. 23.2). The first was a study of parishioners of a Catholic church in the Midwest that found that religious doubt was negatively correlated with self-esteem and positively correlated with trait anxiety and negative mood [27]. The other two were studies of Christian high school and college students that found religious doubt was negatively correlated with life satisfaction [25] and optimism [23].

Other studies provide stronger evidence for the pernicious association between religious doubt and psychological well-being in American adults because they used large probability (i.e., random) samples and controlled for demographic and other

[1] The three studies measured religious doubt with the 1988 Altemeyer scale, which consists of 10 items, including "doubting the existence of God because of suffering or death"; "feeling that religion doesn't really make people better"; "feeling people who go to church … pretend they are better," and" feeling that religious teachings are contradictory or that they don't make very much sense."

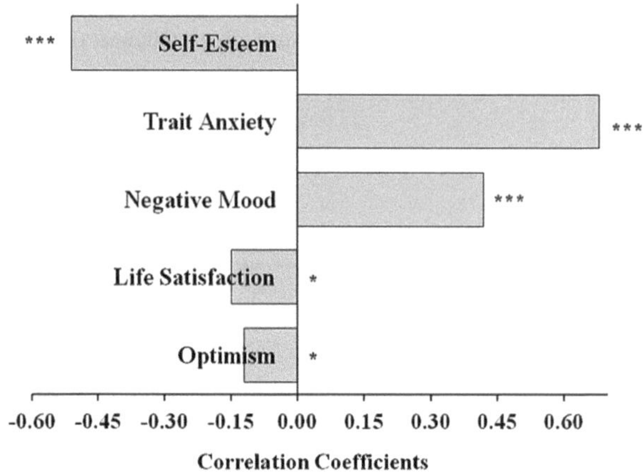

Fig. 23.2 Correlation of religious doubt with psychological well-being in three convenience samples of religious Americans; $*p < .01$; $***p < .001$

variables [28–33]. The results of these studies are shown in Fig. 23.3. The first one is an early study by Chris Ellison of a national sample of American adults which found that religious doubts, arising from concerns about evil in the world, the conflict between faith and science, or lack of meaning in life, had a pernicious association with life satisfaction and happiness. A later study by Neal Krause and Chris Ellison and their colleagues found that religious doubt had a pernicious association with positive and negative affect in a national sample of members of the Presbyterian Church (USA) [31]. That study also found that the adverse effects of religious doubt decreased with age. The third study, which was also conducted by Chris Ellison [30], found a pernicious association between religious doubt and psychological distress (as measured by the K6 [34]) in a national sample of American adults.

Another study by Neal Krause [33], which surveyed a random sample of practicing American Christians in 2001 and 2004, examined the association of religious doubt with self-esteem [35], optimism [36], and life satisfaction [37], controlling for demographic characteristics. The study used a measure of religious doubt which included items that Krause developed through extensive qualitative research [38].[2] That study found that all three measures of psychological well-being decreased from 2001 to 2004 and that the decrease was significantly associated with religious doubt. Because the study measured the psychological outcomes at two points in time, it provides strong evidence that religious doubt had a causal connection with the observed decline in psychological well-being.

[2] The measure included the following items: "having doubts about your religious or spiritual beliefs"; "having doubts about things that you learned at the church"; "doubting that solutions to your problems can be found in the Bible"; "doubting whether your prayers make a difference"; and "doubting that God is directly involved in your daily life."

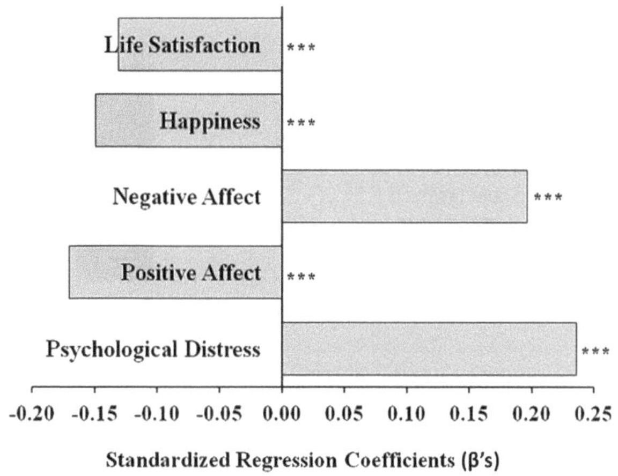

Fig. 23.3 Association of religious doubt with psychological well-being in three national probability samples of Americans; ****p* < .001

23.3 Religious Doubt and Psychiatric Symptoms

National and regional studies by Neal Krause [39–41] have found a pernicious association between religious doubt and a well-established measures of depression [42].[3] Fig. 23.4 shows the results of two of these studies, which used identical depression measures and nearly identical measures of religious doubt, with two distinctly different populations (Mexican Americans and Church Congregants).[4] The common characteristic of the two samples was that they were almost entirely Christian. As seen in Fig. 23.4, religious doubt had comparable positive associations with affective and somatic symptoms of depression in both populations, although the associations were somewhat larger in the sample of Church congregants.

The study of church congregants, which was conducted by Neal Krause and Keith Wulff [41], also found that religious doubt had a more pernicious association with depression among those congregants who played a prominent role in their church (such a teaching Sunday school, singing in the choir, assisting with worship services, or having a leadership or administrative role) compared to other congregants. The authors interpreted this finding in terms of Identity Theory, which proposes that people have various social roles in life that form their social/personal identity: such as being a husband or wife, father or mother, a business owner, a little-league coach, a volunteer firemen, a clergyperson or a church congregant [43–45]. The sense of identity that is tied to these multiple social roles provides meaning in life, to varying degrees, and individuals attach greater importance to some roles

[3] The measures of depression were based on the Center for Epidemiologic Studies Depression Scale (CES-D).

[4] One study used a random sample of over 1200 congregants from churches throughout the U.S., and the other study used a random sample of over 1000 older Mexican Americans living in Arizona, California, Colorado, New Mexico, and Texas.

Fig. 23.4 Association between religious doubt and affective and somatic symptoms of depression (Krause and Wulff, 2004 [41]; Krause, 2012 [39]); values are standardized regression coefficients (β's); All associations are statistically significant

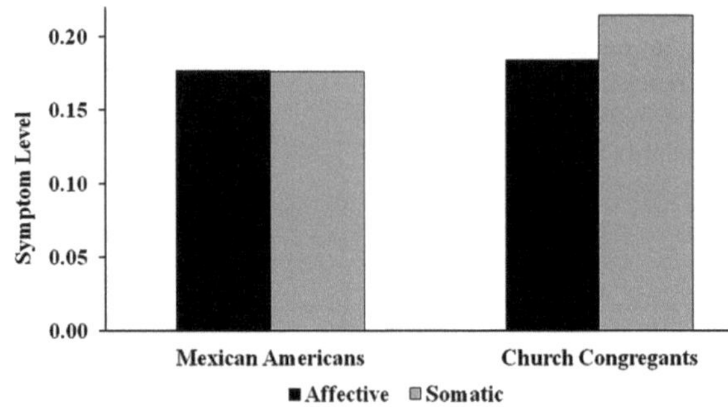

than other roles based on their commitment to and investment in each role. Challenges to these roles can have adverse psychological consequences, especially perceived threats to those roles that one deems to be most important.

Krause and Wulff argued that religious doubt undermines "one of the most fundamental benefits of religion – a sense of meaning in life" [41]. Moreover, religious doubt poses a threat to one's identity as a religious person. Hence, we would expect that religious doubt would have a more adverse effect on individuals who are more invested in and committed to their religion. As it takes commitment and investment for individuals to be a choir member, a Sunday school teacher, etc., Identity Theory predicts that religious doubt will have a more pernicious effect on the psychological well-being of these individuals than on the psychological well-being of other church congregants, which is what Krause and Wulff (2004) found. Two studies by Chris Ellison and his colleagues also found that depression and other psychiatric symptoms were exacerbated in persons with a strong religious identity who had religious doubts, compared to less religious persons who had religious doubts [30, 46].

A 2007 study by Galek et al., using data from National Survey of Religion and Health [47], found that Americans adults who had doubted their religion because of evil and suffering in the world had significantly greater symptoms of general anxiety, paranoid ideation, depression, obsessive-compulsive disorder (OCD), and agoraphobia (see Fig. 23.5), as well as other psychiatric symptoms than people who did not have religious doubts. Like the 1999 study by Krause and this colleagues [31], the Galek study found the adverse effects of religious doubt on mental health decreased with age.

The net effect of religious doubt on all the psychiatric symptoms examined in the Galek study probably reflects the fact that religious doubts undermine the sense of security provided by religious faith. Religious doubts also may lead to fear of retribution from God, and fear that fellow congregants will become aware of one's lack of faith.

A 2015 study by Galek et al. extends the findings of Krause and Ellison and their colleagues [30, 41, 46] in showing that the adverse effects of religious doubt on mental health is more pronounced among persons who have a strong religious commitment [48]. Given Krause and Wulff's [41] premise that religious doubts undermine the sense of meaning provided by religion, Galek thought that the belief that life lacks meaning would be particularly troubling for persons with a strong religious commitment.

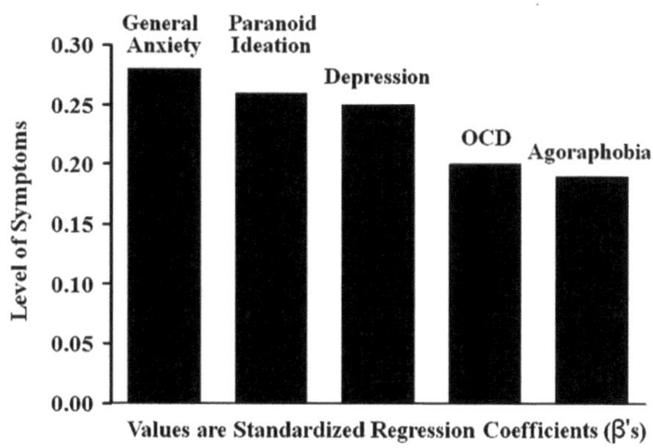

Fig. 23.5 Association between religious doubt and psychiatric symptoms (Galek et al., 2007 [47]); All β's are statistically significant; *OCD* = obsessive-compulsive disorder

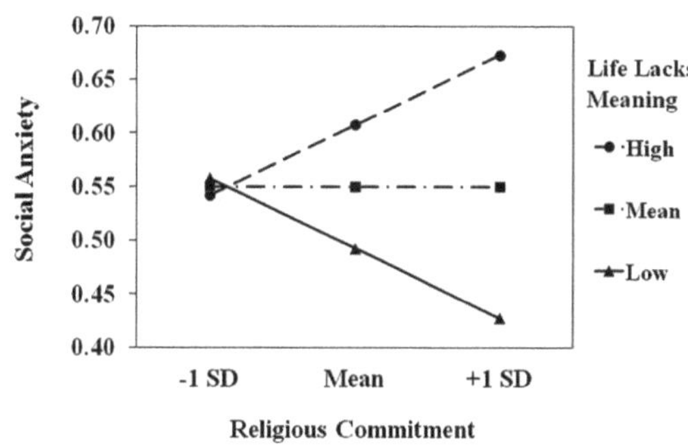

Fig. 23.6 Interaction effect of religious commitment with believing life lacks meaning on social anxiety (Galek et al., 2015) [47]; see reference list for complete citation; used by permission; Copyright © 2015 by the American Psychological Association

The study, which used data from the 2010 Baylor Religion Survey, conducted two sets of regression analyses, controlling for demographic characteristics. The first set of analyses confirmed previous findings that religious doubt has a significant pernicious association with psychological distress, in that it found psychiatric symptoms were significantly associated with the belief that life lacks meaning and purpose: social anxiety (β = .064), paranoid ideation (β = .060), obsession (β = .066), and compulsion (β = .113). The second set of analyses confirmed the specific findings of Ellison [30, 46] and Krause and Wulff [41] that religious doubt had a more pernicious effect on individuals with a strong religious commitment, as indicated by significant interactions of religious commitment with the belief that life lacks meaning and purpose on four types of psychiatric symptoms. Fig. 23.6 illustrates this interaction effect for social anxiety.

Fig. 23.6 shows that believing life lacks meaning had no effect on people with low religious commitment (High, Mean, and Low at −1 SD in the figure). In contrast, people with strong religious commitment who believed life lacks meaning (High at +1 SD in the figure) had high social anxiety, whereas people with strong religious commitment who did not believe life lacks meaning had low social anxiety (Low at +1 SD in the figure). The interaction effects were similar for paranoid ideation, obsession, and compulsion.

Based on Identity Theory, Galek et al. suggested that the belief that life lacks meaning exacerbates psychiatric symptoms among people who have a strong religious commitment because it "threatens their social role within the religious community" (p. 8) [48], which is consistent with ETAS Theory. Moreover, they suggested, from the perspective of ETAS Theory, that such a threat to one's identity represents a direct threat to one's self-esteem, which is one of Baumeister's four basic needs for meaning [49].

23.4 Chapter Highlights and Comments

Doubts about one's religious beliefs can arise from the unworldly nature of the beliefs themselves, the disparate explanations of the world offered by religion and science, and other reasons. Two major sources of religious doubt are (a) disparities between what is practiced and what is preached by religious organizations, clergy, and congregants, and (b) the conflict between the belief that God is good and omnipotent and the existence of evil in the world.

Research has shown that religious doubt is inversely related to measures of religious faith and psychological well-being. Large-scale studies using probability samples of Americans have found that religious doubt has a pernicious association with self-esteem, happiness, life satisfaction, optimism, positive and negative affect, and psychological distress, including psychiatric symptoms. Based on ETAS Theory, the pernicious effects of religious doubt at least partly reflect the fact (a) that doubts undermine the sense of meaning and security provided by religious faith, and (b) that uncertainty about one's beliefs increases anxiety, just as uncertainty about the future increases anxiety. Anxiety and other forms of psychological distress may also result from the fear that fellow congregants will become aware of one's lack of faith and the fear of retribution from God.

Related research has shown the pernicious effects of religious doubt on mental health are particularly troubling for persons who have a strong religious commitment, probably because religious doubt undermines the social identity and threatens the self-esteem of individuals with a strong commitment to their religion and their religious community. A threat to self-esteem has a two-pronged effect on mental health because it has a primary effect of undermining psychological well-being and a secondary effect resulting from the fact that lowered self-esteem makes one more vulnerable to psychological distress from other sources of threat, according to ETAS Theory.

References

1. Exline, J. J. (2002). Stumbling blocks on the religious road: Fractured relationships, nagging vices, and the inner struggle to believe. *Psychological Inquiry, 13*(3), 182–189.
2. Dein, S. (2013). Religious doubts: Implications for psychopathology and psychotherapy. *Bulletin of the Menninger Clinic, 77*(3), 201–221.
3. Hunsberger, B., McKenzie, B., Pratt, M., & Pancer, S. M. (1993). Religious doubt: A social-psychological analysis. *Research in the social scientific study of religion, 5*, 27–51.

4. Beck, J. R. (1990). Doubt. In D. G. Benner (Ed.), *Baker encyclopedia of psychology* (pp. 327–329). Grand Rapids: Baker Book House.
5. Puffer, K. A., Pence, K. G., Graverson, T. M., Wolfe, M., Pate, E., & Clegg, S. (2008). Religious doubt and identity formation: Salient predictors of adolescent religious doubt. *Journal of Psychology & Theology, 36*(4), 270–284.
6. Augustine. (398/1955). *Confessions* (trans: Outler, A. C.). Philadelphia: Westminister Press.
7. Augustine. (398/2008). *The confessions of St. Augustine*. Minneapolis: Filiquarian Publishing.
8. Augustine. (389/2002). *On genesis: A refutation of the Manichees*. Hype Park: New City Press.
9. Augustine. (415/1982). *The literal meaning of Genesis*. Mahwah: Paulist Press.
10. Neil, B. (2006). Exploring the limits of literal exegesis: Augustine's reading of Gen 1:26 *Pacifica, 19*(June), 144–155.
11. Aquinas, T. (1981). *Summa theologica*. Westminister: Christian Classics.
12. Snowden, J. H. (1916). The place of doubt in religious belief. *The Biblical World, 47*(3), 151–155.
13. Tillich, P. (1952). *The courage to be*. New Haven: Yale University Press.
14. Tillich, P. (1957). *The dynamics of faith*. New York: Harper & Row.
15. Fowler, J. W. (1981). *Stages of faith*. New York: HarperCollins.
16. Fowler, J. W. (1996). *Faithful change*. Nashville: Abingdon Press.
17. Craig, W. L. (2003). *Hard questions, real answers*. Wheaton: Crossway Books.
18. Newton, D. (2010). Faith, doubt and biblical criticism: Spiritual survival in the shifting sands. *Evangelical Quarterly, 82*(4), 326–339.
19. Allport, G. W. (1956). *The individual and his religion: A psychological interpretation*. New York: Macmillan.
20. Thang Moe, D. (2015). Sin and evil in Christian and Buddhist perspectives: A quest for theodicy. *Asia Journal of Theology, 29*(1), 22–46.
21. Hunsberger, B., Alisat, S., Pancer, S. M., & Pratt, M. (1996). Religious fundamentalism and religious doubts: Content, connections, and complexity of thinking. *The International Journal for the Psychology of Religion, 6*(3), 201–220.
22. Kooistra, W. P., & Pargament, K. I. (1990). Religious doubting in parochial school adolescents. *Journal of Psychology & Theology, 21*(1), 33–42.
23. Hunsberger, B., Pratt, M., & Pancer, S. M. (2002). A longitudinal study of religious doubts in high school and beyond: Relationships, stability, and searching for answers. *Journal for the Scientific Study of Religion, 41*(2), 255–266.
24. Hunsberger, B., Pratt, M., & Pancer, S. M. (2001). Adolescent identity formation: Religious exploration and commitment. *Identity: An International Journal of Theory and Research, 1*(4), 365–386.
25. Gauthier, K. J., Christopher, A. N., Walter, M. I., Mourad, R., & Marek, P. (2006). Religiosity, religious doubt, and the need for cognition: Their interactive relationship with life satisfaction. *Journal of Happiness Studies, 7*(2), 139–154.
26. Altemeyer, B. (1988). *Enemies of freedom: Understanding right-wing authoritarianism*. San Francisco: Jossey-Bass.
27. Pargament, K. I., Zinnbauer, B. J., Scott, A. B., Butter, E. M., Zerowin, J., & Stanik, P. (1998). Red flags and religious coping: Identifying some religious warning signs among people in crisis. *Journal of Clinical Psychology, 54*(1), 77–89.
28. Ellison, C. G. (1991). Religious involvement and subjective well-being. *Journal of Health and Social Behavior, 32*(1), 80–99.
29. Ellison, C. G., Roalson, L. A., Guillory, J. M., Flannelly, K. J., & Marcum, J. P. (2010). Religious resources, spiritual struggles, and mental health in a nationwide sample of PCUSA clergy. *Pastoral Psychology, 59*(3), 287–304.
30. Ellison, C. G., & Lee, J. (2010). Spiritual struggles and psychological distress: Is there a dark side of religion? *Social Indicators Research, 98*(3), 501–517.
31. Krause, N., Ingersoll-Dayton, B., Ellison, C. G., & Wulff, K. M. (1999). Aging, religious doubt, and psychological well-being. *The Gerontologist, 39*(5), 525–533.

32. Ellison, C. G., Bradshaw, M., Storch, J., Marcum, J. P., & Hill, T. D. (2011). Religious doubts and sleep quality: Findings from a nationwide study of Presbyterians. *Review of Religious Research, 53*(2), 119–136.
33. Krause, N. (2006). Religious doubt and psychological well-being: A longitudinal investigation. *Review of Religious Research, 50*(Special Issue), 94–110.
34. Kessler, R. C., Andrews, G., Colpe, L. J., Hiripi, E., Mroczek, D. K., Normand, S.-L. T., et al. (2002). Short screening scales to monitor population prevalences and trends in non-specific psychological distress. *Psychological Medicine, 32*(6), 959–976.
35. Rosenberg, M. (1965). *Society and the adolescent self image* (Rev. ed.). Princeton: Princeton University Press.
36. Scheier, M. F., & Carver, C. S. (1985). Optimism, coping, and health: Assessment and implications of generalized outcome expectancies. *Health Psychology, 4*(3), 219–247.
37. Neugarten, B. L., Havighurst, R. J., & Tobin, S. S. (1961). The measurement of life satisfaction. *Journal of Gerontology, 16*, 134–143.
38. Krause, N. (2002). A comprehensive strategy for developing closed-ended survey items for use in studies of older adults. *Journals of Gerontology. Series B, Psychological Sciences and Social Sciences, 57*(5), S263–S274.
39. Krause, N. (2012). Religious doubt, financial strain, and depressive symptoms among older Mexican Americans. *Mental Health, Religion and Culture, 15*(4), 335–348.
40. Krause, N. (2003). A preliminary assessment of race differences in the relationship between religious doubt and depressive symptoms. *Review of Religious Research, 45*(2), 93–115.
41. Krause, N., & Wulff, K. M. (2004). Religious doubt and health: Exploring the potential dark side of religion. *Sociology of Religion, 65*(1), 35–56.
42. Radloff, L. S. (1977). The CES-D scale: A self-report depression scale for research in the general population. *Applied Psychological Measurement, 1*(3), 385–401.
43. Stets, J. E., & Burke, P. J. (2000). Identity theory and social identity theory. *Social Psychology Quarterly, 63*(3), 224–237.
44. Burke, P. J. (1991). Identity process and social stress. *American Sociological Review, 56*, 836–849.
45. Thoits, P. A. (1991). On merging identity theory and stress research. *Social Psychology Quarterly, 54*, 101–112.
46. Ellison, C. G., Fang, Q., Flannelly, K. J., & Steckler, R. A. (2013). Spiritual struggles and mental health: Exploring the moderating effects of religious identity. *The International Journal for the Psychology of Religion, 23*, 214–229.
47. Galek, K., Krause, N., Ellison, C. G., Kudler, T., & Flannelly, K. J. (2007). Religious doubt and mental health across the lifespan. *Journal of Adult Development, 14*, 16–25.
48. Galek, K., Flannelly, K. J., Ellison, C. G., Silton, N. R., & Jankowski, K. R. B. (2015). Religion, meaning and purpose, and mental health. *Psychology of Religion and Spirituality, 7*(1), 1–12.
49. Baumeister, R. F. (1991). *Meaning of life*. New York: Guiford Press.

Chapter 24
Belief in Divine Forgiveness, Evil, and Biblical Literalism and Mental Health

Abstract The chapter discusses research on mental health and a few religious beliefs that have received little attention. The findings described in this chapter mainly come from a handful of large national studies. One of these studies, which investigated the association of psychiatric symptoms with belief in Divine forgiveness and belief in human evil found: (a) belief in forgiveness from God was associated with lower anxiety-related symptoms, (b) the belief that human nature is basically evil was associated with higher anxiety-related symptoms, and (c) that belief in Divine forgiveness countered the pernicious association of belief in human evil on anxiety-related symptoms. Other findings reported in the chapter are that belief in Divine forgiveness has a salubrious association with psychological well-being and depression and that belief in Satan has a pernicious association with psychiatric symptoms. From the perspective of ETAS Theory, the belief one has been forgiven by God implies belief in a benevolent God who is involved one's life, which provides a sense of safety that reduces psychiatric symptoms. Beliefs in Satan and human evil imply direct threats of harm from human and supernatural beings, both of which increase psychiatric symptoms. The interaction between belief in human evil and belief in Divine forgiveness confirms the ETAS Theory proposition that beliefs interaction with one another in their effects on psychiatric symptomology. Finally, the chapter discusses evidence that belief in Biblical literalism influences whether people seek help for psychiatric problems from clergy or mental-health professionals and examines the association between Biblical literalism and psychiatric symptomology.

Keywords Agoraphobia • Aquinas • Augustine • Divine forgiveness • Biblical literalism • ETAS Theory • Evil • Help seeking • Mental-health assistance • Psychiatric symptoms • Psychological well-being • Satan • Threat

The present chapter discusses some religious beliefs that have received relatively little research attention, but appear to have important implications for mental health. The first is belief in Divine forgiveness. The second is the belief that there is evil in the world, including the belief that human nature is basically evil and belief in Satan. The third is the belief that the Bible, particularly the Old Testament of the Bible, is literally true.

K.J. Flannelly, *Religious Beliefs, Evolutionary Psychiatry, and Mental Health in America*, Religion, Spirituality and Health: A Social Scientific Approach 1,
DOI 10.1007/978-3-319-52488-7_24

24.1 Belief in Divine Forgiveness and Mental Health

Extensive research has found a salubrious association between forgiveness and physical and mental health. The salubrious association between forgiveness and health appears to be due to the fact that forgiveness of others reduces feelings of hostility that have an adverse effects on health and subjective well-being [1, 2]. Although several books have been published that describe research on the association between forgiveness and mental health [3–5], most of this research has examined the relationship between mental health and forgiving others for their transgressions. Relatively few published studies have examined belief in Divine forgiveness and mental health.

The earliest research on Divine forgiveness and mental health is a series of studies using convenience samples of U.S. college students that were published in 1988 by psychologists P. J. Watson, Ronald J. Morris, and Ralph W. Hood [6–8]. This research consisted of surveys of a half dozen samples of undergraduates attending a state university and one sample from a small religious college.[1] Between 85.3% and 93.6% of the students in the state university and 95.6% of the students in the religious college were Christians. The studies reported consistent negative correlations between symptoms of depression and belief in Divine forgiveness of sin among state university students (r's = −.18 to −.34), with undergraduates at the religious college exhibiting the strongest negative correlation between depressive symptoms and belief in Divine forgiveness ($r = -.39$). The correlations between Divine forgiveness and general anxiety and social anxiety, which were measured in some of the studies, were inconsistent.

Two subsequent national studies of Divine forgiveness in samples of American adults were published in 2001 and 2003 [9, 10]. The first was a study of more than 1300 U.S. adults that examined the association of belief in Divine forgiveness with psychological distress and life satisfaction in different age groups [9].[2] The independent variable was participants' average ratings of the degree to which they agreed with two statements: "I know God forgives me" and "Knowing that I am forgiven for my sins gives me the strength to face my faults and be a better person" (p. 251) [9]. I assume these two statements capture the participants' beliefs that they have been forgiven by God, rather than their actual knowledge.

The study reported that belief in Divine forgiveness varied by age, controlling for demographic variables and other religious variables. Belief in Divine forgiveness had no association with psychological distress or life satisfaction among people over 65 years of age, and it had only a marginally significant association with psychological distress ($\beta = -.07$) and life satisfaction ($\beta = .09$) among people 18–44 years of age. Participants who were 45–64 years-old exhibited no association

[1] The sample sizes of the surveys of the state university students ranged from 124 to 221 participants and the sample size of the survey of the students in the small religious college was 116 participants.

[2] The age groups were 18–44 years, 45–64 years, and 65 years and older.

between belief in forgiveness and psychological distress, but a significant negative association was found between belief in forgiveness and life satisfaction ($\beta = -.18$).

The second study, which was conducted by Neal Krause and Chris Ellison [10], examined the association of life satisfaction and affective and somatic symptoms of depression with the degree to which study participants agreed with the statement: "I believe God has forgiven me for things I've done wrong" (p. 83) [10]. The study analyzed the responses of a random sample of over 1200 U.S. Christians who were 66 years of age or older, controlling for other religious variables and several demographic variables. The analyses found study participants who more strongly believed that they had been forgiven by God had significantly higher life satisfaction ($\beta = -.07$), and significantly lower affective symptoms of depression ($\beta = -.08$) than other participants. However, belief in Divine forgiveness was not significantly associated with somatic symptoms of depression ($\beta = -.02$).

The only other research I know that has examined the relationship between belief in Divine forgiveness and mental health is a study I worked on with my sociologist colleagues Jeremy Uecker, Chris Ellison, and Amy Burdette, which used data from the National Study of Religion and Health (NSRH) [11]. This study examined the association of psychiatric symptoms with belief in Divine forgiveness, as well as belief in human evil, which I will discuss in the next section of this chapter.

The independent variable in our regression analyses[3] was participants' response to the question: "How often have you known that God has forgiven you?" Once again, I assume that "knowing" one has been forgiven by God really means "believing" one has been forgiven by God.[4] Although this study included eight dependent variables [11], Fig. 24.1 only shows the results for the five key variables from the NSRH that I have mentioned in the previous chapters.

The figure shows that belief in Divine forgiveness had significant negative associations with depression, OCD, agoraphobia, and general anxiety. Belief in Divine forgiveness had a non-significant negative association with paranoid ideation. Overall, I think these results offer good evidence that believing one has been forgiven by God has a salutary association with mental health in the U.S. general population, even after controlling for the sense of safety provided by social support. I think believing you have been forgiven by God implies the belief that God is involved in your life and that you have a good relationship with God, both of which should provide a sense of safety, and hence, lower psychiatric symptoms. It also implies that God is benevolent, not punitive, which should also lower anxiety and related symptoms. Finally, obtaining forgiveness from God may be considered a form of protection, as God chose to forgive you rather than to punish you.

---

[3] The regression analyses controlled for frequency of private prayer and attending religious services, demographic variables, social support, life stressors, and belief in human evil.

[4] The response options ranged from "never" to "many times" on a 5-point scale.

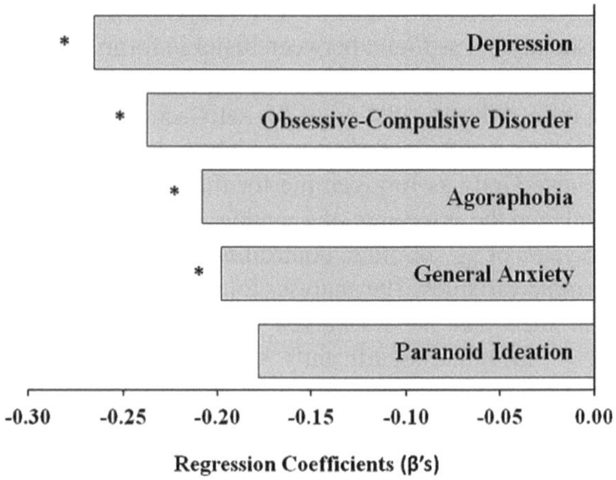

Fig. 24.1 Association of belief in Divine forgiveness with five types of psychiatric symptoms (Uecker et al. 2016 [11]); * $p < .05$

24.2 Belief in Evil and Mental Health

The belief that there is evil in the world can lead to doubts about one's religious beliefs, which in turn, may undermine mental health, as discussed in Chap. 23. This section of the chapter presents evidence that belief in evil can directly affect mental health.

Christianity, Judaism, and other world religions traditionally recognize two sources of evil in the world, human beings and malevolent supernatural beings [12–17]. This theological perspective defines human evil as acting contrary to God's will or God's laws [13, 18, 19]. Although the Hebrew Bible accepted the idea that humans were capable of doing good and evil [13, 20], human evil is more problematic for Christianity, which proposes that all of God's creations reflect God's goodness [21, 22]. The 5th Century theologian Aurelius Augustine provided a solution to this dilemma, claiming that despite the inherent goodness of humanity, the capacity of "free will" makes it possible for individuals to choose between good and evil [13, 23, 24]. Thomas Aquinas incorporated Augustine's explanation of human evil into his influential 13th Century treatise on Christian theology *Summa Theologica* [22].

Over the centuries, western philosophers and theologians have debated whether human nature is basically good or basically evil [25, 26]. Psychologists joined the debate in the 20th Century, with some psychologists arguing that human nature is inherently good (e.g., Carl Rogers) and others (e.g., Sigmund Freud) arguing it is inherently evil [13, 26, 27]. The fact that at least three books have been published since 2000 that contain the phrase "psychology of good and evil" in their titles is evidence that human evil is still a topic of interest in modern psychology [28–30]. However, 21st Century psychologists and other social scientists generally agree that human nature is not inherently good or evil, and that evil is the product of experiential and situational factors.

24.2.1 Belief in Human Evil and Mental Health

Although a number of studies have explored the psychology of evil, few have investigated the connection between evil and mental health. Indeed, to the best of my knowledge, just three published studies have explicitly examined the relationship between believing human nature is basically evil and mental health. Two of the three studies analyzed data from the General Social Survey (GSS) [31, 32].[5] The first study found that belief in human evil had a significant pernicious association with life satisfaction ($\beta = .14$) [31] and the second found that belief in human evil had a marginally significant pernicious association with anxiety ($\beta = .05$) [32].

The third study used data from the NSRH to examine the relationship between belief in human evil and psychiatric symptoms.[6] This is the same 2016 study by Uecker et al. [11], which was described in the preceding section of this chapter about Divine forgiveness and psychiatric symptoms. Figure 24.2 shows the results for the same five classes of psychiatric symptoms that were presented that section, but the names of some of the symptom classes have been shortened.

Believing that human nature is basically evil had significant pernicious associations with all five classes of psychiatric symptoms shown in Fig. 24.2. Belief in human evil had the strongest association with paranoid ideation, which might be expected on a priori grounds, as paranoia is essentially a distrust of people. The second highest association was between belief in human evil and depression. To the extent that depression represents a reaction to loss of social status, social rejection, or the termination of social relationships [33–38], as discussed in Chap. 12, believing that people are basically evil might be expected to increase depressive symptoms since interacting with evil people may yield any of these negative outcomes. The reasons for the variations in the strength of the other associations are not obvious to me. In any case, these results are also consistent with ETAS Theory, as evil people obviously pose a threat of harm; hence, the belief that people are basically evil should increase anxiety-related symptoms.

[5] One study used data from the 1987 GSS and the other used data from the 1996 GSS. The belief that human nature is basically evil was measured in both studies by combining respondents' agreement with the statements: "Human nature is fundamentally perverse and corrupt," and "Human nature is basically good," which was reversed scored. Both studies controlled for demographic characteristics, adverse life events, and religious variables.

[6] Belief in human evil was measured by combining respondents' agreement with the statements: "Human nature is basically evil," and "Human nature is basically good" (reversed scored).

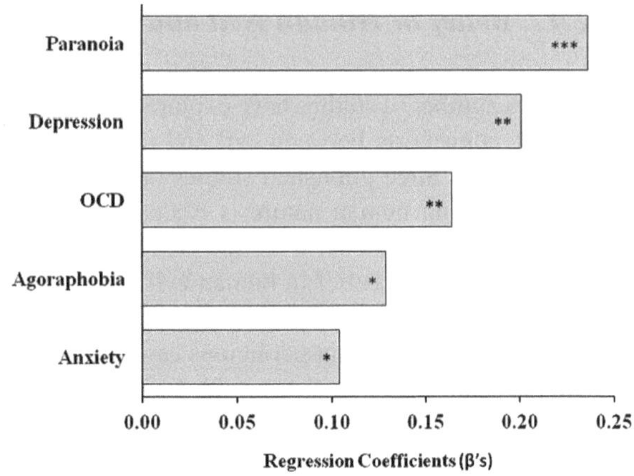

Fig. 24.2 Association of believing human nature is basically evil with five types of psychiatric symptoms (Uecker et al. 2016 [11]); * $p < .05$ ** $p < .01$ *** $p < .001$

24.2.2 *Belief in Human Evil and Divine Forgiveness and Psychiatric Symptoms*

Human evil tends to be subsumed under the concept of sin in Judeo-Christian theology, especially Christian theology [39, 40]. Sigmund Freud, the founder of psychoanalysis, argued that belief in sin, or that one has committed a sin, leads to guilt, which increases anxiety [41, 42]. A 1962 book by Albert Ellis, an American clinical psychologist, went further than Freud in claiming that all "neurotic disturbances" (neuroticism encompasses trait anxiety and other persistent expressions of negative affect [43, 44]) were the direct or indirect result of the concept of sin [45]. Christian writers of the time countered that the guilt associated with sin did not automatically lead to psychological disturbances because of the Christian belief that God forgives sinners, and that the beneficial effects of this belief can offset the adverse effects of guilt on psychological well-being [6].

Some of the studies on forgiveness by Watson, Morris, and Hood, which were described earlier in the chapter, provided evidence that guilt is associated with symptoms of depression and anxiety in college students [6–8], but no study until recently, has investigated whether belief in Divines forgiveness offsets the negative effects of belief in sin on mental health. The one study to do so is the same 2016 study by Uecker et al. that I already have mentioned in this chapter with respect to belief in forgiveness and belief in human evil, the latter of which is conceptually the same as sin in Christian theology [11].

As described above, the Uecker et al. study [11] asked a large sample of American adults about (a) the degree to which they believed that human nature is basically evil and (b) how often they believed that they had been forgiven by God. The net effects of each of the these two independent variables on psychiatric symptoms were presented in Figs. 24.1 and 24.2. Their third set of analyses of these data is of interest to us here. These analyses examined the degree to which belief in Divine forgiveness moderated the pernicious association between belief in human evil and psychiatric symptoms.

The study found that believing one has been forgiven by God significantly moderated the association between belief in human evil and agoraphobia ($\beta = -.11$), general anxiety ($\beta = -.14$), and paranoid ideation ($\beta = .13$). This moderation effect is illustrated for agoraphobia in Fig. 24.3. As one can see clearly in the left side of the figure, individuals who did not believe in human evil had low levels of agoraphobia, regardless of their belief in Divine forgiveness. However, as seen in the right side of the Fig. 24.3, whereas symptoms of agoraphobia were low among individuals who strongly believed in both human evil and Divine forgiveness (Highest Divine Forgiveness), individuals who strongly believed in human evil, but did not believe in Divine forgiveness (Lowest Devine Forgiveness) had significantly higher levels of agoraphobia. The pattern of results was very similar for general anxiety and paranoid ideation.

As already discussed, the net effects of belief and human evil and belief in Divine forgiveness are consistent with ETAS Theory in illustrating that beliefs that heighten fears about the dangerousness of the world and beliefs that provide a sense of safety are associated, respectively, with higher and lower levels of psychiatric symptoms. Uecker's results that belief in Divine forgiveness mediates the pernicious effect of belief in human evil on psychiatric symptoms are consistent with the proposition of ETAS Theory that positive and negative beliefs about the nature of the world (including the behavior of God) interact with each other to produce their net effect on psychiatric symptoms.

24.2.3 Belief in Satan and Psychiatric Symptoms

The second source of evil in Christian theology, as previously mentioned, is malevolent supernatural beings. The major source of supernatural evil in the Christian Bible is Satan, who is mentioned many times and many places in the New Testament. Although Satan is mentioned in several books of the Hebrew Bible (or Old Testament) and later Jewish writings [15, 46, 47], he does not have the same "demonic" status he has in Christian theology [15, 16, 47, 48]. Satan, who is also known to Christians as Lucifer and The Devil, is the personification of evil in Christianity, tempting people to commit sins that destroy themselves spiritually, physically harm others, and aid Satan in his battle against God [16, 49].

Although Catholicism and most Protestant denominations have down-played Satan's role in the world [47, 50, 51], many Americans believe Satan exists. For example, the 2005 Baylor Religious Survey found that 58% of American adults "absolutely" believed that Satan/The Devil exists and another 17% believed Satan/The Devil "probably" exists [52]. Moreover, 70% believe that some type of evil demons exists.

To the extent that individuals believe Satan or other demons exist, we would expect them to believe in the danger these malevolent supernatural beings pose to themselves and other people. Hence, belief in malevolent supernatural beings

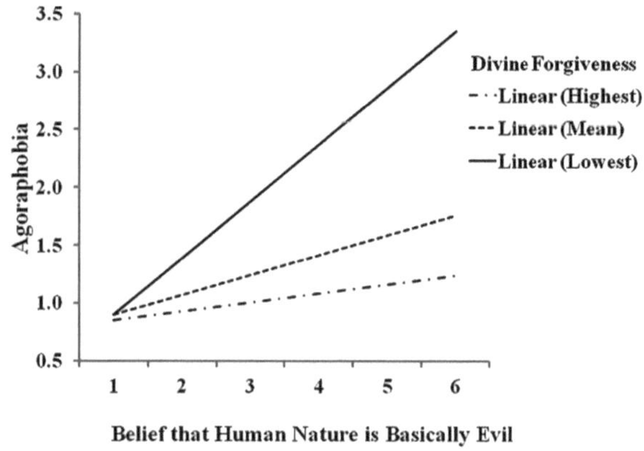

Fig. 24.3 Moderating effect of belief in Divine forgiveness on the association between agoraphobia and the belief that human nature is basically evil (Uecker et al. 2016 [11], *Review of Religious Research*; see reference list for complete citation; used by permission)

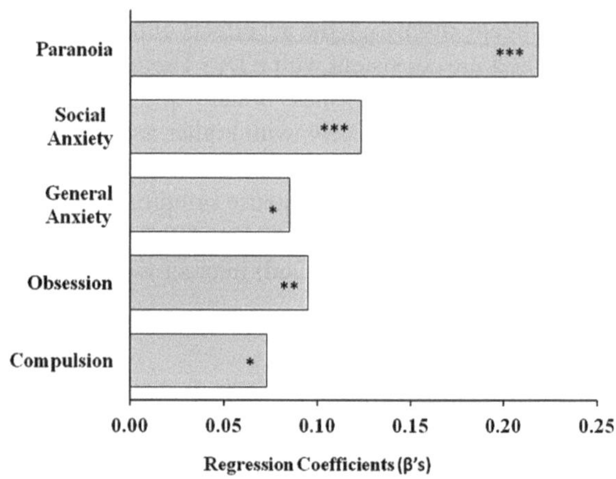

Fig. 24.4 Association of belief in Satan with five types of psychiatric symptoms from the 2010 Baylor Religion Survey; * $p < .05$ ** $p < .01$ *** $p < .001$

should increase psychiatric symptoms. A 2011 study by Flannelly et al. [53] provides some support for this hypothesis, and therefore, ETAS Theory. The study analyzed the association between psychiatric symptoms and a combined measure of people's belief in Satan and their belief in other demons, using data from the 2010 Baylor Religion Survey.

I decided to reanalyze the data from the 2011 Flannelly et al. study to focus solely on belief in Satan, controlling for age, gender, race, and frequency of private prayer and attending religious services. As seen in Fig. 24.4, the independent variable, belief in Satan, had a significant pernicious association with all five types of psychiatric symptoms. By far, the strongest association was between belief in Satan and paranoid ideation, probably because Satan acts through people to cause harm. The fact that Satan acts through people may also account for the association of the belief in Satan with social anxiety; however, social anxiety is mainly a fear of being embarrassed or rejected rather than a fear of actual physical harm, so one might expect a weaker association than that observed for paranoia. Belief in Satan probably had weaker associations with the other three dependent variables because they entail fears of more amorphous sources of danger.

24.3 Belief in Biblical Literalism and Seeking Help for Mental-Health Problems

Clergy are often called the “frontline workers” of the U.S. mental-health system [54, 55], and there is a good reason for this. The Epidemiologic Catchment Area Study, which was conducted by the National Institute of Mental Health in 1980–1985, found that Americans are more likely to seek help from clergy for serious mental-health problems than they are to seek help from psychologists or psychiatrists [56]. This result was confirmed by the 1990–1992 National Comorbidity Survey (NCS). The NCS found: (a) that roughly 25% of U.S. adults who sought treatment for mental-health problems, sought help from clergy; and (b) that nearly 25% of those who sought help from clergy had a serious mental-health disorder. Moreover, most of the persons who sought help from clergy did not seek help from mental-health professionals or other health-care professionals [57].

Naturally, people who are more religious are more likely to seek help from clergy for mental-health problems [58]. A 2006 study by Chris Ellison, me, and some colleagues found that several aspects of religion influence whether people think they should seek mental-health assistance from clergy [59].[7] For example, individuals who attended religious services more often were significantly more likely to recommend clergy as a primary source of mental-health assistance. However, this effect varied by religious denomination. Catholics were more likely to recommend clergy as a primary source of assistance than were all other survey respondents except Protestants. Protestants were more likely than Catholics to recommend clergy, and Conservative Protestants (i.e., Evangelical and Fundamentalist Protestants) were more likely than other Protestants to recommend clergy. After controlling for both church attendance and religious denomination, individuals who believed that the Bible was literally true were significantly more likely than other individuals to recommend clergy as a primary source of assistance for mental-health problems.

Unlike Catholic priests, Protestant clergy provide pastoral counseling to congregants on a wide range of personal and family issues [55, 59–62], which probably accounts for the differences between Protestant and Catholics about recommending clergy. In addition, Conservative Protestant denominations are more likely than other Protestant denominations to profess the belief that mental-health problems are spiritual problems, and that mental illness results from human sinfulness and immorality [63, 64]; thus, members of these religious denominations are naturally more likely to seek help for mental-health problems from their clergy. Furthermore, research also suggests that Conservative Protestants may avoid seeking help from mental-health professionals because they think mental-health professionals do not

[7] The study analyzed data from the 1996 GSS.

share their values [65], and they are concerned that mental-health professionals may try to change their values and beliefs [64].

Belief in Biblical literalism is associated with: (a) belief in the ubiquity of sin [66], which underlies the belief that mental illness is a spiritual problem, and (b) the belief that the Bible is the ultimate source of authority [66], which undermines the acceptance of scientific explanations of the world, including mental illness [66, 67]. Therefore, individuals who believe in Biblical literalism should be less likely to seek help from mental-health providers, whose professional practice is based upon science. Although belief in Biblical literalism is a central tenant of Fundamentalist and Evangelical Protestantism [59, 68], as individuals vary in their degree of belief, some Conservative Protestants in the 2006 Ellison et al. study may have had a stronger belief in Biblical literalism than others, which may be why Biblical literalism had a significant net effect on preferring mental-health assistance from clergy, above that which was accounted for by belonging to a Conservative Protestant denomination. Unfortunately, I am not aware of any published studies that have specifically investigated the association between belief in Biblical literalism and mental health, per se.

24.4 Belief in Biblical Literalism and Psychiatric Symptoms

Although I do not know of any published study that has specifically investigated the association between belief in Biblical literalism and mental health, I came across a 2015 article by David Hayward and Neal Krause that examined depression in older Mexican Americans who were either Evangelical Protestants or Roman Catholics [69]. The study, which surveyed more than 1.500 people, found that the Evangelical Protestants reported significantly fewer depressive symptoms than did the Catholics. As Evangelical Protestants are much more likely than Catholics to believe that the Bible in literally true [70], Evangelical Protestantism may be considered to be a proxy belief for Biblical literalism.

The 2010 Baylor Religion Survey contains one item that measures Biblical literalism, one item that measures Evangelicalism, and one item that provides a crude measure of depression.[8] Therefore, I decided to see if I could separate the apparent effects of Evangelical Protestantism on depression from the possible effects of belief in Biblical literalism. Bivariate correlations indicated that depression had a

[8] Biblical literalism was measured by a participant's response to the question, "Which one statements comes closest to your personal belief about the Bible?": 4 ("The Bible means exactly what it says. It should be taken literally, word-for-word, on all subjects."); 3 ("The Bible is perfectly true but it should not be taken literally, word-for-word. We must interpret its meaning."); 2 ("The Bible contains some human error."), and 1 ("The Bible is an ancient book of history and legend.").

Evangelicalism was measured by a participant's response to the following question. "How well do the following terms describe your religious identity?" Over a dozen terms were listed, including "Evangelical." The response categories were: 4 ("Very well"); 3 ("Somewhat well"); 2 ("Not very well"), and 1 ("Not at all").

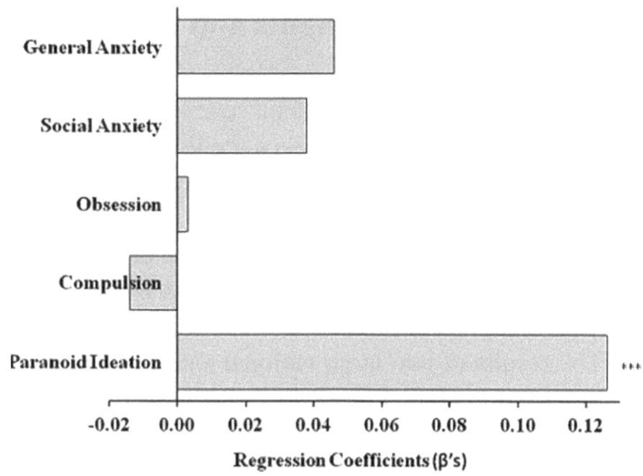

Fig. 24.5 Association of belief in Biblical literalism with five types of psychiatric symptoms in the 2010 Baylor Religion Survey; *** $p < .001$

significant negative relationship with both Evangelicalism ($r = -.074$) and believing in Biblical literalism ($r = -.093$). Therefore, I decided to see if these associations were significant when I used the same regression model I used earlier in this chapter to test the effects of belief in Satan. Separate regression models performed on Evangelicalism and belief in Biblical literalism found that neither had a significant association with depression. These results indicated that the bivariate analyses had probably captured the effects of frequency of prayer or attending religious services on depression, not Evangelicalism or belief in Biblical literalism, per se.

I decided to test the net effects of belief in Biblical literalism on psychiatric symptoms, using the same regression model and the same dependent variables I used in my analyses of belief in Satan (general anxiety, obsession, compulsion, social anxiety, and paranoia), with data from the Baylor Religion Survey. I found belief in Biblical literalism had a fairly large pernicious association with paranoid ideation, but none of the other associations even approached statistical significance (see Fig. 24.5). I suspect the paranoid symptoms reported by persons who believe the Bible is literally true may be attributable to the threats posed to their religious beliefs and cultural values by science and various aspects of modern American culture [66, 67, 71–74]. I think the response to these threats may be expressed as paranoia because the source of the threats is personified as evil people from outside their religious group.

Depression was measured by the question: "During the past 30 days, how many days have you felt sad, blue, or depressed? The response categories were: 4 ("All 30 days"); 3 ("21–29 days"); 2 ("11–20 day"), and 1 ("1–10 days") and 0 ("None").

24.5 Chapter Highlights and Comments

This chapter presents findings on several diverse but inter-related topics. The major findings related to ETAS Theory are the association of psychiatric symptoms with belief in (a) Divine forgiveness, (b) human evil, (c) Satan, and (d) Biblical literalism, and (e) the interaction of belief in human evil and Divine forgiveness. An equally important finding, which is not directly related to ETAS Theory, is that belief in Biblical literalism influences personal attitudes about who to seek for help for psychological problems.

The results of two large national studies of U.S. adults demonstrated that belief in Satan and the belief that human nature is basically evil had significant pernicious associations with all the psychiatric symptoms they measured. These findings are consistent with ETAS Theory in that people who believe in Satan and human evil should also believe that Satan and evil people pose direct threats of harm, which is likely to activate the "aversive amplification circuit" that is known to increases the amygdala's response to potential threats, and therefore, increases fear and anxiety. These two studies found that paranoia had the strongest association with belief in human evil and belief in Satan possibly because these beliefs imply there are evil people who intend to do you harm and that Satan does harm by working through people.

In contrast to the pernicious association between mental health and the three religious beliefs I just mentioned, belief in Divine forgiveness has been found to have a salubrious associated with depression and other psychiatric symptoms in convenience and national samples of Americans. Moreover, these national studies found that belief in Divine forgiveness directly counters the pernicious effect of belief in human evil on depression, anxiety disorders, and other psychiatric symptoms. This interaction of belief in human evil and belief in Divine forgiveness confirms the prediction of ETAS Theory that beliefs interact with one another in determining their net effects on psychiatric symptoms. Believing that you have been forgiven by God implies you believe (a) that God is benevolent, (b) that God is involved your life, and (c) that you have a good relationship with God. All of these beliefs should provide a sense of safety that reduces psychiatric symptoms.

My own analyses of the association between belief in Biblical literalism and psychiatric symptoms found that it had a pernicious association only with paranoia. I think this can be explained, consistent with ETAS Theory, by the fact that science poses a direct threat to belief in Biblical literalism and aspects of modern American culture pose a threat to other religious and cultural beliefs of individuals who believe the Bible is literally true. Because the source of these threats is personified as evil outsiders, the reaction to the threats is paranoia.

References

1. Lutjen, L. J., Silton, N. R., & Flannelly, K. J. (2012). Religion, forgiveness, hostility and health: A structural equation analysis. *Journal of Religion and Health, 51*(2), 468–478.
2. Silton, N. R., Flannelly, K. J., & Lutjen, L. J. (2013). It pays to forgive! Aging, forgiveness, hostility, and health. *Journal of Adult Development, 20*(4), 222–231.
3. McCullough, M. E., Pargament, K. I., & Thoresen, C. E. (2000). *Forgiveness: Theory, research, and practice*. New York: Guilford Press
4. McCullough, M. E. (2008). *Beyond revenge: The evolution of the forgiveness instinct*. San Francisco: Jossey-Bass.
5. Worthington, E. L., Jr. (Ed.). (1998). *Dimensions of forgiveness: Psychological research & theological perspectives*. Philadelphia: Templeton Foundation Press.
6. Watson, P. J., Morris, R. J., & Hood, R. W. (1988). Sin and self-functioning: I. Grace, guilt, and self-consciousness. *Journal of Psychology and Theology, 16*, 254–269.
7. Watson, P. J., Morris, R. J., & Hood, R. W. (1988). Sin and self-functioning: II. Grace, guilt, and psychological adjustment. *Journal of Psychology and Theology, 16*, 270–281.
8. Watson, P. J., Morris, R. J., & Hood, R. W. (1988). Sin and self-functioning: III. The psychology and ideology of irrational beliefs. *Journal of Psychology and Theology, 16*, 348–361.
9. Toussaint, L. L., Williams, D. R., Musick, M. A., & Everson, S. A. (2001). Forgiveness and health: Age differences in a U.S. probability sample. *Journal of Adult Development, 8*, 249–257.
10. Krause, N., & Ellison, C. G. (2003). Forgiveness by God, forgiveness of others, and psychological well-being in late life. *Journal for the Scientific Study of Religion, 42*, 77–93.
11. Uecker, J. E., Ellison, C. G., Flannelly, K. J., & Burdette, A. M. (2016). Belief in human sinfulness, belief in experiencing divine forgiveness, and psychiatric symptoms. *Review of Religious Research. 58*(1), 1–26.
12. Kolakowski, L. (2004). Leibniz & Job: The metaphysics of evil and the experience of evil. *The New Criterion, 22*(5), 18–23.
13. Buchholz, E. S., & Mandel, J. K. (2000). Reaching for virtue, stumbling on sin: Concepts of good and evil in a postmodern era. *Journal of Religion and Health, 39*(2), 123.
14. Martinez, B. (2013). Is evil good for religion? The link between supernatural evil and religious commitment. *Review of Religious Research, 55*(2), 319–338.
15. Pagels, E. (1991). The social history of Satan, the "intimate enemy": A preliminary sketch. *Harvard Theological Review, 84*(2), 105–128.
16. Perry, M. (1990). Taking Satan seriously. *The Expository Times, 101*(4), 105–112.
17. Atran, S., & Norenzayan, A. (2004). Religion's evolutionary landscape: Counterintuition, commitment, compassion, communion. *Behavioral and Brain Sciences, 27*(6), 713–730.
18. Peels, R. (2010). The effects of sin upon human moral cognition. *Journal of Reformed Theology, 4*(1), 42–69.
19. Thang Moe, D. (2015). Sin and evil in Christian and Buddhist perspectives: A quest for theodicy. *Asia Journal of Theology, 29*(1), 22–46.
20. King James Holy Bible (1611/1999). Dayton: Greyden Press.
21. Webster, J. (2015). *God without measure: Working papers in Christian theology* (Vol. 1). New York: Bloomsbury Publishing.
22. Aquinas, T. (1981). *Summa theologica*. Westminister: Christian Classics.
23. Augustine (398/2008). *The confessions of St. Augustine*. Minneapolis: Filiquarian Publishing LLC.
24. Augustine, A. (2010). *On the free choice of will, on grace and free will, and other writings*. Cambridge: Cambridge University Press.
25. Kelly, J. F. (2002). *The problem of evil in the Western tradition*. Collegeville: The Liturgical Press.
26. Boa, K. (2004). *Augustine to Freud: What theologians and psychologists tell us about human nature*. Nashville: B & H Publishing.

27. Martin, J. D., Blair, G. E., Nevels, R. M., & Brant, M. M. (1987). A study of the relationship between a personal philosophy of human nature (good or evil) and self-esteem. *Psychological Reports, 61*(2), 447–451.
28. Staub, E. (2003). *The psychology of good and evil: Why children, adults, and groups help and harm others*. Cambridge: Cambridge University Press.
29. Miller, A. G. (Ed.). (2004). *The social psychology of good and evil*. New York: Guilford Press.
30. Dilman, I. (2005). *The self, the soul, and the psychology of good and evil*. New York: Routledge.
31. Musick, M. A. (2000). Theodicy and life satisfaction among black and white Americans. *Sociology of Religion, 61*(3), 267–287.
32. Ellison, C. G., Burdette, A. M., & Hill, T. D. (2009). Blessed assurance: Religion, anxiety, and tranquility among US adults. *Social Science Research, 38*(3), 656–667.
33. Price, J. S., Gardner, R., Jr., Wilson, D. R., Sloman, L., Rohde, P., & Erickson, M. (2007). Territory, rank and mental health: The history of an idea. *Evolutionary Psychology, 5*(3), 531–554.
34. Price, J. S., Gardner, R., Jr., & Erickson, M. (2004). Can depression, anxiety and somatization be understood as appeasement displays? *Journal of Affective Disorders, 79*(1–3), 1–11.
35. Sloman, L., Gilbert, P., & Hasey, G. (2003). Evolved mechanisms in depression: The role of attachment and social rank in depression. *Journal of Affective Disorders, 74*(2), 107–121.
36. Panksepp, J. (2010). Affective neuroscience of the emotional BrainMind: Evolutionary perspectives and implications for understanding depression. *Dialogues in Clinical Neuroscience, 12*(4), 533–544.
37. Watson, P. J., & Andrews, P. W. (2002). Toward a revised evolutionary adaptationist analysis of depression: The social navigation hypothesis . *Journal of Affective Disorders, 72*(1), 1–14.
38. Welling, H. (2003). An evolutionary function of the depressive reaction: The cognitive map hypothesis. *New Ideas in Psychology, 21*(2), 147–156.
39. Richardson, A., & Bowden, J. (Eds.). (1983). *The Westminister dictionary of Christian theology*. Philadelphia: The Westminister Press.
40. Lotker, M. (2004). *A Christian's guide to Judaism*. Mahwah: Paulist Press.
41. Freud, S. (1939). *Moses and monotheism*. London: The Hogarth Press.
42. Freud, S. (1939/1962). *Civilization and its discontents*. New York: W.W. Norton & Company.
43. Lahey, B. B. (2009). Public health significance of neuroticism. *American Psychologist, 64*(4), 241–256.
44. Ormel, J., Rosmalen, J., & Farmer, A. (2004). Neuroticism: A non-informative marker of vulnerability to psychopathology. *Social Psychiatry and Psychiatric Epidemiology, 39*(11), 906–912.
45. Ellis, A. (1962). *Reason and emotion in psychotherapy*. Secaucus: Lyle Stuart.
46. Tate, M. E. (1992). Satan in the old testament. *Review and Expositor, 89*(4), 461–474.
47. Mallowe, M. (1995). Is evil just the devil in disguise? *U.S. Catholic*, 60, 6–13.
48. Lenchak, T. A. (2009). What's biblical about … the devil? *Bible Today, 47*(4), 277–279.
49. Russell, J. B. (1977). *The devil: Perceptions of evil from anitquity to primitive Christianity*. Ithaca: Cornell University Press.
50. Camille, A. (2003). Where have all the demons gone? *U.S. Catholic, 68*(2), 45–47.
51. Quay, P. M. (1981). Angels and demons: The teaching of IV Lateran. *Theological Studies, 42*(1), 20–45.
52. Baker, J. (2008). Who believes in religious evil? An investigation of sociological patterns of belief in Satan, hell, and demons. *Review of Religious Research, 50*(2), 206–220.
53. Flannelly, K. J., Galek, K., Jankowski, K. R. B., Ellison, C. G., & Silton, N. R. (2011). Angels and demons and psychiatric symptoms. Paper presented at the Annual meeting of the Association for Psychological Science, Washington, DC.
54. Oppenheimer, J., Flannelly, K., & Weaver, A. (2004). A comparative analysis of the psychological literature on collaboration between clergy and mental-health professionals – Perspectives from secular and religious journals: 1970–1999. *Pastoral Psychology, 53*(2), 153–162.

55. Weaver, A. J., Flannelly, K. J., Flannelly, L. T., & Oppenheimer, J. E. (2003). Collaboration between clergy and mental-health professionals: A review of professional health-care journals from 1980 to 1999. *Counseling and Values, 47*, 162–171.
56. Hohmann, A. A., & Larson, D. B. (1993). Psychiatric factors predicting use of clergy. In E. L. Worthington, Jr. (Ed.), *Psychotherapy and religious values* (pp. 71–84). Grand Rapids: Baker House.
57. Wang, P., Berglund, P., & Kessler, R. (2003). Patterns and correlates of contacting clergy for mental disorders in the United States. *Health Services Research, 38*(2), 647–673.
58. Abe-Kim, J., Gong, F., & Takeuchi, D. (2004). Religiosity, spirituality, and help-seeking among Filipino Americans: Religious clergy or mental health professionals? *Journal of Community Psychology, 32*(6), 675–689.
59. Ellison, C. G., Vaaler, M. L., Flannelly, K. J., & Weaver, A. J. (2006). The clergy as a source of mental health assistance: What Americans believe. *Review of Religious Research, 48*(2), 190–211.
60. Moran, M., Flannelly, K., Weaver, A., Overvold, J., Hess, W., & Wilson, J. (2005). A study of pastoral care, referral, and consultation practices among clergy in four settings in the New York City area. *Pastoral Psychology, 53*(3), 255–266.
61. Clemens, N. A., Corradi, R. B., & Wasman, M. (1978). The parish clergy as a mental health resource. *Journal of Religion and Health, 17*(4), 227–232.
62. Bell, R. A., Morris, R. R., Holzer, C. E., 3rd, & Warheit, G. J. (1976). The clergy as a mental health resource: Part I. *Journal of Pastoral Care, 30*(2), 103–108.
63. Wesselmann, E. D., Day, M., Graziano, W. G., & Doherty, E. F. (2015). Religious beliefs about mental illness influence social support preferences. *Journal of Prevention & Intervention in the Community, 43*(3), 165–174.
64. McLatchie, L. R., & Draguns, J. G. (1984). Mental health concepts of Evangelical Protestants. *Journal of Psychology, 118*(2), 147.
65. Chaddock, T. P., & McMinn, M. R. (1999). Values affecting collaboration among psychologists and evangelical clergy. *Journal of Psychology and Theology, 27*(4), 319–328.
66. Ellison, C. G., & Musick, M. A. (1995). Conservative Protestantism and publice opinion toward science. *Review of Religious Research, 36*(3), 245.
67. Evans, J. H. (2011). Epistemological and moral conflict between religion and science. *Journal for the Scientific Study of Religion, 50*(2), 707–727.
68. Marsden, G. M. (2006). *Fundamentalism and American culture*. New York: Oxford University Press.
69. Hayward, R. D., & Krause, N. (2015). Evangelical group membership, depression, and well-being among older Mexican Americans: A comparison with older non-Hispanic Whites. *Mental Health, Religion and Culture, 18*(4), 273–285.
70. Steensland, B., Robinson, L. D., Wilcox, W. B., Park, J. Z., Regnerus, M. D., & Woodberry, R. D. (2000). The measure of American religion: Toward improving the state of the art. *Social Forces, 79*(1), 291–318.
71. Evans, J. H. (2013). The growing social and moral conflict between conservative Protestantism and science. *Journal for the Scientific Study of Religion, 52*(2), 368–385.
72. Sherkat, D. E., & Ellison, C. G. (1997). The cognitive structure of a moral crusade: Conservative Protestantism and opposition to pornography. *Social Forces, 75*(3), 957–980.
73. Bartkowski, J. P., & Ellison, C. G. (1995). Divergent models of childrearing in popular manuals: Conservative Protestants vs. the mainstream experts. *Sociology of Religion, 56*(1), 21–34.
74. Ellison, C. G., & Nybroten, K. A. (1999). Conservative protestantism and opposition to state-sponsored lotteries: Evidence from the 1997 Texas poll. *Social Science Quarterly, 80*(2), 356–369.

Part V
Summary, Conclusions, and Recommendations for Future Research

Chapter 25
The Historical Development of Theories of Organic Evolution

Abstract This chapter reviews most of the major points made in Part 1 of the book. The first chapter of Part I (Chap. 2) describes the philosophical and theological beliefs held in the Western world from the 5th Century (BCE) through the 13th Century (AD) that were impediments to the recognition of organic evolution. The Protestant Reformation, which began in the early part of the 16th Century, rejected Scholasticism (which had dominated Christian theology and learning), and stressed the supremacy of the *Holy Scriptures* in Christian theology and the belief that the *Scriptures* were literally true. As Chap. 3 notes, this context transformed the study of Natural History into Natural Theology, which became a mechanism to understand God through his creations. Although some areas of science flourished during this time, religious orthodoxy hampered evolutionary thought. The Age of Enlightenment, which began in the late 17th Century, questioned accepted beliefs about the world, opening the door, ever so slightly, for scientific explanations of the origin of the universe and the origin of life. The latter part of this chapter (which covers portions of Chaps. 3 and 4) summarizes the contributions of the Enlightenment thinkers Georges-Louis Leclerc Buffon, Dr. Erasmus Darwin, and Jean-Baptiste Lamarck to the development of the theory of organic evolution, and presents conclusions to be drawn from Part I.

Keywords Aristotle • Augustine • Bible • Buffon • Common ancestor • Darwin • Evolution • Intelligent design • Lamarck • Natural Theology

25.1 Historical Background from the Greeks to the Enlightenment

Part I of the book traced the development of theories of organic evolution before Charles Darwin. The prevailing philosophical and theological beliefs held in the Western world from the 5th Century (BCE) through the 13th Century (AD) were not conducive to the development of a theory of organic evolution or even the idea of organic evolution. Philosophers and theologians mainly believed in a static world created by God or some other higher power, such as Plato's divine creator or Aristotle's prime mover. The keystone of the static-world view in Christianity was

K.J. Flannelly, *Religious Beliefs, Evolutionary Psychiatry, and Mental Health in America*, Religion, Spirituality and Health: A Social Scientific Approach 1,
DOI 10.1007/978-3-319-52488-7_25

the Bible's *Book of Genesis* that described how God created the universe, the earth, and all its inhabitants in 6 days. Although a literal interpretation of the *Book of Genesis* strongly implies that God's creatures have not changed since God made them, the 5th Century (AD) theologian, Augustine of Hippo, thought the 6 days of creation described in the *Book of Genesis* should not be taken literally and that the *Book of Genesis* did not necessarily preclude the possibility that the animals and plants that God created could not change in form [1–3]. Although few Christian theologians before the 20th Century embraced Augustine's idea that plant and animal forms could change over time, Augustine's critique of the *Book of Genesis* [2, 3] undermined the belief that the *Holy Scriptures* are the literal word of God, as early as the 5th Century AD.

Both Aristotle and Plato's philosophical ideas influenced Christian thought about the nature of God, humans, and the world at large. Their belief in an unchanging world and their belief in teleology – that everything in the world exists for a purpose – reinforced the Christian belief that the *Book of Genesis* was literally true and that the apparent harmony and purposiveness of nature was exclusively the work of God. Their beliefs satisfied the goal of Thomas Aquinas and Scholasticism to demonstrate that Christian faith is consistent with reason [1], but it gave scientific credence to religious beliefs that were inconsistent with the recognition that plants and animals, and the earth itself, changed over time, and therefore, hampered the development of theories of organic evolution.

There were two key Christian beliefs that became barriers to the development of evolutionary theory. The first belief was that the world and the plants and animals that inhabit it were created by God as described in the *Book of Genesis*. The second related belief was that plants and animals have not changed since they were created by God – the belief than plant and animal species are immutable.

The Protestant Reformation, which began in the early part of the 16th Century, rejected Scholasticism, and stressed the supremacy of the *Holy Scriptures* in Christian theology [1, 4]. It stressed, among other things, that all Christians should read the Old Testament (the Hebrew Bible) and that the *Book of Genesis*, like the rest of the Bible, was literally true. The Reformation coincided with an increased interest in Natural History [5] and its rejection of Scholasticism may have spurred this interest [6, 7]. Many Protestant ministers actively pursued the study of nature [5], turning Natural History into Natural Theology, as a way to understand God through his creations [6]. Religious beliefs were expressed in the writings of many 16th Century Naturalists [8, 9], the most prominent of which was John Ray, whose book, *The Wisdom of God Manifested in the Works of Creation*, discussed how God had fashioned each kind animal so that it is ideally suited, or adapted, to the environment in which it lives [10–12]. According to Ray, each species was created by God to be perfectly matched to its environment; hence, it must have remained the same as it was on the day of its creation. The belief that the earth was only several thousand years old also made it difficult imagine that animals had changed since God created them.

The evolutionary biologist Ernst Mayr has said that belief in Divine design was the only possible explanation, at the time, of the fit between an animal and its environment because there was no other plausible explanation of why each animal species is so well adapted to its environment [6]. Swiss naturalist Carl von Linnė (better known as Linnaeus) spent much of his life systematically classifying plants and animals based on the assumption of Divine creation and design. Although Linnaeus' taxonomic system contributed directly to the advancement of biology, and perhaps, indirectly to the development of evolutionary theory, Ernst Mayr thought it hampered evolutionary thought more than it helped it, because Linnaeus' belief that species were immutable made organic evolution a scientific problem that it would not have been otherwise [6].

The Age of Enlightenment, which began in the late 17th Century [13, 14], was a time during which thoughtful people tried to understand the reason behind everything and questioned accepted beliefs about the world and traditional institutions, including governments and religions [6, 13–15]. "To the extent that Christianity was based on divine revelation rather than human reason, it lost its credibility among enlightened thinkers" (p. 13) [15].

25.2 Three Enlightenment Thinkers and Their Thoughts About Evolution

Georges-Louis Leclerc Buffon, Erasmus Darwin, and Jean-Baptiste de Monet Lamarck were three major Enlightenment thinkers who questioned accepted religious beliefs about nature of the world. By challenging the concept of the immutability of species that had become ingrained in Christian theology and science, they laid the philosophical and scientific groundwork for the modern theory of organic evolution [16, 17].

Buffon introduced the readers of his widely popular *Historie Naturelle* to every major topic that Charles Darwin discussed in his 1859 book on evolution, and Buffon's writings thereby set the stage for Charles Darwin and other 19th Century evolutionary theorists [16, 18]. Buffon's major contributions to evolutionary thought were: (1) the concept of "degeneration," which was comparable to the concept of evolution; (2) that degeneration reflected descent from a common ancestor; (3) that degeneration results from physical changes that occur in wild animals as they adapt to changes in their environments; and (4) that these gradual changes in wild animals and their offspring over vast amounts of time led to the development of different species, much as domestic animals can be bred to create different varieties and breeds of animals [18].

Dr. Erasmus Darwin, Charles Darwin's grandfather, had ideas about organic evolution that were similar, in many ways, to Buffon's ideas. Like Buffon, he believed animals evolved to adapt to their environments, but he went beyond Buffon ideas about evolution by suggesting that evolution was driven by three basic "wants" or needs: the need for self-protection ("security"), the need for nourishment ("hunger"), and the need to reproduce ("mating"). Changes in animals that arose to meet these needs resulted in improvements in their ability to survive that were passed onto offspring over successive generations. Over generations, more and more improvements would be reflected in more and more changes in morphology and behavior, which would make the descendents a different species than their common ancestor. Like Buffon, Dr. Darwin thought that domestication provided evidence for the evolution of different species from a common ancestor through very gradual steps, and that the great age of the earth made it possible for vast changes to occur in both plants and animals over time. However, he went much farther than Buffon in explicitly proposing that all plants and animals have descended from a common primitive form of life.

In 1802, seven years before Jean-Baptiste Lamarck published his book on evolution, the prominent Anglican priest and theologian William Paley published a book in England titled *Natural Theology; or Evidences of the Existence and Attributes of the Deity, Collected from the Appearances of Nature* [19]. *Natural Theology* expanded on John Ray's themes in *The Wisdom of God*, which claimed that God designed each plant and animal species to fit perfectly into the habitat in which it lives. *Natural Theology* included the frequently repeated analogy that the parts of the body are like the parts of a watch, which are so complicated and inter-related that they must be the product of an "intelligent and designing Creator" (p. 154) or "an intelligent, designing mind" (p. 280) [20]. Although the book was popular among the British public as well as British academics, who rejected the possibility of organic evolution, European academics were more open to evolutionary ideas, and by the early 19th Century, naturalists and intellectuals in Germany, Italy, and France were discussing the possibility of organic evolution [21–23]. Thus, the time was right on the Continent, if not in Britain, for a comprehensive theory of organic evolution [23].

Jean-Baptiste Lamarck is recognized as the founder of evolutionary theory because his 1809 book *Philosophie Zoologique* [24] contains the first thorough formulation of the causes of organic evolution and the first attempt to trace a possible path of descent from a common ancestor across the animal kingdom [1, 25–28]. Like the Comte de Buffon and Erasmus Darwin before him, Lamarck believed the earth was very old and that the dramatic changes that humans can produce in domesticated animals through selective breeding provided evidence that wild animals could change dramatically in behavior, shape, size, and other characteristics over vast amounts of time [29]. Over time, species of animals could transform into entirely new species; species could change so much that they could form new genera, and new genera could change so much they could form new families of animals, and so on. Given enormous amounts of time, families could form new orders and new orders could form new classes of animals.

Lamarck had two theories of evolution. The first theory was that lower forms of life progressed into higher forms in terms of complexity and perfection [24, 29] because there is a natural force in living things that drive them to perfect themselves [26, 29–31]. His second theory is famously known as the "the theory of the inheritance of acquired characteristics" [26, 27]. Both theories were eventually refuted and neither was every widely accepted [26].

Several theories of evolution were proposed between Lamarck's 1809 *Philosophie Zoologique* and Darwin's 1859 *Origins of Species*. Though none of them was accepted by the scientific community, these theories demonstrate that the concept of organic evolution was "in the air," so to speak. While no theory of evolution had yet attained scientific acceptance, the 1844 book *Vestiges of the Natural History of Creation* [32] created popular interest in Britain about the possibility of evolution. The book summarized the existing geological evidence of the time to argue that life on earth had gradually evolved as Lamarck had proposed over an extremely long period of time. Even thought the *Vestiges* was renounced by British intellectuals and condemned by British theologians as Godless and heretical, it became a best seller in Britain [6, 16], which suggests that the general public may have been more open to the idea of organic evolution than were British theologians of intellectuals.

25.3 Conclusions

Early theological and philosophical thought did not provide fertile ground for the emergence of ideas about organic evolution, and by the end of 13th Century AD both religion and science in Europe accepted two basic beliefs that were barriers to the development of evolutionary theory: (1) that the world and the plants and animals that inhabit it were created by God as described in the *Book of Genesis*; and (2) that plants and animals have not changed since they were created by God – the belief than plants and animals species are immutable.

Theories of organic evolution began to appear in the middle of the 18th Century, but religion, science, and society at large were not receptive to them. Little had changed by the beginning of beginning of the 19th Century when Lamarck published his theories of evolution. Lamarck's theories were dismissed in favor of the accepted doctrine that species were immutable and that God had designed each and every creature so that it fit perfectly into its habitat. However, evidence was mounting that organic evolution occurs and it is clear that a theory of evolution much like Charles Darwin's would have been published by the end of the 19th Century even if Darwin had not published his *Origin of Species*.

References

1. Sedgwick, W. T., Tyler, H. W., & Bigelow, R. P. (1939). *A short history of science* (Revised ed.). New York: MacMillan.
2. Augustine (389/2002). *On Genesis: A refutation of the Manichees*. Hype Park: New City Press.
3. Augustine (415/1982). *The literal meaning of Genesis*. Mahwah: Paulist Press.
4. Selden, J. (1984). Aquinas, Luther, Melanchthon, and biblical apologetics. *Grace Theological Journal, 5*(2), 181–195.
5. Miall, L. C. (1912). *The early naturalists, their lives and work (1530–1789)*. New York: Macmillan.

6. Mayr, E. (1982). *The growth of biological thought*. London: Belknap Press.
7. Harrison, P. (1998). *The Bible, Protestantism, and the rise of natural science*. Cambridge: Cambridge University Press.
8. Ley, W. (1968). *Dawn of zoology*. Englewood Cliffs: Prentice-Hall.
9. Ogilvie, B. W. (2008). Nature's Bible: Insects in seventeenth-century art and science. *Tidsskrift for Kulturforskning, 7*(3), 5–21.
10. Bowler, P. J. (2003). *Evolution: The history of an idea*. Berkeley/Los Angeles: University of California Press.
11. Bowler, P. J., & Morus, I. R. (2005). *Making modern science: A historical survey*. Chicago: University of Chicago Press.
12. Huxley, R. (2007). John Ray: The english aristotle. In R. Huxley (Ed.), *The great naturalists* (pp. 92–97). London: Thames & Hudson.
13. Reill, P. H., & Wilson, E. J. (2004). *Encyclopedia of the enlightenment* (Revised ed.). New York: Book Builders.
14. Venn, C. (2006). The enlightenment. *Theory, Culture and Society, 23*(2–3), 477–498.
15. Larson, E. J. (2004). *Evolution: The remarkable history of a scientific theory*. New York: The Modern Library.
16. Eiseley, L. (1961). *Darwin's century: Evolution and the men who discovered it*. Garden City: Anchor Books.
17. Dendy, A. (1915). Progressive evolution and the origin of species. *The American Naturalist, 49*(579), 149–182.
18. Eiseley, L. (1970). The dawn of evolutionary theory. In L. B. Young (Ed.), *Evolution on man*. New York: Oxford University Press.
19. Ferre, F. (2001). William Paley. In P. B. Dematteis, & P. S. Fosi (Eds.), *Dictionary of literary biography: British philosophers, 1500–1799* (Vol. 252, pp. 299–306). Farington Hills: The Gale Group.
20. Paley, W. (1802/1881). *Natural theology*. New York: American Trust Society.
21. Osborn, H. F. (1894). *From the Greeks to Darwin*. New York: MacMillan.
22. Corsi, P. (2005). Before Darwin: Transformist concepts in European natural history. *Journal of the History of Biology, 38*(1), 67–83.
23. Corsi, P. (1988). *The age of Lamarck: Evolutionary theories in France 1790–1830* (J. Mandelbaum, Trans.). Berkeley: University of California Press.
24. Lamarck, J. B. (1809/1873). *Philosophie zoologique*. Paris: Librairie F. Savy.
25. Curtis, W. C. (1922). *Science and human affairs from the viewpoint of biology* New York: Harcourt, Brace and Company.
26. Mayr, E. (1972). Lamarck revisited. *Journal of the History of Biology, 5*(1), 55–94.
27. Butler, S. (1879). *Evolution, old and new; or, the theories of Buffon, Dr. Erasmus Darwin, and Lamarck, as compared with that of Mr. Charles Darwin*. London: Hardwicke and Bogue.
28. Misra, K. K. (2011). Philosophie zoologique – 200: Lamarck in retrospect. *Science and Culture, 77*(5–6), 198–207.
29. Lamarck, J. B. (1809/1914). *Zoological philosophy* (H. Elliot, Trans.). London: MacMillan and Company.
30. Gillispie, C. C. (2006). The formation of Lamarck's theory. *Transactions of the American Philosophical Society, 65*(5), 47–62.
31. Burkhardt, R. W. (1972). The inspiration of Lamarck's belief in evolution. *Journal of the History of Biology, 5*(2), 413–438.
32. Anonymous (1844). *Vestiges of the natural history of creation*. London: John Churchill.

Chapter 26
Darwin's Books About Evolution and Reactions to Them

Abstract This chapter provides a précis of Part II of the book, including a brief discussion of Charles Darwin's basic ideas about evolution, and the major theories presented in his three books on evolution: the theory of common descent (or descent with modification), the theory of natural selection, the theory of sexual selection, and the theory of continuity of mind. The chapter explains that Darwin's ideas about evolution were rapidly and widely accepted by the general public in the U.K. and U.S., with the exception of Conservative Christians in the U.S. The chapter also briefly describes the reactions of American psychology and the development of Evolutionary Psychology, as well as the development of Ethology in Europe. The scientific concepts of ultimate causes and proximate causes are discussed and several examples of proximate causes (or proximate mechanisms) are given in the section titled Ultimate Causes and Proximate Mechanisms. The final section of the chapter highlights the key conclusions to be drawn from Part II of the book.

Keywords Darwin • Continuity of mind • *Descent of Man* • Ethology • Evolution • *Expression of Emotions* • Natural Selection • *Origin of Species* • Proximate cause • Ultimate cause

26.1 Darwin's Basic Ideas

By 1837, Charles Darwin had become convinced that species evolved [1], and he formulated the mechanism by which this happens (Natural Selection) the following year [2, 3]. Yet, he did not publish anything about evolution until his 1859 book, *The Origin of Species* [2], apparently because he wanted to amass as many facts as he could to support his theory [4], since he knew the concept of evolution was controversial [2, 4, 5]. He might not have even published *The Origin of Species* in 1859 were it not for the fact that the naturalist Alfred Russell Wallace had independently developed a theory of organic evolution that was astonishingly similar to his own theory [3, 6].

Like his grandfather Erasmus Darwin, and the Comte de Buffon and Jean-Baptiste Lamarck, Charles Darwin made his argument for evolution by explaining that it was analogous to the selective breeding of domesticated plants and animals;

K.J. Flannelly, *Religious Beliefs, Evolutionary Psychiatry, and Mental Health in America*, Religion, Spirituality and Health: A Social Scientific Approach 1,
DOI 10.1007/978-3-319-52488-7_26

but unlike his predecessors, Charles Darwin had a mechanism of evolution (his theory of Natural Selection). The analogy of selective breeding was well-suited for his British audience because many British people were familiar with breeding plants and pigeons and the British gentry were particularly familiar with the breeding of livestock, hounds, and horses [2].

According to Charles Darwin, Natural Selection works solely by preserving variations in individual characteristics (such as structures) that, by chance, increase the likelihood that an individual will survive and reproduce. Since these beneficial characteristics are inherited by an individual's offspring, they make successive generations of offspring better suited (or better adapted) to their environment. As further modifications in beneficial or adaptive characteristics accumulate over successive generations, individuals tend to diverge from their ancestral forms, which is called the theory of "common descent" or "descent with modification." In addition to demonstrating the feasibility of evolution and presenting a plausible mechanism of evolution, *The Origin of Species* undermined the central tenants of Natural Theology that each animal is perfectly designed and ideally suited for the world in which it lives [2, 7].

26.2 Reaction to the Darwin's *Origin of Species*

When Darwin's *Origin of Species* was published in 1859, it was immediately controversial in religious and scientific circles [8]. By the 1870s, however, Darwin's "theory of descent with modification" was widely accepted among scientists in Britain and the U.S. [2, 9], and some say evolution was accepted as a scientific fact by then [10]. However, many biologists were not convinced that Darwin's "theory of Natural Selection" was the mechanism of evolution until the 20th Century [2, 11], when the science of genetics was able to explain the sources of variation (i.e., genes) in characteristics and the inheritance of characteristics.

As the scientific community came to endorse evolution, the Roman Catholic Church and most Protestant denominations also came to accept, or at least tolerate it, claiming that God used evolution as a means to create the diversity of life on earth [12, 13]. However, American Christians who believed the Old Testament (the *Book of Genesis*, in particular) was literally true sought to ban the teaching of evolution in American public schools [2, 13]. This movement has continued in different forms since the 1920s, such as "Creation Science" [12–15] and "Intelligent Design" [12, 14–17].

26.3 Darwin's *Descent of Man* and *The Expression of Emotions*

Darwin's two later books about evolution were *The Descent of Man* [18], which was published in 1871 and *The Expression of Emotions in Man and Animals* [19], which was published one year later. *The Descent of Man* formally extended the theory of common descent to humans and described Darwin's theory of sexual selection. In it, Darwin claimed that humans not only shared a common ancestor with other animals, but that humans and animals have similar mental faculties or abilities, such as curiosity, imitation, attention, memory, reason, and some form of language. To the extent that humans and animals differ in their mental abilities, Darwin believed, the differences were only a matter of degree. This concept has come to be known as the theory of "continuity of mind" [20, 21].

The Expression of Emotions [19], which has been called the first book on "evolutionary psychiatry" [22], extended the idea that animals and humans have similar mental faculties to include emotions. The book covers a wide range of emotions in animals and humans, with several chapters concentrating on anger and fear, and to a lesser extent, joy, love, and pain. The book attempted to demonstrate the similarity of emotional expressions across animals and humans.

26.4 Reactions to *The Descent of Man* and *The Expression of Emotions*

The Descent of Man did not create the controversy one might have expected because two colleagues of Darwin had already published books that claimed that humans had evolved from other primates (e.g., apes and monkeys). The publication of *The Expression of Emotions* led, directly or indirectly, to the development of several schools of thought and scientific fields, including comparative psychology. However, the reaction of American psychology to Darwin's *Expression of Emotions* and evolutionary theory, in general, has been inconsistent. Some prominent American psychologists embraced Darwin's theory of evolution around the beginning of the 20th Century [23]. However, Behaviorism, which dominated American psychology from the second decade of the 1900s until the 1970s, essentially dismissed the study of the consciousness in animals or humans, denied that humans had instincts, cared little about the study of emotion, and mainly ignored the theory of evolution.

Evolution did not become a topic of interest in American psychology again until the 1990s, in the form of Evolutionary Psychology." However, several basic assumptions of Evolutionary Psychology have been the subject of criticism. One such assumption is that the past 1.8 years of the earth's history is the critical period in human evolution that has had the greatest influence of human behavior. This assumption minimizes the importance of the adaptations of our animal ancestors that occurred during vast periods of geological time before then [24]. Another assumption is that human adaptations for addressing social relationships are primarily cognitive, which ignores the interplay between emotional and cognitive brain systems [24].

In Europe, *The Expression of Emotions* and the theory of evolution, in general, led to the development of the modern science of Ethology, which primarily studies the instinctive behavior of animals. Ethologists devote a great deal of time to observing animals in their natural habitat to make detailed descriptions of the animal in its world [25–27], before they conduct studies to examine how the instinctive behaviors of different species of animals are adaptive [27]. Most of the research in ethology involves the study of instinctive (i.e., inherited) behaviors that are rigidity performed in sequences of behavior called fixed-action patterns [27–30]. Fixed-action-patterns are used for many types of functions, including nest-building, grooming, courtship and mating, and agonistic behaviors (e.g., attack, threat, defense, and submission). Although our behavior is far less rigid, we still have some behaviors that are instinctive, and the same brain regions that controlled these kinds of behavior in our animal ancestors still affect our behavior.

26.5 Ultimate Causes and Proximate Mechanisms

As the behavioral branch of biology [27], a key question in ethology is [27, 29]: What is a given behavior for? The answer to this question corresponds to Aristotle's final cause – its purpose. In modern terminology, Aristotle's final cause [31, 32] is called the ultimate cause or distal cause of something. Within biology, including ethology, another way of expressing this question is: How is this characteristic (a structure or behavior) adaptive for an animal? Another type of question one may ask about a behavior or other characteristic is: How does it work? This type of question refers to what is called a proximate cause of something. Just as Aristotle proposed different ways of considering the cause of something, so do modern biologists. The proximate causes of modern science (also called proximate mechanisms) are grossly similar to Aristotle's first three causes in that they define how an ultimate cause is achieved.

For example, one might ask the question: Why do male animals of the same species fight each other? Based on Darwin's theory of sexual selection, the ultimate cause is to secure access to females in order to reproduce. However, the proximate causes, at different levels of explanation, may be: (a) to defend their territory; (b) because they respond aggressively to the sight or odor of nearby males; (c) increased testosterone levels at certain times of the year make them aggressive; (d) the presence of another male activates the part of the brain that elicits aggression; or (e) part of their brain is genetically programmed to attack another male. A question more common to our ordinary experience might be: Why do we eat? The ultimate cause is to obtain the nourishment we need to live. However, the proximate causes may be: (a) the sight and smell of food; (b) our blood sugar is low; (c) we feel a sense of hunger; (d) a part of the brain that monitors blood sugar triggers hunger; or (e) part of the brain is genetically programmed to trigger hunger when our blood sugar is low.

In humans, proximate mechanisms that have the ultimate goal of ensuring survival may give rise to physical and mental health problems. The proximate mechanisms that initiate eating, for example, tend to override the proximate mechanism that stop eating; thus, many people in developed countries where there is ample access to food become overweight. Other people may develop psychiatric problems related to trying to overcome the failure of the proximate mechanisms to stop eating (e.g., anorexia).

26.6 Conclusions

Charles Darwin's *Origin of Species* explains how animals and plants could change in form over time by a process he called Natural Selection. This process applies not only to the emergence of different species, but also to the emergence of different genera, families, orders, classes, etc., as adaptations accumulate over time. This process forms the basis for both the concept of evolution, in general, and the concept of descent from a common ancestor. The fact that Alfred Russell Wallace developed a theory of evolution that was very similar to Charles Darwin's theory made it inevitable that a theory of organic evolution would have been published in the 19th Century even if Darwin had not published his *Origin of Species*.

Darwin's theory of common descent was accepted rather quickly by society and the scientific community, although his theory of Natural Selection was not accepted by scientists until the development of genetics demonstrated how characteristics varied and how they were inherited. The reader should keep in mind that scientists continue to react to Darwin's theories of evolution by proposing new ideas about how evolution operates. For instance, whereas Charles Darwin proposed that evolution is a very gradual process, more recent theories have proposed that evolution is a sporadic process in which very little change in species may occur over long periods of time until some dramatic environmental change provides the opportunity for new species to proliferate [33, 34]. On the other hand, some groups of religious individuals continue to react to evolutionary theory by denying that evolution is real.

Darwin's *The Descent of Man* [18] and *The Expression of Emotions* [19] included humans in the chain of evolution (the theory of common descent) and introduced the idea that humans and animals have similar mental abilities (the theory of continuity of mind), creating the framework for Evolutionary Psychiatry. Ethology, the biology of behavior, has made significant contributions to our understanding of the evolution of behavior in animals, which have important implications for understanding the relationship between the brain and behavior, including the proximate mechanisms that underlie psychiatric symptoms.

References

1. Sulloway, F. J. (1982). Darwin's conversion: The *Beagle* voyage and its aftermath. *Journal of the History of Biology, 15*(3), 325–396.
2. Larson, E. J. (2004). *Evolution: The remarkable history of a scientific theory*. New York: The Modern Library.
3. Francis, K. A. (2007). *Charles Darwin and The Origin of Species*. Westport: Greenwood Press.
4. Richards, R. J. (1983). Why Darwin delayed, or interesting problems and models in the history of science. *Journal of the History of the Behavioral Sciences, 19*(1), 43–53.
5. Endersby, J. (2009). Sympathetic science: Charles Darwin, Joseph Hooker, and the passions of Victorian naturalists. *Victorian Studies, 51*(2), 299–320.
6. Osborn, H. F. (1894). From the Greeks to Darwin. New York: MacMillan.
7. Darwin, C. (1859). *On the origin of species by means of natural selection, or the preservation of favoured races in the struggle for life*. London: John Murray.
8. Colp, R., Jr. (1986). The relationship of Charles Darwin to the ideas of his grandfather, Dr. Erasmus Darwin. *Biography, 9*(1), 1–24.
9. Bowler, P. J. (2004). The specter of Darwinism: The popular image of Darwinism in early twentieth century Britain. In A. Lustig, R. J. Richards, & M. Ruse (Eds.), *Darwinian heresies*. Cambridge: Cambridge University Press.
10. Huxley, T. H. (1880). The coming of age of The Origin of Species. *Science, 1*(2), 15–17, 20.
11. Waller, J. (2005). Evolution's inside man: Other people could have had Darwin's insights, but no one else could have gotten them accepted by the establishment. *New Scientist, 187*(2513), 42–44.
12. Pennock, R. T. (2003). Creationism and intelligent design. *Annual Review of Genomics & Human Genetics, 4*(1), 143–163.
13. Dixon, T. (2009). America's difficulty with Darwin. *History Today, 59*(2), 22–28.
14. Bailey, D. H. (2010). Creationism and intelligent design: Scientific and theological difficulties. *Dialogue: A Journal of Mormon Thought, 43*(3), 62–87.
15. Brown, S. (2014). The evolution of creationism. *Church & State, 67*(3), 9–12.
16. Wald, D. (2000). Special section on intelligent design: The new creationism. *Skeptic, 8*(2), 12.
17. Melott, A. L. (2002). Intelligent design is creationism in a cheap tuxedo. *Physics Today, 55*(6), 48.
18. Darwin, C. (1871). *The descent of man and selection in relation to sex* (Vol. 1). London: John Murray.
19. Darwin, C. (1872). *The expression of emotions in man and animals*. London: John Murray.
20. Bolhuis, J. J., & Wynne, C. D. L. (2009). Can evolution explain how minds work? *Nature, 548*, 832–833.
21. Hauser, M. (2009). The mind. *Scientific American, 301*(3), 44–51.
22. O'Connell, H. P. (2008). 150 years of evolutionary theory. *British Journal of Psychiatry, 193*, 258–259.
23. Green, C. D. (2009). Darwinian theory, functionalism, and the first American psychological revolution. *American Psychologist, 64*(2), 75–83.
24. Panksepp, J., & Panksepp, J. B. (2000). The seven sins of evolutionary psychology. *Evolution and Cognition, 6*(2), 108–131.
25. von Uexkull, J. (1975). A stroll through the world of animals and men. In C. H. Schiller (Ed.), *Instinctive behavior: The development of the modern concept* (pp. 5–80). New York: International Universities Press.
26. Tinbergen, N. (1975). Preface. In C. H. Schiller (Ed.), *Instinctive behavior: The development of the modern concept* (pp. 15–19). New York: International Universities Press.
27. Tinbergen, N. (1963). On the aims and methods of ethology. *Zeitschrift furTierpsychologie, 26*, 410–433.
28. Thorpe, W. H. (1973). Ethology as a new branch of biology. In M. W. Fox (Ed.), *Readings in ethology and comparative psychology* (pp. 5–23). Monterey: Books/Cole.

29. Lorenz, K. (1981). *The foundations of ethology*. New York: Spinger-Verlag.
30. Moltz, H. (1965). Contemporary instinct theory and the fixed-action pattern. *Psychological Review, 72*(1), 27–47.
31. Aristotle. (1961). *Aristotle's physics* (R. Hope, Trans.). Lincoln: University of Nebraska Press.
32. Aristotle. (1991). *The metaphysics* (J. H. McMahon, Trans.). Buffalo: Prometheus Books.
33. Simpson, G. G. (1944/1984). *Tempo and mode in evolution*. New York: Columbia University Press.
34. Gould, S. J., & Eldredge, N. (1977). Punctuated equilibria: The tempo and mode of evolution reconsidered. *Paleobiology, 3*(2), 115–151.

Chapter 27
Evolutionary Psychiatry and ETAS Theory

Abstract This chapter covers all the chapters in Part IV of the book in abbreviated form, including the material contained in each section and subsection of the chapters. The first portion of the chapter briefly describes the general timeframe of the evolution of the brain stem, the basal ganglia, the limbic system, and the neocortex in vertebrates, and the function of these brain areas in self defense and threat assessment. Special attention is given to the role of the amygdala (which is part of the limbic system) in the generation of fear and the role of the prefrontal cortex (PFC) in modulating fear generated by the amygdala. The next section explains the adaptive functions of psychiatric symptoms associated with fear of small animals, acrophobia, panic attack and agoraphobia, obsessive-compulsive disorder (OCD), general anxiety, social anxiety, depression, somatization, and paranoia, and the estimated times in our evolutionary history that the proximate mechanisms underlying them developed. The nature of beliefs (including "folk beliefs") and the relationship between dysfunctional beliefs and psychiatric symptoms are discussed next. The remaining sections describe the degree to which the brain stem, the basal ganglia, the limbic system, and the PFC are involved in fear of small animals, panic attack, OCD, general anxiety, social anxiety, depression, and paranoia, and the operation of evolutionary threat assessment systems, especially the role of the ventromedial PFC in assessing threats and safety and the influence on beliefs on its assessments.

Keywords Amygdala • Basal ganglia • Brain • Brain stem • Causal beliefs • Emotions • ETAS Theory • Evolutionary Psychiatry • Folk beliefs • Limbic system • PFC • Proximate mechanisms • Psychiatric symptoms • Safety • Threat

27.1 Brain Evolution and Emotions

The gross structure of the modern mammalian brain roughly reflects the evolutionary development of the brain from fish through reptiles and mammals. The brain stem, which is the most primitive part of the brain, probably evolved in early fish [1] to regulate and coordinate reflexes. The basal ganglia, which evolved in later fish [2], are the main brain structures in early amphibians and reptiles [2], and their elaboration in reptiles probably increased their behavioral repertoire [2]. The limbic

K.J. Flannelly, *Religious Beliefs, Evolutionary Psychiatry, and Mental Health in America*, Religion, Spirituality and Health: A Social Scientific Approach 1,
DOI 10.1007/978-3-319-52488-7_27

system existed in a rudimentary form in reptiles, amphibians, and some fish [1, 3, 4], and it is closely connected to the brain stem [5] and the basal ganglia. As the limbic system evolved further in early mammals, it incorporated some of the functions of the basal ganglia [6], including the regulation of instinctive behaviors related to mating, territoriality, and self-defense [7]. The limbic system is extensively involved in emotions, which provide mammals with greater flexibility to respond to threats of harm and other life challenges [4] because stimuli elicit an emotion instead of a specific behavior, and emotions are able to activate an array of possible responses. The neocortex (which evolved extensively in mammals [4, 8]), like the limbic system before it, added greater flexibility for responding to the environment [4]; this flexibility is partly achieved because cortical structures can inhibit the instinctive responses of subcortical structures [4].

27.2 Fear in the Brain

The periaqueductal gray, which is part of the brain stem, is known to be involved in self-defense and to activate innate reactions to threats, including freezing and flight [9–11]. The basal ganglia are also involved in defensive behaviors in animals [3, 12], but it is not clear that they serve the same function in humans.

Emotions probably did not exist before the evolution of the limbic system, and fear may not have existed before the evolution of the amygdala, which is a part of the limbic system [13, 14]. The amygdala generates fear as a warning of potential threats of harm, and its reaction to certain threats is unconscious [15–17] and automatic [15]. It also reacts to ambiguous stimuli as if they are dangerous [18, 19], and it treats unpredictability and the lack of control over current events and uncertainty about future events as forms of threat [18, 20–23].

A part of the neocortex called the prefrontal cortex (PFC) modulates fear by modulating the activity of the amygdala in animals [24–26] and humans [27, 28]. The ventromedial portion of the PFC (vmPFC) in humans is known to inhibit amygdala activity [29, 30], and therefore, fear [27, 31]. Moreover, the vmPFC makes it own threat assessments, which can over-ride the threat assessments of the amygdala.

27.3 Psychiatric Disorders as Evolutionary Adaptations

Randolph M. Nesse and other psychiatrists and clinical psychologists in the 1980s tried to explain the evolutionary roots of psychiatric symptoms. Nesse thought that anxiety disorders are expressions of proximate brain mechanisms that are adaptive for survival [32–34] because the fears they entail evolved to protect us from various sources of danger [32, 33]. An important point to remember is that the number of people who experience psychiatric symptoms is far greater than the number of people who are diagnosed as having psychiatric disorders because their symptoms are not severe enough to warrant a diagnosis.

27.3.1 Fear of Small Animals

Fear of small animals serves an obvious survival function because many kinds of small animals can cause us harm. Thus, animal phobias are very common [35, 36]. Fear of snakes and spiders are especially common, but snakes and spiders are so different in their appearance, behaviors, and habitats, we probably evolved different proximate mechanisms to protect us from each of them. Indeed, it has been suggested that the fear of snakes evolved in primates about 20 million years ago [37], whereas the fear of small animals and insects evolved in humans about 70,000 years ago [38].

We tend to have a fear of small animals despite the fact that many small animals are not dangerous to us. This is because the proximate mechanisms that protect us from harm do not differentiate between what animals are harmful or harmless, they only provide algorithms (or rules) for identifying animals that can cause harm. As some small animals can be harmful, the mechanisms tend to treat all small animals as being potentially harmful, since it is better for survival to treat a harmless animal as if it is dangerous ("a false positive") than to treat a dangerous animal as if it is harmless ("a false negative").

27.3.2 Acrophobia (Fear of Heights)

The function of acrophobia (fear of heights) is obvious; it is a mechanism for avoiding high places from which we could fall and suffer serious injury or death. The survival value of acrophobia presumably accounts for the fact that it is the second most common phobia in the U.S., after the fear of small animals [39, 40].

27.3.3 Panic Attack and Agoraphobia

Panic attack entails a feeling of extreme fear even though no potential source of physical harm is present [33, 41]. Many symptoms of panic attack are similar to the "fight or flight" reaction to threat, and it is thought that panic attack may reflect an adaption to predatory threats that may have arisen in early mammals, which evolved roughly 280 million years ago [8], or in modern mammals, which evolved about 100 million years ago [42, 43].

About half of the individuals who have had repeated panic attacks develop agoraphobia [44], but many people who suffer from agoraphobia have never had a panic attack [45]. It has been suggested that agoraphobia, like panic attacks, represents a fear of being harmed when outside the safety of one's home-range or territory [34, 46]. If this is true, its evolutionary roots could be very ancient, since most lizards and some fish exhibit territoriality.

27.3.4 Obsessive-Compulsive Disorder (OCD)

OCD consists of obsessive thoughts that harm will occur if an individual does not perform certain behaviors, which are called compulsions or compulsive acts. Obsessive thoughts are associated with anxiety and compulsive acts are performed to reduce the anxiety [47]. The evolutionary psychiatrist Martin Brune draws a parallel between human compulsive acts and animal behaviors called "displacement activities." Displacement activities are seemingly irrelevant fixed-action patterns that are performed when an animal is faced with two competing motivations, such a fight or flight. This could explain why some compulsive acts have no immediately obvious survival value in relation to the situation in which they are exhibited.

27.3.5 General Anxiety

Nesse thought general anxiety probably evolved to deal with threats that could not be clearly defined [34], which is consistent with Sigmund Freud's idea that anxiety is "free-floating fear," in which we cannot identify our fear with particular threat of danger [48]. One function of general anxiety is to increase vigilance to recognize potential threats of harm in our surroundings [34].

27.3.6 Social Phobia (Social Anxiety)

Social anxiety mainly entails the fear of acting in ways that will make us less attractive to others, and it seems to stem from the fear of being rejected by a social group [49, 50]. As the evolution of social groups has been particularly important for the success of primates [51], the evolutionary origin of social anxiety may date back to the evolution of monkeys over 50 million years ago, or at least back to the split between monkeys and apes around 20 million years ago [52, 53].

27.3.7 Depression

Major depressive disorder (MDD) is defined as having five or more of nine types of symptoms, which include feeling sad or empty, having a reduced interest in anything, unintended weight loss or weight gain, insomnia or hypersomnia, psychomotor agitation or retardation, fatigue, feeling worthless or guilty, an inability to concentrate, and frequent thoughts about death [54, 55]. Though it might seem unlikely that such a cluster of symptoms could be adaptive, over a half dozen theoretical articles have proposed that depression is adaptive [56–63]. Most of these theories propose that depression mainly evolved to deal with social losses, including the loss of social status, social rejection, and the termination of social relationships. The American psychologist and neuroscientist Jaak Panksepp believes depression is associated with an innate "GRIEF" system in the brain that evolved more than 100 million years ago to regulate social relationships, including infant-parent attachment, and that depressive symptoms are triggered when social bonds are broken [64].

27.3.8 Somatization

Somatization is one type of a class of psychiatric disorders called somatoform disorders [54, 55]. Somatization, which was originally called hysteria and hysterical neurosis, entails having symptoms of pain, as well as gastrointestinal and other somatic symptoms, which that cannot be traced to a physical cause. There are two evolutionary theories of somatization. The first theory proposes that somatization is related to social competition [57] and the other proposes that it is an adaptation to detect internal rather than external threats of harm [65].

27.3.9 Paranoid Ideation

Paranoid ideation reflects a basic distrust of people, which is typically expressed as the belief that people (or someone in particular) intend to deceive, exploit, or harm you, or that they are actively doing so, when there is no actual evidence that this belief is true. False beliefs, such as these, are called delusions when they reflect a severe break from reality [54, 55]. The two most common types of paranoid delusions are persecutory delusions and jealousy delusions of sexual infidelity. Chapter 12 discusses the possible evolutionary roots of persecutory and jealous paranoid ideation.

27.3.10 Problems with Proximate Mechanisms

The fact that psychiatric disorders result from the operation of proximate brain mechanisms that are adaptive does not mean that psychiatric disorders themselves are adaptive [58, 66]. The symptoms may be adaptive for survival generally, but the fact that symptoms can become so severe, so frequent, or so prolonged that they interfere with a person's life is not an evolutionary adaptation.

The frequent occurrence of anxiety and related symptoms is a side effect of the operating characteristics of the brain mechanisms that detect threats of harm. Since the detection and assessment of potential threats must be rapid to ensure protection from harm, the brain's decisions about what poses a threat are biased towards identifying danger even when none exists.

The prolonged duration of symptoms may be attributable to at least two causes. Since proximate mechanisms for detecting threats have evolved to react to immediate short-term threats, their prolonged activation can be problematic [4]. This is not a problem for most animals because once a threat no longer exists the mechanism returns to its normal baseline. However, because humans have the ability to think about the past and future, they can activate self-defense mechanisms when no potential threat exists [66, 67]. The other cause of the prolonged activation of symptoms may be that there is no "off-switch" for our threat detection mechanisms. Since the identification of threat is often based on ambiguous stimuli and little evidence [68], the proximate mechanisms of threat assessment systems rarely get definitive feedback that no threat actually exists, so anxiety tends to persist over time [69].

Finally, it is possible that some proximate mechanisms for detecting threats are no longer adaptive, but they are not harmful either, at least from an evolutionary perspective. Paul Gilbert suggests this might be the case for the mechanisms underlying social anxiety. As humans evolved to live in small, relatively stable social groups similar to many primates, our mechanisms for detecting social threats may not function well in the larger societies we live in now, in which we have more extensive social interactions [70–72].

27.4 The Nature of Beliefs

Historically, beliefs have been considered to be propositions or statements about the nature of the world that can be true or false [73–76], and it was considered irrational for a person to hold two contradictory beliefs simultaneously [76–78]. However, many scholars and researchers now think (1) that beliefs often consist of mental representations [79–82] or mental models of the world that are not linguistic [81, 83, 84], and (2) that individuals may rationally hold contradictory beliefs with varying degrees of certainty [78, 85–89].

27.4.1 Folk Beliefs

Research has shown that very young children have implicit mental models or basic beliefs about the nature of world [90]. These mental models are beliefs about physical, psychological, and biological phenomena, which have come to be called "naïve" or "folk" physics, psychology, and biology, respectively [91–93]. For example, folk physics includes beliefs about the motion and physical characteristics of objects and causation [91, 93–96], whereas folk psychology includes the belief that other beings have beliefs and desires that are similar to our own [91–93, 97–99] and that animals and other humans have the power of agency, i.e., the ability to perform intentional acts [97, 99].

Folks beliefs are what British evolutionary biologist Lewis Wolpert called strong causal beliefs, which he thought are preprogrammed in our brains [100]. Wolpert thought strong causal beliefs about nature and the world began to evolve in humans when we began to make tools [100]. As such, folk physics presumably evolved first, followed by other causal beliefs that helped us to understand the causes of everything we observe in our world.

27.4.2 Religious Beliefs as Folk Beliefs

It has been suggested that some religious beliefs reflect the human tendency to presume that actions or events are caused by agents, even when no agent is apparent [92, 93, 101]. These folk beliefs about agency assume that harmful supernatural agents (e.g., angry ancestors or demons) are the cause of negative life events, and beneficent supernatural agents (e.g., supportive ancestors or gods) are the cause of positive life events [92, 93]. Moreover, humans tend to create causal explanations (or beliefs) based on very little information about the actual causes of events [92, 93].

27.5 Beliefs and Psychiatric Symptoms

Aaron T. Beck and his colleagues found that anxious patients are sensitive to stimuli that might signal potential dangers and that they constantly experience "false alarms" that keep them in a constant state of emotional distress [67]. Their fears are partly driven by their belief that the world is a dangerous place. Such "dysfunctional beliefs" [102] contribute to many psychiatric disorders, including social anxiety [49, 50, 103], obsessive-compulsive disorder [104–106], panic attack [107, 108], and paranoia [109, 110].

27.6 Beliefs and the Brain

The brain has been called a belief-generating machine [93, 111]; yet, it is unclear where beliefs are stored in the brain. Nevertheless, at least one specific area of the brain has been found to be involved in the processing of beliefs, that is, the vmPFC [112–114]. This research indicates that the vmPFC is involved in the processing of both religious and non-religious beliefs.

27.7 Evolutionary Threat Assessment Systems Theory

A 2007 article by me and my colleagues proposed that the proximate mechanisms underlying psychiatric disorders involve neural circuits (Evolutionary Threat Assessment Systems) connecting the basal ganglia, the limbic system, and the prefrontal cortex (PFC) [115]. A number of subsequent articles have endorsed the basic premise of ETAS Theory that psychiatric symptoms are the product of threat assessment systems that evolved for self-protection [69, 116–122]. The unique feature of ETAS Theory, which differentiates it from other theoretical models of threat assessment, is that ETAS Theory explains how beliefs influence psychiatric systems by influencing the brain systems that make threat assessments.

27.7.1 Brain Regions Involved in Different Psychiatric Disorders

I conducted an extensive literature review of brain imaging studies that examined the involvement of the PFC, the limbic system, the basal ganglia, and the brain stem in different psychiatric disorders. Consistent with ETAS Theory, the review found that these four brain areas were involved in several of the psychiatric disorders covered by the review for which sufficient data were available. The best evidence available implicates all four brain areas in panic attack, social anxiety, and major depression, and the PFC, limbic system, and basal ganglia in paranoid ideation. However, only the PFC and the limbic system have been implicated in general anxiety and animal phobia. There are fewer studies on general anxiety that one might expect, so the evidence is limited, but there have been numerous studies on small animal phobia, particularly fear of snakes and spiders. The finding that the basal ganglia and brain stem are not involved in small animal phobia aligns with the notion that fear of small animals is a relatively recent adaptation (70,000 thousand to 20 million years ago)

Obsessive-compulsive disorder (OCD) is the only anxiety disorder that does not seem to involve the amygdala, even though the amygdala is thought to be the major, if not the sole, source of fear in humans. The basal ganglia are clearly involved in

OCD, and there is strong evidence that the brain stem plays some part in OCD. The fact that the amygdala does not appear to be involved in OCD could be because its evolutionary roots date back further than the evolution of the amygdala.

27.7.2 The vmPFC in Deductive Reasoning and the Influence of Beliefs

The PFC is involved in inductive and deductive reasoning or logic [123–127]. Two brain systems are involved in deductive logic in humans [128, 129]. One system uses language and abstract reasoning [129], whereas the other does not. Indeed, the second system is not strictly logical and it can be influenced by beliefs [129–131]. This second system involves areas of the PFC [132, 133], including the vmPFC [134].

27.7.3 Threat, Safety, and the vmPFC

Paul Gilbert claims that a sense of safety is not just the absence of threat, and that the human brain contains both a threat system and a safety system, the latter of which evolved in the context of social relationships, especially mother-infant relationships [135]. He says that relationships with people who are supportive and helpful promote a sense of safety [135], which alters the processing of potential threats so that someone who feels safe assesses potentially dangerous stimuli as being less threatening [136]. Research has shown that the vmPFC is responsive to safety cues [137] and suggests that the vmPFC may be involved in Gilbert's proposed safety system [138–143].

Other theorists think there is an interplay between safety and threat across the spectrum of anxiety disorders [144, 145], and that safety is provided not only by social relationships, but also by situations and other aspects of human experience. A person's home, for example, is a source of safety that inhibits fear in persons with agoraphobia just as an animal's territory seems to provide a sense of safety or security [146].

Psychological characteristics of individuals, such as self-esteem and self-efficacy, also provide a sense of personal safety because they enhance the belief that an individual has the personal resources to deal with adverse life events effectively [147, 148]. Thus, like social support, self-esteem and self-efficacy buffer against the anxiety produced by various threats of harm encountered in the world.

27.7.4 The Role of the PFC in Threat Assessment

The vmPFC plays a critical role in threat assessment in that it independently assesses both safety and threat. Thus, when the vmPFC makes a different threat assessment than subcortical brain areas do, it can override their threat assessments and suppress the activity of the amygdala, thereby reducing fear and psychiatric symptoms related to fear. As the vmPFC is (a) involved in the processing of beliefs [113, 114] and deductive reasoning [129, 131, 134], and (b) the deductions of the vmPFC are influenced by beliefs about the world [129, 131], it seems that (c) its decisions about the degree to which something poses a threat of harm are influenced by beliefs about the world.

Although I have focussed on the vmPFC because the best evidence indicates that it is involved in threat assessment and the processing of both fear and beliefs, other areas of the PFC may play a role in all three of these brain activities. The orbitofrontal portion of the PFC (the OFC) is a case in point, as discussed in Chap. 14. Chapter 14 also discusses recent findings about the dorsomedial PFC (dmPFC) that are important for ETAS Theory because the dmPFC is a key component of an "aversive amplification circuit" [149, 150], which "is associated with elevated threat processing" (p. 295) [150] and appears to enhance fear by priming the amygdala to be more sensitive to potential threats [149].

27.7.5 Description of ETAS Functioning

The brain stem, the basal ganglia, the limbic system, and the PFC are all thought to be involved in the threat assessments that underlie psychiatric symptoms. Since they evolved in different points in time, they make assessments through different mechanisms: the brain stem and basal ganglia use instinctive processing of information, the limbic system uses affective processing of information, and the PFC uses cognitive processing of information [115, 151, 152]. The threat assessments of the brain stem, the basal ganglia, and the limbic system (i.e., the amygdala) are automatic and mainly made outside of awareness [15, 57, 115], and they are biased toward deciding a stimulus poses a threat even when it may not be a threat.

The PFC integrates information from subcortical structures and any cortical areas that may have been activated by them [57, 69], and the vmPFC makes its own threat assessment based on cognition. The cognitive threat assessments made by the vmPFC are particularly important because the vmPFC can override the threat assessments of the amygdala and inhibit amygdala activity [29, 153], thereby reducing fear. When the vmPFC makes its threat assessments, it takes belief about the world into account in assigning a probability that a stimulus is threatening. It also takes personal safety into account, including social support, and situations and beliefs that provide a sense of safety. If the vmPFC decides that something is not threatening, it decreases the activity of the amygdala, which decreases anxiety and related symptoms. Thus, the vmPFC acts as a gating system that sets a threshold for what is and what is not a threat of harm. Generally, given its ability to reduce the activity of the amygdala, the vmPFC appears to raise the threshold of what constitutes a threat.

The dmPFC, on the other hand, is a key element of the so-called "aversive amplification circuit" [149, 150], which "is associated with elevated threat processing" (p. 295) [150]. As the "aversive amplification circuit" appears to enhance fear by priming the amygdala to be more sensitive to potential threats [149], the dmPFC may lower the threshold of what constitutes a threat.

References

1. Aboitiz, F., & Montiel, J. (2007). *Origin and evolution of the vertebrate telencephalon, with special reference to the mammalian neocortex*. New York: Springer.
2. Reiner, A., Medina, L., & Veenman, C. L. (1998). Structural and functional evolution of the basal ganglia in vertebrates. *Brain Research Reviews, 28*(3), 235–285.
3. MacLean, P. D. (1990). *The triune brain in evolution: Role in paleocerebral functions*. New York: Plenum Press.
4. Panksepp, J. (1998). *Affective neuroscience: The foundations of human and animal emotions*. New York: Oxford University Press.
5. Price, J. L. (2003). Comparative aspects of amygdala connectivity. *Annals of the New York Academy of Sciences, 985*, 50–58.
6. Laberge, F., Muhlenbrock-Lenter, S., Grunwald, W., & Roth, G. (2006). Evolution of the amygdala: New insights from studies in amphibians. *Brain, Behavior and Evolution, 67*, 177–187.
7. Sokolowski, K., & Corbin, J. G. (2012). Wired for behaviors: From development to function of innate limbic system circuitry. *Frontiers in Molecular Neuroscience, 5*(55), 1–15.
8. Kaas, J. H. (2011). Neocortex in early mammals and its subsequent variations. *Annals of the New York Academy of Sciences, 1225*, 28–36.
9. McNaughton, N., & Corr, P. J. (2044). A two-dimensional neuropsychology of defense: Fear/anxiety and defensive distance. *Neuroscience & Biobehavioral Reviews, 28*(3), 285–305.
10. Morgan, M. M., & Clayton, C. C. (2005). Defensive behaviors evoked from the ventrolateral periaqueductal gray of the rat: Comparison of opioid and GABA disinhibition. *Behavioural Brain Research, 64*, 61–66.
11. Vianna, D. M. L., Graeff, F. G., Brandao, M. L., & Landeira-Fernandez, J. (2001). Defensive freezing evoked by electrical stimulation of the periaqueductal gray: Comparison between dorsolateral and ventrolateral regions. *Neuroreport, 12*(18), 4109–4112.
12. Baxter, L. R. (2003). Basal ganglia systems in ritualistic social displays: Reptiles and humans; function and illness. *Physiology & Behavior, 79*, 451–460.
13. Panksepp, J. (2011). The basic emotional circuits of mammalian brains: Do animals have affective lives? *Neuroscience & Biobehavioral Reviews, 35*(9), 1791–1804.
14. Panksepp, J., Fuchs, T., & Iacobucci, P. (2011). The basic neuroscience of emotional experiences in mammals: The case of subcortical FEAR circuitry and implications for clinical anxiety. *Applied Animal Behaviour Science, 129*(1), 1–17.
15. Öhman, A. (2005). The role of the amygdala in human fear: Automatic detection of threat. *Psychoneuroendocrinology, 30*(10), 953–958.
16. Zald, D. H. (2003). The human amygdala and the emotional evaluation of sensory stimuli. *Brain Research Reviews, 41*(1), 88–123.

17. Lipka, J., Miltner, W. H. R., & Straube, T. (2011). Vigilance for threat interacts with amygdala responses to subliminal threat cues in specific phobia. *Biological Psychiatry, 70*(5), 472–478.
18. Rosen, J. B., & Donley, M. P. (2006). Animal studies of amygdala function in fear and uncertainty: Relevance to human research. *Biological Psychology, 73*(1), 49–60.
19. Zaretsky, M., Mendelsohn, A., Mintz, M., & Hendler, T. (2010). In the eye of the beholder: Internally driven uncertainty of danger recruits the amygdala and dorsomedial prefrontal cortex. *Journal of Cognitive Neuroscience, 22*(10), 2263–2275.
20. Sarinopoulos, I., Grupe, D. W., Mackiewicz, K. L., Herrington, J. D., Lor, M., Steege, E. E., et al. (2010). Uncertainty during anticipation modulates neural responses to aversion in human insula and amygdala. *Cerebral Cortex, 20*(4), 929–940.
21. Grupe, D. W., & Nitschke, J. B. (2013). Uncertainty and anticipation in anxiety: An integrated neurobiological and psychological perspective. *Nature Reviews: Neuroscience, 14*(7), 488–501.
22. Thompson, S. C. (1981). Will it hurt less if I can control it? A complex answer to a simple question. *Psychological Bulletin, 90*(1), 89–101.
23. Williams, L. E., Oler, J. A., Fox, A. S., McFarlin, D. R., Rogers, G. M., Jesson, M. A. L., et al. (2015). Fear of the unknown: Uncertain anticipation reveals amygdala alterations in childhood anxiety disorders. *Neuropsychopharmacology, 40*(6), 1428–1435.
24. Sotres-Bayon, F., Sierra-Mercado, D., Pardilla-Delgado, E., & Quirk, G. J. (2012). Gating of fear in prelimbic cortex by hippocampal and amygdala inputs. *Neuron, 76*(4), 804–812.
25. Charney, D. S. (2003). Neuroanatomical circuits modulating fear and anxiety behaviors. Neuroanatomical circuits modulating fear and anxiety behaviors. *Acta Psychiatrica Scandinavica, 108*, 38.
26. Kalin, N. H. (2002). The neurobiology of fear. *Scientific American, 12*(1), 72–81.
27. Quirk, G. J., & Beer, J. S. (2006). Prefrontal involvement in the regulation of emotion: Convergence of rat and human studies. *Current Opinion in Neurobiology, 16*, 723–727.
28. Stern, C. A. J., Do-Monte, F. H., Gazarini, L., Carobrez, A. P., & Bertoglio, L. J. (2010). Anxiety disorders and anxiolytics – Anxiety disorders (basic): Ventromedial prefrontal cortex activity is required for anxiety expression: Distinct neurochemical mechanisms evidence. *European Neuropsychopharmacology, 20*(Supplement 3), S538–S539.
29. Greenberg, T., Carlson, J. M., Cha, J., Hajcak, G., & Mujica-Parodi, L. R. (2013). Ventromedial prefrontal cortex reactivity is altered in generalized anxiety disorder during fear generalization. *Depression and Anxiety, 30*(3), 242–250.
30. Motzkin, J. C., Philippi, C. L., Wolf, R. C., Koenigs, M., & Baskaya, M. K. (2015). Ventromedial prefrontal cortex is critical for the regulation of amygdala activity in humans. *Biological Psychiatry, 77*(3), 276–284.
31. Berkowitz, R. L., Coplan, J. D., Reddy, D. P., & Gorman, J. M. (2007). The human dimension: How the prefrontal cortex modulates the subcortical fear response. *Reviews in the Neurosciences, 18*(3–4), 191–208.
32. Nesse, R. (1998). Emotional disorders in evolutionary perspective. *British Journal of Medical Psychology, 71*(4), 397–415.
33. Nesse, R. M. (1990). Evolutionary explanations of emotions. *Human Nature, 1*(3), 261–289.
34. Marks, I. M., & Nesse, R. M. (1994). Fear and fitness: An evolutionary analysis of anxiety disorders. *Ethology & Sociobiology, 15*(5–6), 247–261.
35. Merckelbach, H., de Jong, P. J., Muris, P., & van den Hout, M. A. (1996). The etiology of specific phobias: A review. *Clinical Psychology Review, 16*(4), 337–361.
36. Fredrikson, M., Annas, P., Fischer, H., & Wik, G. (1996). Gender and age differences in the prevalence of specific fears and phobias. *Behaviour Research and Therapy, 34*(1), 33–39.
37. Isbell, L. A. (2009). *The fruit, the tree and the serpent*. Cambridge, MA: Harvard University Press.

38. Bracha, H. S. (2006). Human brain evolution and the "Neuroevolutionary Time-depth Principle:" Implications for the Reclassification of fear-circuitry-related traits in DSM-V and for studying resilience to warzone-related posttraumatic stress disorder. *Progress in Neuro-Psychopharmacology and Biological Psychiatry, 30*(5), 827–853.
39. LeBeau, R. T., Glenn, D., Liao, B., Wittchen, H. U., Beesdo-Baum, K., Ollendick, T., & Craske, M. G. (2010). Specific phobia: A review of DSM-IV specific phobia and preliminary recommendations for DSM-V. *Depression and Anxiety, 27*, 148–167.
40. Curtis, G. C., Magee, W. J., Eaton, W. W., Wittchen, H.-U., & Kessler, R. C. (1998). Specific fears and phobias: Epidemiology and classification. *British Journal of Psychiatry, 173*, 212–217.
41. Nesse, R. M. (1984). An evolutionary perspective on psychiatry. *Comprehensive Psychiatry, 25*(6), 575–580.
42. Seiffert, E. R. (2012). Early primate evolution in Afro-Arabia. *Evolutionary Anthropology, 21*(6), 239–253.
43. Luo, Z.-X. (2007). Transformation and diversification in early mammal evolution. *Nature, 450*(7172), 1011–1019.
44. Eaton, W. W., Kessler, R. C., Wittchen, H. U., & Magee, W. J. (1994). Panic and panic disorder in the United States. *American Journal of Psychiatry, 151*(3), 413–420.
45. Horwath, E., Lish, J. D., Johnson, J., Hornig, C. D., & Weissman, M. M. (1993). Agoraphobia without panic: Clinical reappraisal of an epidemiologic finding. *American Journal of Psychiatry, 150*(10), 1496–1501.
46. Lelliott, P., Marks, I., McNamee, G., & Tobena, A. (1989). Onset of panic disorder with agoraphobia: Toward an integrated model. *Archives of General Psychiatry, 46*(11), 1000–1004.
47. Brune, M. (2006). The evolutionary psychology of obsessive-compulsive disorder: The role of cognitive metarepresentation. *Perspectives in Biology and Medicine, 49*(3), 317–329.
48. Freud, S. (1920). *A general introduction to psychoanalysis*. New York: Horace Liveright.
49. Moscovitch, D. A. (2009). What is the core fear in social phobia? A new model to facilitate individualized case conceptualization and treatment. *Cognitive and Behavioral Practice, 16*(2), 123–134.
50. Gilbert, P. (2001). Evolution and social anxiety. The role of attraction, social competition, and social hierarchies. *Psychiatric Clinics of North America, 24*(4), 72–51.
51. Boesch, C. (2012). The ecology and evolution of social behavior and cognition in primates. In J. Vonk, & T. K. Shackelford (Eds.), *The Oxford handbook of comparative evolutionary psychology* (pp. 489–503). Oxford: Oxford University Press.
52. Barras, C. (2013). Humanity's earliest cousin. *New Scientist, 218*(2920), 8–9.
53. Jaeger, J.-J., & Marivaux, L. (2005). Shaking the earliest branches of anthropoid primate evolution. *Science, 310*(5746), 244–245.
54. American Psychiatric Association. *Diagnostic and statistical manual of mental disorders* (1994). (4th ed.). Washington, DC: American Psychiatric Association.
55. American Psychiatric Association. *Diagnostic and statistical manual of mental disorders* (2013). (5th ed.). Washington, DC: American Psychiatric Association.
56. Price, J. S., Gardner, R., Jr., Wilson, D. R., Sloman, L., Rohde, P., & Erickson, M. (2007). Territory, rank and mental health: The history of an idea. *Evolutionary Psychology, 5*(3), 531–554.
57. Price, J. S., Gardner, R., Jr., & Erickson, M. (2004). Can depression, anxiety and somatization be understood as appeasement displays? *Journal of Affective Disorders, 79*(1–3), 1–11.
58. Sloman, L., Gilbert, P., & Hasey, G. (2003). Evolved mechanisms in depression: The role of attachment and social rank in depression. *Journal of Affective Disorders, 74*(2), 107–121.
59. Watson, P. J., & Andrews, P. W. (2002). Toward a revised evolutionary adaptationist analysis of depression: The social navigation hypothesis. *Journal of Affective Disorders, 72*(1), 1–14.
60. Welling, H. (2003). An evolutionary function of the depressive reaction: The cognitive map hypothesis. *New Ideas in Psychology, 21*(2), 147–156.

61. Nettle, D. (2004). Evolutionary origins of depression: A review and reformulation. *Journal of Affective Disorders, 81*(2), 91–102.
62. Nesse, R. M. (2000). Is depression an adaptation? *Archives of General Psychiatry, 57*(1), 14–20.
63. Gilbert, P. (2006). Evolution and depression: Issues and implications. *Psychological Medicine, 36*(3), 287–297.
64. Panksepp, J. (2010). Affective neuroscience of the emotional BrainMind: Evolutionary perspectives and implications for understanding depression. *Dialogues in Clinical Neuroscience, 12*(4), 533–544.
65. Dantzer, R. (2005). Somatization: A psychoneuroimmune perspective. *Psychoneuroendocrinology, 30*(10), 947–952.
66. Gilbert, P. (2001). Evolutionary approaches to psychopathology: The role of natural defences. *Australian and New Zealand Journal of Psychiatry, 35*(1), 17–27.
67. Beck, A. T., Emery, G., & Greenberg, R. L. (1985). *Anxiety disorders and phobias: A cognitive perspective*. New York: Basic Books.
68. Woody, E. Z., & Szechtman, H. (2011). Adaptation to potential threat: The evolution, neurobiology, and psychopathology of the security motivation system. *Neuroscience and Biobehavioral Reviews, 35*(4), 1019–1033.
69. Eilam, D., Izhar, R., & Mort, J. (2011). Threat detection: Behavioral practices in animals and humans. *Neuroscience and Biobehavioral Reviews, 35*(4), 999–1006.
70. Gilbert, P. (1998). Evolutionary psychopathology: Why isn't the mind designed better than it is? *British Journal of Medical Psychology, 71(* Pt 4*)*, 353–373.
71. Gilbert, P. (1998). The evolved basis and adaptive functions of cognitive distortions. *British Journal of Medical Psychology, 71(* Pt 4*)*, 447–463.
72. Gilbert, P. (2002). Evolutionary approaches to psychopathology and cognitive therapy. *Journal of Cognitive Psychotherapy: An International Quarterly, 16*(3), 263–294.
73. Smith, G. F., Benson, P. G., & Curley, S. P. (1991). Belief, knowledge, and uncertainty: A cognitive perspective on subjective probability. *Organizational Behavior and Human Decision Processes, 48*(2), 291–321.
74. Leben, D. (2014). When psychology undermines beliefs. *Philosophical Psychology, 27*(3), 328–350.
75. McKinsey, M. (1999). The semantics of belief ascriptions. *Nous, 33*(4), 519–557.
76. Egan, A. (2008). Seeing and believing: Perception, belief formation and the divided mind. *Philosophical Studies, 140*(1), 47–63.
77. Priest, G. (1985–1986). Contradiction, belief and rationality. *Proceedings of the Aristotelian Society, 86*, 99–116.
78. Leitgeb, H. (2014). The stability theory of belief. *Philosophical Review, 123*(2), 131–171.
79. Nichols, S. (2006). Just the imagination: Why imagining doesn't behave like believing. *Mind & Language, 21*(4), 459–474.
80. Green, D. W. (1993). Mental models: Rationality, representation and process. *Behavioral and Brain Sciences, 16*(2), 352–353.
81. Johnson-Laird, P. N., & Byrne, R. M. J. (1993). Precis of deduction. *Behavioral and Brain Sciences, 16*(2), 323–380.
82. Malt, B. C. (1990). Features and beliefs in the mental representation of categories. *Journal of Memory and Language, 29*(3), 289–315.
83. Bara, B. G. (1993). Toward a developmental theory of mental models. *Behavioral and Brain Sciences,* 16(2), 336.
84. Gilbert, D. T. (1991). How mental systems believe. *American Psychologist, 46*(2), 107–119.
85. Koriat, A., & Adiv, S. (2012). Confidence in one's social beliefs: Implications for belief justification. *Consciousness and Cognition, 21*, 1599–1616.
86. Kyburg, H. E. (2003). Are there degrees of belief? *Journal of Applied Logic, 1*(3), 139–149.
87. Enoch, D., & Schechter, J. (2008). How are basic belief-forming methods justified? *Philosophy and Phenomenological Research, 76*(3), 547–579.

88. Over, D. (1993). Deduction and degrees of freedom. *Behavioral and Brain Sciences, 16*(2), 361–362.
89. Zynda, L. (2000). Representation theorems and realism about degrees of belief. *Philosophy of Science, 67*(1), 45–69.
90. Atran, S. (1998). Folk biology and the anthropology of science: Cognitive universals and cultural particulars. *Behavioral & Brain Sciences, 21*(4), 547–609.
91. Wellman, H. M., & Gelman, S. A. (1992). Cognitive development: Foundational theories of core domains. *Annual Review of Psychology, 43*, 337–375.
92. Atran, S., & Norenzayan, A. (2004). Religion's evolutionary landscape: Counterintuition, commitment, compassion, communion. *Behavioral and Brain Sciences, 27*(6), 713–730.
93. Boyer, P. (2001). *Religion explained: The evolutionary origins of religious thought*. New York: Basic Books.
94. Bertamini, M., & Casati, R. (1993). False beliefs and naive beliefs: They can be good for you. *Behavioral and Brain Sciences, 16*(2), 512–513.
95. Reiner, M., Slotta, J. D., Michelene, T. H. C., & Resnick, L. B. (2000). Naive physics reasoning: A commitment to substance-based conceptions. *Cognition and Instruction, 18*(1), 1–34.
96. Markman, K. D., & Guenther, C. L. (2007). Psychological momentum: Intuitive physics and naive beliefs. *Personality and Social Psychology Bulletin, 33*(6), 800–812.
97. Arico, A., Fiala, B., Nichols, S., & Goldberg, R. F. (2011). The folk psychology of consciousness. *Mind and Language, 26*(3), 327–352.
98. Greenwood, D. J. (Ed.). (1991). *The future of folk psychology*. Cambridge: Cambridge University Press.
99. Christensen, S. M., & Turner, D. R. (Eds.). (1993). *Folk psychology and the philosophy of mind*. Hillsdale: Lawrence Erlbaum.
100. Wolpert, L. (2007). *Six impossible things before breakfast: The evolutionary origins of beliefs*. New York: W.W. Norton & Co.
101. Bloom, P. (2007). Religion is natural. *Developmental Science, 10*(1), 147–151.
102. Beck, A. T., & Freeman, A. (1990). *Cognitive therapy of personality disorders*. New York: Guilford Press.
103. Gumley, A., O'Grady, M., Power, K., & Schwannauer, M. (2004). Negative beliefs about self and illness: A comparison of individuals with psychosis with or without comorbid social anxiety disorder. *Australian and New Zealand Journal of Psychiatry, 38*(11/12), 960–964.
104. Chik, H. M., Calamari, J. E., Rector, N. A., & Riemann, B. C. (2010). What do low-dysfunctional beliefs obsessive-compulsive disorder subgroups believe? *Journal of Anxiety Disorders, 24*, 837–846.
105. Moulding, R., Anglim, J., Nedeljkovic, M., Doron, G., Kyrios, M., & Ayalon, A. (2011). The Obsessive Beliefs Questionnaire (OBQ): Examination in nonclinical samples and development of a short version. *Assessment, 18*(3), 357–374.
106. Taylor, S., Abramowitz, J. S., McKay, D., Calamari, J. E., Sookman, D., Kyrios, M., et al. (2006). Do dysfunctional beliefs play a role in all types of obsessive-compulsive disorder? *Journal of Anxiety Disorders, 20*(1), 85–97.
107. Wenzel, A., Sharp, I. R., Brown, G. K., Greenberg, R. L., & Beck, A. T. (2006). Dysfunctional beliefs in panic disorder: The panic belief inventory. *Behaviour Research and Therapy, 44*(6), 819–833.
108. Hoppe, L. J., Ipser, J., Gorman, J. M., & Stein, D. J. (2012). Panic disorder. In T. E. Schaepfer, & C. B. Nemeroff (Eds.), *Handbook of clinical neurolology: Neurobiology of psychiatric disorders* (2012/05/23 ed., Vol. 106, pp. 363–374). Amsterdam: Elsevier.
109. Fenigstein, A. (1984). Self-consciousness and the overperception of self as a target. *Journal of Personality and Social Psychology, 47*(4), 860–870.
110. Fenigstein, A., & Vanable, P. A. (1992). Paranoia and self-consciousness. *Journal of Personality and Social Psychology, 62*(1), 129–138.
111. Alcock, J. E. (1995). The belief engine. *The Skeptical Inquirer, 19*(3), 14–18.

112. Han, S., Mao, L., Gu, X., Zhu, Y., Ge, J., & Ma, Y. (2008). Neural consequences of religious belief on self-referential processing. *Social Neuroscience, 3*(1), 1–15.
113. Harris, S., Kaplan, J. T., Curiel, A., Bookheimer, S. Y., Iacoboni, M., & Cohen, M. S. (2009). The neural correlates of religious and nonreligious belief. *PloS One, 4*(10), e0007272–e0007272.
114. Harris, S., Sheth, S. A., & Cohen, M. S. (2008). Functional neuroimaging of belief, disbelief, and uncertainty. *Annals of Neurology, 63*(2), 141–147.
115. Flannelly, K. J., Koenig, H. G., Galek, K., & Ellison, C. G. (2007). Beliefs, mental health, and evolutionary threat assessment systems in the brain. *Journal of Nervous and Mental Disease, 195*(12), 996–1003.
116. Canteras, N. S., Mota-Ortiz, S. R., & Motta, S. C. (2012). What ethologically based models have taught us about the neural systems underlying fear and anxiety. *Brazilian Journal of Medical and Biological Research, 45*, 321–327.
117. Fiddick, L. (2011). There is more than the amygdala: Potential threat assessment in the cingulate cortex. *Neuroscience and Biobehavioral Reviews, 35*(4), 1007–1018.
118. Neuberg, S. L., Kenrick, D. T., & Schaller, M. (2011). Human threat management systems: Self-protection and disease avoidance. *Neuroscience and Biobehavioral Reviews, 35*(4), 1042–1051.
119. Stein, D. J., & Nesse, R. M. (2011). Threat detection, precautionary responses, and anxiety disorders. *Neuroscience & Biobehavioral Reviews, 35*(4), 1075–1079.
120. Woody, E., & Boyer, P. (2011). Threat-detection and precaution: Introduction to the special issue. *Neuroscience & Biobehavioral Reviews, 35*(4), 989–990.
121. Graeff, F. G. (2011). Defense-related emotions in humans. *Psychology & Neuroscience, 4*(2), 183–189.
122. Brune, M., Belsky, J., Fabrega, H., Feierman, H. R., Gilbert, P., Glantz, K., et al. (2012). The crisis of psychiatry – insights and prospects from evolutionary theory. *World Psychiatry, 11*(1), 55–57.
123. Jia, X., Liang, P., Lu, J., Yang, Y., Zhong, N., & Li, K. (2011). Common and dissociable neural correlates associated with component processes of inductive reasoning. *NeuroImage, 56*, 2292–2299.
124. Bunge, S. A., Wendelken, C., Badre, D., & Wagner, A. D. (2005). Analogical reasoning and prefrontal cortex: Evidence for separable retrieval and integration mechanisms. *Cerebral Cortex, 15*(3), 239–249.
125. Fuster, J. (2008). *The prefrontal cortex*. London: Academic Press.
126. Goel, V., & Dolan, R. J. (2004). Differential involvement of left prefrontal cortex in inductive and deductive reasoning. *Cognition, 93*(3), B109–B121.
127. Waltz, J. A., & Knowlton, B. J. (1999). A system for relational reasoning in human prefrontal cortex. *Psychological Science, 10*(2), 119.
128. Evans, J. S. B. T., & Over, D. E. (2013). Reasoning to and from belief: Deduction and induction are still distinct. *Thinking and Reasoning, 19*(3–4), 267–283.
129. Evans, J. S. B. T. (2003). In two minds: Dual-process accounts of reasoning. *Trends in Cognitive Sciences, 7*(10), 454–459.
130. Trippas, I., Handley, S. J., & Verde, M. F. (2014). Fluency and belief bias in deductive reasoning: New indices for old effects. *Frontiers in Psychology, 5*(June), Article 631. Retrieved from: http://journal.frontiersin.org/article/10.3389/fpsyg.2014.00631/full.
131. Goel, V., & Dolan, R. J. (2003). Explaining modulation of reasoning by belief. *Cognition, 87*(1), B11–B22.
132. Monti, M. M., Osherson, D. N., Martinez, M. J., & Parsons, L. M. (2007). Functional neuroanatomy of deductive inference: A language-independent distributed network. *NeuroImage, 37*, 1005–1016.
133. Kroger, J. K., Nystrom, L. E., Cohen, J. D., & Johnson-Laird, P. N. (2008). Distinct neural substrates for deductive and mathematical processing. *Brain Research, 1243*, 86–103.

134. Houde, O., Zago, L., Crivello, F., Moutier, S., Pineau, A., Mazoyer, B., et al. (2001). Access to deductive logic depends on a right ventromedial prefrontal area devoted to emotion and feeling: Evidence from a training paradigm. *NeuroImage, 14*(6), 1486–1492.
135. Gilbert, P. (1993). Defence and safety: Their function in social behaviour and psychopathology. *British Journal of Clinical Psychology, 32(* Pt 2*)*, 131–153.
136. Gilbert, P. (2007). Evolved minds and compassion in the therapeutic relationship. In P. Gilbert, & R. L. Leahy (Eds.), *The therapeutic relationship in cognitive behavioural psychotherapies* (pp. 107–142). London: Routledge.
137. Eisenberger, N. I., Master, S. L., Inagaki, T. K., Taylor, S. E., Shirinyan, D., Lieberman, M. D., et al. (2011). Attachment figures activate a safety signal-related neural region and reduce pain experience. *Proceedings of the National Academy of Sciences, 108*(28), 11721–11726.
138. Coria-Avila, G. A., Manzo, J., Garcia, L. I., Carrillo, P., Miguel, M., & Pfaus, J. G. (2008). Neurobiology of social attachments. *Comparative Biochemistry and Physiology: Toxicology & Pharmacology, 148*(4), 401–410.
139. Minagawa-Kawai, Y., Matsuoka, S., Dan, I., Naoi, N., Nakamura, K., & Kojima, S. (2009). Prefrontal activation associated with social attachment: Facial-emotion recognition in mothers and infants. *Cerebral Cortex, 19*(2), 284–292.
140. Moutsiana, C., Fearon, P., Murray, L., Cooper, P., Goodyer, I., Johnstone, T., et al. (2014). Making an effort to feel positive: Insecure attachment in infancy predicts the neural underpinnings of emotion regulation in adulthood. *Journal of Child Psychology & Psychiatry, 55*(9), 999–1008.
141. Noriuchi, M., Kikuchi, Y., & Senoo, A. (2008). The functional neuroanatomy of maternal love: Mother's response to infant's attachment behaviors. *Biological Psychiatry, 63*(4), 415–423.
142. Vrticka, P., Sander, D., Vuilleumier, P., & Bondolfi, G. (2012). The neural substrates of social emotion perception and regulation are modulated by adult attachment style. *Social Neuroscience, 7*(5), 473–493.
143. Vrticka, P., & Vuilleumier, P. (2012). Neuroscience of human social interactions and adult attachment style. *Frontiers in Human Neuroscience, 6*, 212.
144. Rachman, S. (1984). Agoraphobia-A safety-signal perspective. *Behaviour Research and Therapy, 22*(1), 59–70.
145. Woody, S., & Rachman, S. (1994). Generalized anxiety disorder (GAD) as an unsuccessful search for safety. *Clinical Psychology Review, 14*(8), 743–753.
146. Flannelly, K. J., Flannelly, L., & Blanchard, R. J. (1984). Adult experience and the expression of aggression: A comparative analysis. In K. J. Flannelly, R. J. Blanchard, & D. C. Blanchard (Eds.), *Biological perspectives on aggression*. New York: Alan R. Liss.
147. Martens, A., Greenberg, J., & Allen, J. J. B. (2008). Self-esteem and autonomic physiology: Parallels between self-esteem and cardiac vagal tone as buffers of threat. *Personality and Social Psychology Review, 12*(4), 370–389.
148. Karademas, E. C., Kafetsios, K., & Sideridis, G. D. (2007). Optimism, self-efficacy and information processing of threat- and well-being-related stimuli. *Stress and Health, 23*(5), 285–294.
149. Vytal, K. E., Overstreet, C., Charney, D. R., Robinson, O. J., & Grillon, C. (2014). Sustained anxiety increases amygdala-dorsomedial prefrontal coupling: A mechanism for maintaining an anxious state in healthy adults. *Journal of Psychiatry & Neuroscience, 39*(5), 321.
150. Robinson, O. J., Krimsky, M., Lieberman, L., Allen, P., Vytal, K., & Grillon, C. (2014). Towards a mechanistic understanding of pathological anxiety: The dorsal medial prefrontal-amygdala "aversive amplification" circuit in unmedicated generalized and social anxiety disorders. *The lancet. Psychiatry, 1*(4), 294.
151. Marshall, R. D., Bryant, R. A., Amsel, L., Suh, E. J., Cook, J. M., & Neria, Y. (2007). The psychology of ongoing threat: Relative risk appraisal, the September 11 attacks, and terrorism-related fears. *American Psychologist, 62*(4), 304–316.

152. Leahy, R. L. (2002). Pessimism and the evolution of negativity. *Journal of Cognitive Psychotherapy, 16*, 295–316.
153. Cha, J., Greenberg, T., Hajcak, G., Mujica-Parodi, L. R., Carlson, J. M., & DeDora, D. J. (2014). Circuit-wide structural and functional measures predict ventromedial prefrontal cortex fear generalization: Implications for generalized anxiety disorder. *Journal of Neuroscience, 34*(11), 4043–4053.

Chapter 28
Belief in Life-After-Death and Mental Health

Abstract This chapter summarizes all the major research findings presented in Chaps. 16, 17, and 18 about the association of belief in life-after-death with death anxiety, psychological well-being, psychological distress, and psychiatric symptoms among American adults. The chapter describes (a) the capacity of belief in an afterlife to buffer against the pernicious effects of adverse life events on psychological distress, (b) how pleasant and unpleasant beliefs about the afterlife have differential effects on psychiatric symptomology, and (c) that belief in life-after-death may indirectly affect psychiatric symptoms by affecting our beliefs about the nature of the world. The chapter interprets the major findings in light of Evolutionary Threat Assessment Systems Theory (ETAS Theory) and contrasts ETAS Theory with Terror Management Theory (TM Theory) in several respects, including (a) their predictions about the effects of mortality salience on psychiatric symptoms; (b) the reason why ETAS Theory, but not TM Theory, can explain why certain beliefs about life-after-death can decrease anxiety-related psychiatric symptoms, whereas other beliefs about life-after-death can increase them; and (c) the superior ability of ETAS Theory to explain why psychiatric symptoms exist at all. Finally, the chapter describes how, according to ETAS Theory, social support directly influences psychological distress by providing a sense of safety that alters the brain's perception of potential threats of harm.

Keywords Afterlife • Death anxiety • ETAS Theory • Life-after-death • Psychiatric symptoms • Psychological distress • Psychological well-being • Terror Management Theory

28.1 Background

A larger proportion of people in the U.S. believe in life-after-death than the proportion of people who belief in life-after-death in almost any other country in the world. In fact, the percentage of people in the U.S. who believe in an afterlife is comparable to the percentages reported in the predominantly Catholic countries of Ireland and Poland [1]. According to data from the General Social Survey (GSS), most Americans believe that the afterlife will be a place of peace and tranquility and that

K.J. Flannelly, *Religious Beliefs, Evolutionary Psychiatry, and Mental Health in America*, Religion, Spirituality and Health: A Social Scientific Approach 1,
DOI 10.1007/978-3-319-52488-7_28

it entails union with God and reunion with relatives [2]. Despite the high rate of the belief in life-after-death among Americans, very little research has explored whether belief in an afterlife contributes to mental health, aside from studies on death anxiety.

28.2 Belief in Life-After-Death and Death Anxiety

Terror Management Theory (TM Theory) claims the primary function of religion is to reduce fear of death by offering a sense of security and the possibility of immortality through life-after-death [3, 4]. Indeed, U.S. research of convenience samples of mainly Christian adults and college students generally shows that belief in life-after-death is inversely related to death anxiety (i.e., fear of death) [5]. However, people have many different fears about death, including fear of the dying process, fear for the well-being of surviving loved ones, and fear of not knowing what happens after death [6]. So, a study by psychologist Nava Silton and her colleagues examined the extent to which belief in life-after-death (and other aspects of religion) was associated with fear of dying in pain, fear of dying alone, fear of leaving loved ones' behind, and fear of not knowing what happens after death [7]. The study, which used data from a large national sample of American Christians, found that belief in life-after-death had a significant salutary association with fear of not knowing what happens after death. However, it did not have a significant association with any of the other fears.

28.3 Belief in Life-After-Death and Psychological Well-Being

Two studies by Chris Ellison and his colleagues examined the association between belief in an afterlife and psychological distress and well-being in American adults, using large probability (i.e., random) samples [8, 9]. Both studies (which were published in 2001 and 2009) found salutary associations between belief in an afterlife and their two outcome measures, but the net effects of belief in an afterlife were statistically significant only for the measures of psychological well-being, controlling for other religious and demographic variables.

Three other findings from these studies are of particular interest. First, the studies found that adverse life events (i.e., poor health and financial problems) had significant pernicious associations with both psychological well-being and psychological distress. Second, the studies found that belief in life-after-death buffered against the pernicious effects of poor health and financial problems on well-being and distress. This means that belief in life-after-death was particularly beneficial for individuals dealing with these adverse life effects. Third, the 2001 study [8] found a significant salutary association between social support and psychological distress, consistent with ETAS Theory's proposition that social support provides a sense of personal safety. Although belief in life-after-death provides a sense of security by reducing uncertainty about the future, social support seems to provide an immediate sense of security regarding one's current circumstances that may exert a stronger influence on mental health than the security proved by belief in life-after-death.

From the perspective of ETAS Theory, poor health poses a threat to one's life, and poor health and financial problems both pose a threat to one's way of life. They also create uncertainty about the future, and uncertainty is known to produce anxiety [10, 11]. Hence, it is not surprising that these adverse life events were associated with higher levels of psychological distress in these studies, which both used anxiety as an outcome measure. The results of the studies suggest that belief in life-after-death quells the anxiety posed by these threats and/or the uncertainty they create.

A third study by Ellison and his colleague Matt Bradshaw [12] examined the degree to which belief in life-after-death buffers against the psychological distress produced by financial hardship. Although belief in an afterlife did not have a main effect on psychological distress, people experiencing financial hardship who believed in life-after-death reported significantly lower levels of psychological distress than those who did not believe in life-after-death. These findings confirm that belief in an afterlife buffers against the psychological distress associated with adverse life events.

Ellison and his colleagues suggested that the salubrious association of belief in an afterlife with psychological distress and well-being was the product of a worldview within which individuals interpret their personal circumstances in a larger context. Since people who believe in life-after-death view their earthly existence as being temporary, they view their earthly problems as temporary, which provides a sense of calm, and reduces worry, fear, and other negative feelings [9].

28.4 Belief in an Afterlife and Psychiatric Symptoms

A 2006 national study by me, Chris Ellison, and our colleagues [13] examined the association between belief in life-after-death and six classes of psychiatric symptoms: agoraphobia, depression, general anxiety, obsessive-compulsive disorder, paranoid ideation, and somatization. Belief in life-after-death had significant salubrious associations with all six classes of psychiatric symptoms, controlling for other religious variables and demographic variables. The association was strongest for agoraphobia, probably because many people with agoraphobia also suffer from panic attacks, which often include fear of imminent death. The association was nearly as strong for general anxiety, which involves fear of unspecified or unknown threats of harm.

I think these results suggest that part of the net effect of belief in life-after-death on psychiatric symptoms is that it provides a sense of certainty about the future. Behavioral studies have shown that uncertainty about life is associated with anxiety [14, 15], and neuro-physiological studies have shown that the amygdala responds to uncertainty with fear as if uncertainty poses a threat of harm [10, 11]. Hence, feeling secure about what will happen in the future should reduce anxiety and other psychiatric symptoms related to fears about the dangerousness of the world.

Although TM Theory proposes that the "terror of death" underlies much of human behavior, I tend to side with the Dutch psychologist Kees van den Bos [16] and Uncertainty Management Theory that uncertainty about the future, including such things as health and financial well-being, are more common human concerns than death. I readily concede, however, that death is the major existential uncertainty of humans, which is why I think believing in eternal life reduces fears about present and future circumstances. I think this notion is compatible with Ellison's interpretation of the effects of belief in an afterlife on psychological distress in that belief in an afterlife provides certainty about a future life as well as putting one's present life in an eternal perspective.

28.5 Different Afterlife Beliefs and Psychiatric Symptoms

A 2008 article by me, Chris Ellison, and our colleagues analyzed the same dataset used in the 2006 study to examine the association between psychiatric symptoms and various beliefs about life-after-death [17]. I grouped the afterlife beliefs into two categories (four pleasant and two unpleasant beliefs) in Chap. 18 to analyze the degree to which two these categories of beliefs were associated with five of the six classes of psychiatric symptoms studied in 2006. The four pleasant beliefs were: "Union with God," "Reunion with family and loved ones," "A life of peace and tranquility," and "A paradise of pleasures and delights." The two unpleasant beliefs were: "Reincarnation into another life form" and "A pale, shadowy form of life, hardly life at all." The five psychiatric symptoms were agoraphobia, depression, general anxiety, obsessive-compulsive disorder, and paranoid ideation.

The study found pleasant beliefs about life-after-death had a significant salubrious association with four of the five classes of psychiatric symptomology. Once again, the largest association was found for agoraphobia. No significant association was found between pleasant afterlife beliefs and depression, probably because the pleasant beliefs about the afterlife were more likely to tap into symptoms of anxiety than depression.

Unpleasant beliefs about the experience of life-after-death had a significant net effect on all five dependent measures. Although far fewer study participants believed in the unpleasant beliefs than the pleasant beliefs about the afterlife, unpleasant beliefs apparently have a substantial pernicious affect on the mental health of those who do believe them.

28.6 Beliefs About the Afterlife, the World, and Psychiatric Symptoms

A 2012 study by me and my colleagues, including Chris Ellison, provides evidence that belief in life-after-death may influence psychiatric symptoms by altering the way we think about life [18]. We used data from a national sample of American adults, which we analyzed by structural equation modeling (SEM). Five classes of psychiatric symptoms served as the dependent variables (general anxiety, social anxiety, paranoid ideation, obsession, and compulsion). The SEM model included the latent variables religious commitment, belief in a pleasant afterlife, belief in a cynical world, and belief in an equitable world. Separate models were conducted for each dependent variable. The SEM hypothesized that: (1) religious commitment is positively associated with pleasant beliefs about life-after-death; that pleasant beliefs about life-after-death are (2) positively associated with the belief that the world is equitable and (3) negatively associated with the belief that the world is cynical; and that (4) belief in an equitable world are negatively associated with psychiatric symptoms, whereas (5) belief in a cynical world are positively associated with psychiatric symptoms.

The analyses confirmed all the hypotheses to some extent. As predicted, religious commitment had a strong positive association with pleasant beliefs about life-after-death, and pleasant beliefs about life-after-death had a positive association with belief in an equitable world and a negative association with belief in a cynical world. However, belief in an equitable world had salubrious associations with only two of the four classes of psychiatric symptoms (i.e., general anxiety and obsession), whereas belief in a cynical world had significant pernicious associations with all five types of psychiatric symptoms. I think these results provide support for Ellison's premise that belief in life-after-death influences psychological distress by altering the way we think about the temporal world.

28.7 Terror Management Theory and Psychiatric Symptoms

Some proponents of TM Theory contend that anxiety-related disorders result from the inability of individuals to manage their terror of death [19]. However, there is no evidence that this is true. Moreover, TM Theory, unlike ETAS Theory, does not explain why many different classes of psychiatric symptoms exist – which is explained by their evolutionary functions, as discussed in Chaps. 11 and 12. Nor do the TM Theory proponents of this hypothesis even attempt to explain how fear of death could produce such a variety of psychiatric symptoms [19].

The "mortality salience" hypothesis, which is a central element of TM Theory [20, 21], proposes that things that remind people of death will increase their anxiety [22]. A 2014 study by Chris Ellison, me, and a colleague investigated the degree to which mortality salience (a heighted awareness of one's own mortality) moderated the association of beliefs about the afterlife with selected psychiatric symptoms [23]. The study found that the effect of mortality salience was influenced by one's beliefs about what the afterlife will be, not just the belief that there is an afterlife. For people who believed the afterlife will be a pleasant experience, mortality salience decreased anxiety-related symptoms; whereas, for people who believed the afterlife will be an unpleasant experience, mortality salience increased anxiety-related symptoms. These findings are consistent with ETAS Theory, but not with TM Theory, which proposes that mortality salience increases anxiety and related psychiatric symptoms.

28.8 Conclusions

The research results summarized in this chapter show that belief in life-after-death has a salutary association with death anxiety, psychological well-being, psychological distress, and several classes of psychiatric symptoms. Moreover, they indicate that belief in life-after-death buffers against the pernicious effects of the adverse life events on psychological well-being and distress, including psychiatric symptoms. According to ETAS Theory, at least part of the reason for the overall salubrious effect of belief in an afterlife on psychological distress, and its stress buffering effects, are that belief in an afterlife reduces uncertainty about one's future existence. This effect is due to the fact that the amygdala is known to produce fear in response to uncertainty, just as it does to threats of harm; hence, reducing uncertainty reduces anxiety. I tend to think fear about the future is a more common concern among most people than the fear of death itself, as TM Theory claims.

The pleasant afterlife beliefs we tested ("union with God" and "reunion with relatives") provide reassurance about the future in the afterlife, whereas the unpleasant beliefs we tested ("a pale shadowy place, hardy life at all" and "reincarnation into another life form") raise uncertainties about the afterlife. Therefore, morality salience reduces anxiety when one has pleasant beliefs about the afterlife, but increases anxiety when one has unpleasant beliefs about the afterlife. This proposition, which follows from ETAS Theory, differs from TM Theory's more simplistic proposition that mortality salience increases anxiety. Although some advocates of TM Theory claim that the terror of death can lead to anxiety and associated disorders, they do not provide a mechanism by which this can happen, nor do they explain how fear of death could produce the variety of psychiatric symptoms that people commonly experience. ETAS Theory, in contrast, explains that the variety of existing psychiatric symptoms are linked to proximate mechanisms that evolved to promote survival, as described in Chaps. 11 and 12.

The notion that belief in life-after-death reduces anxiety by providing certainty about the future differs from, but is consistent with, Ellison's explanation that belief in an afterlife may reduce anxiety by putting people's worldly problems in the broader perspective of eternal life. The results of the 2012 study on beliefs about the afterlife, beliefs about the world, and psychiatric symptoms [18] are important because they support Ellison's notion that belief in life-after-death may reduce psychological distress, in part, by altering the way we think about temporal problems in the context of an external life.

Finally, the results of the 2001 study by Ellison [8] are important because they show that social support has a salubrious association with psychological distress, which is consistent with ETAS Theory's proposition that social support provides a sense of personal safety. Although most researchers who study healthcare think social support has an indirect effect on physical and mental health, ETAS Theory proposes that part of the effect of social support on health is its ability to directly reduce the anxiety produced by threats of harm, by providing a sense of safety or security that makes the threat of illness, injury, or other source of harm seem less threatening. Specifically, the sense of safety assessed by the ventromedial prefrontal cortex (vmPFC) causes the vmPFC to reduce the activity of the amygdala, which produces fear in response to perceived threats of harm (including uncertainty).

References

1. Smith, A. (2008). *Beliefs about God across time and countries*. Chicago: National Opinion Research Board.
2. Greeley, A. M., & Hout, M. (1999). Americans' increasing belief in life after death: Religious competition and acculturation. *American Sociological Review, 64*(6), 813–835.
3. Vail, K. E., 3rd, Rothschild, Z. K., Weise, D. R., Solomon, S., Pyszczynski, T., & Greenberg, J. (2010). A terror management analysis of the psychological functions of religion. *Personality and Social Psychology Review, 14*(1), 84–94.
4. Jonas, E., & Fischer, P. (2006). Terror management and religion: Evidence that intrinsic religiousness mitigates worldview defense following mortality salience. *Journal of Personality and Social Psychology, 91*(3), 553–567.
5. Ellis, L., & Wahab, E. (2013). Religiosity and fear of death: A theory-oriented review of the empirical literature. *Review of Religious Research, 55*(1), 149–189
6. Hoelter, J. W. (1979). Multidimensional treatment of fear of death. *Journal of Consulting and Clinical Psychology, 47*(5), 996–999
7. Silton, N. R., Flannelly, K. J., Ellison, C. G., Galek, K., Jacobs, M. R., Marcum, J. P., et al. (2011). The association between religious beliefs and practices and end-of-life fears among members of the Presbyterian Church (USA). *Review of Religious Research, 53*, 357–370.
8. Ellison, C. G., Boardman, J. D., Williams, D. R., & Jackson, J. S. (2001). Religious involvement, stress, and mental health: Findings from the 1995 Detroit area study. *Social Forces, 80*(1), 215–249.
9. Ellison, C. G., Burdette, A. M., & Hill, T. D. (2009). Blessed assurance: Religion, anxiety, and tranquility among US adults. *Social Science Research, 38*(3), 656–667.
10. Grupe, D. W., & Nitschke, J. B. (2013). Uncertainty and anticipation in anxiety: An integrated neurobiological and psychological perspective. *Nature Reviews: Neuroscience, 14*(7), 488–501.
11. Sarinopoulos, I., Grupe, D. W., Mackiewicz, K. L., Herrington, J. D., Lor, M., Steege, E. E., et al. (2010). Uncertainty during anticipation modulates neural responses to aversion in human insula and amygdala. *Cerebral Cortex, 20*(4), 929–940.
12. Bradshaw, M., & Ellison, C. G. (2010). Financial hardship and psychological distress: Exploring the buffering effects of religion. *Social Science & Medicine, 71*(1), 196–204.

13. Flannelly, K. J., Koenig, H. G., Ellison, C. G., Galek, K., & Krause, N. (2006). Belief in life after death and mental health: Findings from a national survey. *Journal of Nervous and Mental Disease, 194*(7), 524–529.
14. Hirsh, J. B., Mar, R. A., & Peterson, J. B. (2012). Psychological entropy: A framework for understanding uncertainty-related anxiety. *Psychological Review, 119*(2), 304–320.
15. Sorrentino, R. M., Ye, Y., & Szeto, A. C. H. (2009). Uncertainty management: To fear of not to fear? *Psychological Inquiry, 20*(4), 240–244.
16. Van den Bos, K. (2009). Making sense of life: The existential self trying to deal with personal uncertainty. *Psychological Inquiry, 20*(4), 197–217.
17. Flannelly, K. J., Ellison, C. G., Galek, K., & Koenig, H. G. (2008). Beliefs about life-after-death, psychiatric symptomology and cognitive theories of psychopathology. *Journal of Psychology & Theology, 36*, 94–103.
18. Flannelly, K. J., Galek, K., Ellison, C. G., & Silton, N. R. (2012). Belief in life-after-death, beliefs about the world, and psychiatric symptoms. *Journal of Religion and Health, 51*(3), 651–662.
19. Arndt, J., Routledge, C., Cox, C. R., & Goldenberg, J. L. (2005). The worm at the core: A terror management perspective on the roots of psychological dysfunction. *Applied and Preventive Psychology, 11*(3), 191.
20. Greenberg, J., Pyszczynski, T., Solomon, S., Rosenblatt, A., Veeder, M., Kirkland, S., et al. (1990). Evidence for terror management theory II: The effects of mortality salience on reactions to those who threaten or bolster the cultural worldview. *Journal of Personality and Social Psychology, 58*(2), 308–318.
21. Rosenblatt, A., Greenberg, J., Solomon, S., Pyszczynski, T., & Lyon, D. (1989). Evidence for terror management theory: I. The effects of mortality salience on reactions to those who violate or uphold cultural values. *Journal of Personality and Social Psychology, 57*(4), 681–690.
22. Pyszczynski, T., Greenberg, J., & Solomon, S. (1999). A dual-process model of defense against conscious and unconscious death-related thoughts: An extension of terror management theory. *Psychological Review, 106*(4), 835–845.
23. Ellison, C. G., Flannelly, K. J., & Barrie, C. K. (2014, November 1). *Do afterlife beliefs moderate the association between recent serious illness and symptoms of anxiety-related disorders?* Paper presented at the National Meeting of the Society for the Scientific Study of Religion, Indianapolis, IN.

Chapter 29
Beliefs About God and Mental Health

Abstract This chapter highlights the major key findings presented in Chaps. 19, 20, and 21 on beliefs about God and mental health among Americans. The first part of the chapter summarizes evidence that belief in a benevolent God and belief in a malevolent God have, respectively, salubrious and pernicious associations with psychological well-being and distress in convenience samples of Christian college students, and with psychiatric symptoms in national samples of the U.S. general public. The next few sections of the chapter cover findings from small-scale and large-scale studies about (a) different types of religious coping related to one's perceived relationship with God, (b) the belief that one collaborates with God, and (c) their associations with psychological well-being (e.g., optimism, life-satisfaction, self-esteem) and psychological distress (including psychiatric symptoms). Subsequent sections describe the results of small-scale studies of U.S. college students and large national studies that have examined the association of believing one has an attachment relationship with God and psychological well-being and distress. The national studies that focused on psychological distress found that believing one has secure attachment to God has a salutary association with psychological distress, whereas believing one has an anxious attachment to God has a pernicious association with psychological distress. Key findings are interpreted in light of Evolutionary Threat Assessment Systems (ETAS) Theory, including the mediating effects of anxiety on psychological well-being. Results are also presented about the effects of self-esteem on anxiety, which are discussed in terms of ETAS Theory and Terror Management Theory.

Keywords Attachment to God • Attachment theory • Collaboration with God • ETAS theory • God • Happiness • Nature of God • Psychiatric symptoms • Psychological distress • Psychological well-being • Relationship with God • Religious coping • Self-esteem

K.J. Flannelly, *Religious Beliefs, Evolutionary Psychiatry, and Mental Health in America*, Religion, Spirituality and Health: A Social Scientific Approach 1,
DOI 10.1007/978-3-319-52488-7_29

29.1 Background

More than 90% of Americans say "Yes" when asked "Do you believe in God," according to a 2011 telephone survey [1]. Moreover, the percent of Americans who say they believe in God has been higher than 90% since the 1940s [2]. However, it is not necessarily clear what people mean when they say they believe in God [3]. When pressed, some people say they do not believe in God, per se, but they believe in a Higher Power. Others say they believe in God, but they also have doubts about God's existence [1, 4].

Findings from studies of convenience samples of American college students and national surveys of American adults help to paint a picture of what Americans believe about God. My own analyses of data from the Baylor Religion Survey, as well as other survey findings, show that the most common beliefs American hold about God are related to images of God in the New Testament (e.g., fatherly, forgiving, and loving) [5, 6]. Devout Christians are particularly inclined to believe God is involved in their lives [7–9].

Beliefs based on themes from both the Old and New Testaments about God's omnipotence, omniscience, and omnipresence are also common [6, 10–12], as well as the beliefs that God is the creator and judge [12–14]. Beliefs entailing the negative attributes of God, which are associated with the Old Testament (e.g., punitive, severe, and wrathful), are far less common.

29.2 Beliefs About the Nature of God and Mental Health

29.2.1 Beliefs About the Nature of God and Psychological Well-Being

Research on small samples of mainly Christian college students have found that belief in a benevolent God (e.g., forgiving, loving, and merciful) has a strong salubrious association with trait anxiety and self-esteem [15, 16], whereas belief in a malevolent God (e.g., cruel, punishing, and wrathful) has a pernicious association with self-esteem [15–19]. Although this research does not tell us much about the relationship between beliefs about God and anxiety, it provides good evidence that belief in a benevolent God has a salubrious association with self-esteem, whereas belief in a malevolent God has a pernicious association with self-esteem. These findings are important from the perspective of ETAS Theory because several studies indicate that self-esteem buffers against the pernicious effects of the threat of harm on anxiety [20–22], whereas threats to self-esteem, itself, increase anxiety [23–26].

I only know of two other quantitative studies that have examined the relationship between beliefs about the nature of God and psychological well-being. Both studies, which used samples of Christian college students, found that belief in a benevolent God had a salutary association with life satisfaction [19, 27].

29.2.2 Beliefs About the Nature of God and Psychiatric Symptoms

This section summarizes the results of two large national studies on the association between beliefs about the nature of God and psychiatric symptoms among the U.S. general public [28, 29]. The first study, published in 2006, examined the association between six classes of psychiatric symptoms (agoraphobia, depression, general anxiety, OCD, paranoia, and somatization) and three sets of beliefs about God: a close and loving God, and approving and forgiving God, and creating and judging God [30, 31]. Based on ETAS Theory, we hypothesized that belief in a close and loving God would have a salubrious association with psychiatric symptomology because a close and loving God should provide a sense of security. As we thought that belief in a creating and judging God or an approving and forgiving God did not imply safety or security, we hypothesized that these beliefs would not be related to psychiatric symptoms. Finally, based on Dantz's theory that somatization does not involve cognitive input (see Chap. 12) [32], we hypothesized that somatization would not be affected by beliefs. The results generally confirmed all the hypotheses.

The study also found a salubrious association of social support with all of the psychiatric symptoms, which were stronger than the net effects of belief in a close and loving God. According to ETAS Theory, the observed relationship between social support and psychiatric symptomology is due, at least in part, to the fact that close social relationships provide a sense of safety.

The second study, published in 2010 [29], examined the relationship between three different beliefs about the nature of God and the five sets of psychiatric symptoms. The three independent variables were belief in a deistic God (absolute and just), a benevolent God (kind and accepting), and a punitive God (wrathful and punishing), and the psychiatric symptoms were general anxiety, obsession, compulsion, paranoia, and social anxiety. Based on ETAS Theory, we hypothesized that psychiatric symptomology would have no association with a deistic God, a salubrious association with a Benevolent God, and a pernicious association with a punitive God.

As expected, belief in a deistic God was not significantly associated with any of the measures of psychiatric symptomology, whereas belief in a benevolent God had a salubrious association with four of the five types of psychiatric symptoms, and belief in a punitive God had a pernicious association with four of the five types of psychiatric symptoms. The results for a deistic God and a benevolent God were similar to the results of the 2010 study [28], presumably because belief in a benevolent God provides a sense of security and belief in a deistic God does not, according to ETAS Theory. We hypothesized that belief in a punitive God would have a pernicious association with psychiatric symptomology because a wrathful and punishing God poses a direct threat of harm.

29.2.3 Belief in a Harsh God, Psychiatric Symptoms, and Happiness

Though ETAS Theory does not explain the existence of positive emotions, it proposes that psychiatric symptoms influence positive emotions. So, I decided to test if anxiety (i.e., symptoms of anxiety disorders) would mediate the effects of beliefs about God on positive emotions. I used data from the Baylor Religion Survey, which measured several psychiatric symptoms and one positive emotion, i.e., happiness.

My analyses confirmed that symptoms of anxiety mediated the salutary association of belief in a loving God on happiness and the pernicious association of belief in a harsh God on happiness. These findings indicate that positive emotions, such as happiness, are influenced by negative affect linked to psychiatric symptoms, particularly anxiety, and that anxiety mediates the influence of religious beliefs on positive emotions. Hence, it appears that threat assessments and the beliefs that modulate them affect positive emotions. Therefore, the mediation results illustrate that ETAS Theory can help to explain the association of positive and negative beliefs about God with positive emotions, in addition to explaining the association of positive and negative beliefs about God with psychiatric symptoms.

29.3 Beliefs About One's Relationship with God and Mental Health

29.3.1 Background

Although one's relationship with God is a vital element of the Christian experience, [33, 34], this concept received little attention in the social sciences until Melvin Pollner published a 1989 article that argued that one's relationship with God is a form of social relationship [35]. Pollner thought that individuals interacted with God symbolically through prayer and that this interaction had a salutary effect on psychological well-being by providing individuals with a sense of security. Chris Ellison, who tested Pollner's ideas in 1991, found that people who believed they had a close relationship with God and frequently prayed to God were significantly more satisfied with life and somewhat happier, compared to other people [36].

29.3.2 Three Beliefs About One's Relationships with God and Mental Health

A 1988 U.S. study by Ken Pargament of Bowling Green State University and his colleagues identified three styles of religious problem-solving that people use when confronted with stressful situations [37]. The first two (collaborative and deferring styles) involve reliance on God, whereas the third (self-directed problem-solving) assumes that individuals are responsible for solving their own problems [37]. A 1991 study found the belief that one collaborates with or defers to God is associated with lower anxiety, whereas self-directed problem-solving is associated with higher anxiety among Christian college students in the U.S. [16]. Related research with religious American undergraduates found that both deferring and collaborative religious problem-solving have significant salubrious associations with psychological well-being and psychological distress [38]. Other research has confirmed that the deferring and collaborative styles have salubrious associations with mental health in different populations.

29.3.3 Collaboration with God and Mental Health

Neal Krause, a sociologist and a psychologist who was a Professor of Public Health at the University of Michigan for 20 years, explored the concept of collaboration with God (which he calls God-mediated control) in a series of national surveys of U.S. adults [39–44]. The Americans in these studies who embraced the concept of God-mediated control expressed the belief that God controlled their lives, but because they believed they had a close relationship with God, they trusted God would do what is best for them [40, 41, 45]. Their own role in this relationship, therefore, may be seen as following God's guidance about what they should do for themselves. Such studies have reported that collaboration with God has a salutary association with psychological well-being [41] and the belief that life has meaning [43].

29.3.4 Positive and Negative Religious Coping and Mental Health

Other research by Ken Pargament revealed many different methods of religious coping and how they were related to mental health [46–48]. These different coping methods, (which mostly entailed one's relationship with God) [49], were generally classified as positive and negative religious coping. In general, this research found that people who believed they had a good relationship with God had better mental-health outcomes than those who thought they had a poor relationship with God.

The most striking finding was that believing that one has been punished or abandoned by God had a particularly profound pernicious association with mental-health outcomes [50].

This research led to the development of the 14-item Brief RCOPE. The seven positive coping items of the RCOPE reflect the patterns of religious coping one tends to use if individuals believe that they have a secure relationship with God and a spiritual connection with others and that there is meaning in life [47]. The seven negative coping items of the RCOPE reflect the belief that one has "a less secure relationship with God, a tenuous and ominous view of the world, and a religious struggle in search significance " (p. 712) [47].

My own review and analysis of research on the RCOPE indicates that the negative RCOPE (which has been called "spiritual struggles") had a significant pernicious association with psychological well-being and psychological distress. I found, on other hand, that the positive RCOPE had only a small association with psychological well-being and distress. Three major U.S. studies that used the negative RCOPE found that it had a significant pernicious association with psychiatric symptoms and other measures of psychological distress [51–53]. These results confirm behavioral predictions from ETAS Theory that various classes of psychiatric symptoms in the general public are influenced by religious beliefs, in this case, beliefs about one's relationship with God.

In the context of ETAS Theory, the salubrious association of believing one has a good relationship with God and mental health reflects the fact that God provides a sense of safety, which causes ETAS to raise the threshold of what constitutes a threat, thereby lowering anxiety and other forms of psychological distress. In general, because anxiety mediates the relationship between beliefs and psychological well-being, this increases psychological well-being. Having a poor relationship with God reduces this sense of safety, thereby lowering the threshold of what is a threat and increasing psychiatric symptoms and related forms of psychological distress.

29.4 Belief in God as an Attachment Figure and Mental Health

29.4.1 Background

The British psychologist John Bowlby [54–56] developed Attachment Theory based on his research into the mother-infant bond, which he began in the 1940s as a complement to his work as a child psychiatrist [57]. American psychologist Mary Ainsworth, who worked with Bowlby in the early 1950s [57], conducted classic studies that confirmed and extended Attachment Theory, including the classification of three attachment styles exhibited by children: secure, anxious-avoidant, anxious-ambivalent attachment [58, 59]. Anxious-avoidant and anxious-ambivalent attachment came to be known simply as avoidant attachment and anxious attachment, respectively. Kirkpatrick and Shaver [60] applied Attachment Theory to the religion and mental health, contending that religion provides security in a world of uncertainty [61, 62], and that a person's relationship with God can be considered to be an attachment relationship much like the relationship between a parent and child [60, 63, 64].

29.4.2 *Attachment to God and Psychological Well-Being*

Studies of college students in the 1990s found that those who believed they had a secure attachment to God were more satisfied with their lives, and less anxious, lonely, and depressed than those who believed they had an avoidant or anxious attachment to God [63, 65]. Later studies of Christian college students reported that avoidant and anxious attachment were negatively related to self-esteem, life satisfaction, and positive affect [19, 66–68].

29.4.3 *Attachment to God, Psychological Distress, and Psychiatric Symptoms*

Two national studies by Ellison and his colleagues examined the degree to which secure attachment and anxious attachment to God were associated with psychological distress in a national sample of Church members [69, 70]. The first study found that Church members who believed they had a secure relationship with God had a significantly lower level of psychological distress than those who believed they had an anxious relationship with God. The second study, which surveyed the same sample one year later, found that psychological distress decreased during the intervening year among the Church members who believed they had a secure relationship with God. Since the second study compared the net effects of attachment styles over one year, it provides evidence that believing one has a secure attachment with God is causally related to lower levels of psychological distress.

A more recent study by Ellison and his colleagues examined attachment to God and psychiatric symptoms. Bivariate correlations found that believing one has a secure attachment to God had a significant salubrious association with all four classes of anxiety symptoms studied, whereas believing that one has an anxious attachment to God had a significant pernicious association with all four classes of symptoms. The associations remained significant for anxious attachment, but not for secure attachment in the multivariate analyses that controlled for other religious variables and socio-demographic characteristics.

29.4.4 Mediating Effect of Anxiety on the Association Between Attachment to God and Happiness

I used the 2010 Baylor Religious Survey's measure of happiness as a dependent variable to analyze the mediating effect of anxiety-related symptoms on the association between religious beliefs and positive affect. As found in my analysis of the relationship between beliefs about God and happiness in Chap. 19, I found that anxiety symptoms mediated the association of between happiness and both positive and negative beliefs about one's attachment to God. The mediation model showed, consistent with ETAS Theory, that anxiety mediates the influences of religious beliefs on happiness. This strongly implies that threat assessments and the beliefs that modulate them affect positive emotions. Therefore, ETAS Theory can help to explain the association of positive and negative beliefs about God with positive emotions, as well as being able to explain their association with psychiatric symptoms.

29.5 Conclusions

The research described above shows that belief in a benevolent God has a salubrious association with mental health, whereas belief in a malevolent God has a pernicious association with mental health. According to ETAS Theory, the salubrious effects of belief in a benevolent God on anxiety and related symptoms results from the combined effects of the perception of threat and a sense of safety. ETAS Theory claims that belief in a benevolent God causes the ventromedial prefrontal cortex to increase the threshold of what constitutes a threat and suppress amygdala activity, thereby lowering anxiety and other psychiatric symptoms. On the other hand, belief in a malevolent God lowers the threshold of what constitutes a threat because God not only fails to provide protection from harm, but poses a direct threat of harm. The threshold of what constitutes a threat is probably lowered because belief in a malevolent God activates the "aversive amplification circuit," which makes the amygdala more sensitive to threats. Belief in a deistic God has no association with symptomology because it does not provide protection from harm.

Terror Management Theory claims that self-esteem evolved to buffer against anxiety about death because self-esteem provides a sense of security that counters the reality that one will inevitably die (i.e., the terror of death) [71–73]. However, it seems more likely to me that self-esteem evolved in primates long before our ancestors became aware of their own mortality, as a cognitive mechanism to assess one's relative status within a dominance hierarchy. It is equally likely that self-efficacy evolved about the same time as a cognitive mechanism to assess the likelihood that one can succeed in moving up in a dominance hierarchy or maintaining one's place in a dominance hierarchy by defeating one's social rivals.

Thus, both self-esteem and self-efficacy should reduce anxiety and related symptoms because the former provides a sense of safety from potential threats and the latter provides a sense that whatever threats exist can be overcome. Like the sense of safety provided by belief in a benevolent God, the sense of safety provided by self-esteem and self-efficacy presumably raises the threshold of what constitutes a threat, thereby reducing anxiety-related symptoms. On the other hand, threats to self-esteem presumably increase anxiety and related symptoms by reducing the sense of safety from harm that it provides.

The findings of the 2010 Flannelly et al. [28] study showed, consistent with past research, that social support had a significant salubrious association with mental health. However, whereas most researchers believe that social support indirectly affects mental health, ETAS Theory proposes that social support has a direct effect on anxiety and related psychiatric symptoms by providing a sense of security that counters the effects of the perceived threats that cause psychiatric symptomology.

The results presented in Sect. 29.3 demonstrate that many Americans believe they have a relationship God and that many Americans believe they collaborate with God to deal with daily stressors. The evidence is compelling that individuals who believe they collaborate with God have better mental health. In contrast, individuals who believe that they have a poor relationship with God have poorer mental-health outcomes, and this association is even more pronounced among individuals who believe that God has abandoned or punished them. Similarly, believing that one has a secure attachment of God is associated with better mental health, whereas believing one has an anxious attachment to God is associated with poorer mental health, including a variety anxiety-related symptoms.

The salubrious association of mental health with believing one has a good relationship with God reflects the fact that God provides a sense of safety that causes ETAS to raise the threshold of what constitutes a threat, which lowers anxiety and related forms of psychological distress. As anxiety mediates the relationship between religious beliefs and psychological well-being (as demonstrated in Chaps. 19 and 21), believing one has a good relationship with God increases psychological well-being. Having a poor relationship with God reduces this sense of safety, thereby lowering the threshold of what is a threat and increasing psychiatric symptoms and related types of psychological distress. The belief that one has been abandoned by God presumably eliminates any sense of safety God may provide, whereas believing God is punishing you makes God a direct threat of harm.

The belief that one has an attachment relationship with God (Sect. 29.4 and Chap. 21) is a special case of the belief that one has a relationship with God. Thus, believing one has an anxious attachment to God increases anxiety, whereas believing one has a secure attachment to God decreases anxiety, by the same mechanisms, respectively, that believing one has a poor relationship or a good relationship with God do.

References

1. Newport, F. (2011). More than 9 in 10 Americans continue to believe in God. Princeton: Gallup. Retrieved from http://www.gallup.com/poll/147887/americans-continue-believe-god.aspx

2. Piazza, T., & Glock, C. Y. (1979). Images of God and their social meanings. In R. Wuthnow (Ed.), *The religious dimension: New directions in quantitative research*. New York: Academic Press.
3. Cranney, S. (2013). Do people who believe in God report more meaning in their lives? The existential effects of belief. *Journal for the Scientific Study of Religion, 52*(3), 638–646.
4. Sherkat, D. E. (2008). Beyond belief: Atheism, agnosticism, and theistic certainty in the United States. *Sociological Spectrum, 28*(5), 438–459.
5. Hoffman, L., Hoffman, J. L., Dillard, K., Clark, J., Acoba, R., Williams, F., et al. (2008). Diversity and the God image: Examining ethnic differences in the experience of God for a college-age population. *Journal of Psychology & Theology, 36*(1), 26–41.
6. Foster, R. A., & Keating, J. P. (1992). Measuring androcentrism in the Western God-concept. *Journal for the Scientific Study of Religion, 31*(3), 366–375.
7. Hammersla, J. F., Andrews-Qualls, L. C., & Frease, L. G. (1986). God concepts and religious committment among Christian university students. *Journal for the Scientific Study of Religion, 25*(4), 424–435.
8. Froese, P., & Bader, C. D. (2010). *America's four Gods*. New York: Oxford University Press.
9. Noffke, J. L. M. S. H. (2001). Denominational and age comparisons of God concepts. *Journal for the Scientific Study of Religion, 40*(4), 747–756.
10. Gorsuch, R. L. (1968). The conceptualization of God as seen in adjective ratings. *Journal for the Scientific Study of Religion, 7*(1), 56–64.
11. Kunkel, M. A., Cook, S., Meshel, D. S., Daughtry, D., & Hauenstein, A. (1999). God images: A concept map. *Journal for the Scientific Study of Religion, 38*(2), 193–202.
12. Tamayo, A., & Desjardines, L. (1976). Belief systems and conceptual images of parents and God. *Journal of Psychology: Interdisciplinary and Applied, 92*(1), 131–140.
13. Nelsen, H. M., Cheek, N. H., & Au, P. (1985). Gender differences in images of God. *Journal for the Scientific Study of Religion, 24*(4), 396–402.
14. Roof, W. C., & Roof, J. L. (1984). Review of the polls: Images of God among Americans. *Journal for the Scientific Study of Religion, 23*(2), 201–205.
15. Benson, P., & Spilka, B. (1973). God image as a function of self-esteem and locus of control. *Journal for the Scientific Study of Religion, 12*(3), 297–310.
16. Schaefer, C. A., & Gorsuch, R. L. (1991). Psychological adjustment and religiousness: The multivariate belief-motivation theory of religiousness. *Journal for the Scientific Study of Religion, 30*(4), 448–461.
17. Francis, L. J. (2005). God images and self-esteem: A study among 11–18 year olds. *Research in the Social Scientific Study of Religion, 18*(1), 105–121.
18. Francis, L. J., Gibson, H. M., & Robbins, M. (2001). God images and self-worth among adolescents in Scotland. *Mental Health, Religion and Culture, 4*(2), 103–108.
19. Zahl, B. P., & Gibson, N. J. S. (2012). God representations, attachment to God, and satisfaction with life: A comparison of doctrinal and experiential representations of God in Christian young adults. *International Journal for the Psychology of Religion, 22*(3), 216–230.
20. Martens, A., Greenberg, J., & Allen, J. J. B. (2008). Self-esteem and autonomic physiology: Parallels between self-esteem and cardiac vagal tone as buffers of threat. *Personality and Social Psychology Review, 12*(4), 370–389.
21. Baldwin, M. W., & Wesley, R. (1996). Effects of existential anxiety and self-esteem on the perception of others. *Basic and Applied Social Psychology, 18*(1), 75–94.
22. Karademas, E. C., Kafetsios, K., & Sideridis, G. D. (2007). Optimism, self-efficacy and information processing of threat- and well-being-related stimuli. *Stress and Health, 23*(5), 285–294.
23. Gruenewald, T. L., Aziz, N., Fahey, J. L., & Kemeny, M. E. (2004). Acute threat to the social self: Shame, social self-esteem, and cortisol activity. *Psychosomatic Medicine, 66*(6), 915–924.
24. Houston, B. K., Olson, M., & Botkin, A. (1972). Trait anxiety and beliefs regarding danger and threat to self-esteem. *Journal of Consulting and Clinical Psychology, 38*(1), 152.

25. vanDellen, M. R., Campbell, W. K., Hoyle, R. H., & Bradfield, E. K. (2001). Compensating, resisting, and breaking: A meta-analytic examination of reactions to self-esteem threat. *Personality and Social Psychology Review, 15*(1), 51–74.
26. Leary, M. R., Barnes, B. D., & Griebel, C. (1986). Cognitive, affective, and attributional effects of potential threats to self-esteem. *Journal of Social & Clinical Psychology, 4*(4), 461.
27. Steenwyk, S. A. M., Atkins, D. C., Bedics, J. D., & Whitley, B. E., Jr. (2010). Images of God as they relate to life satisfaction and hopelessness. *International Journal for the Psychology of Religion, 20*(2), 85–96.
28. Flannelly, K. J., Galek, K., Ellison, C. G., & Koenig, H. G. (2010). Beliefs about God, psychiatric symptoms, and evolutionary psychiatry. *Journal of Religion and Health, 49*(2), 246–261.
29. Silton, N. R., Flannelly, K. J., Galek, K., & Ellison, C. G. (2014). Beliefs about God and mental health among American adults. *Journal of Religion and Health, 53*(5), 1285–1296.
30. Flannelly, K. J., Koenig, H. G., Ellison, C. G., Galek, K., & Krause, N. (2006). Belief in life after death and mental health: Findings from a national survey. *Journal of Nervous and Mental Disease, 194*(7), 524–529.
31. Flannelly, K. J., Ellison, C. G., Galek, K., & Koenig, H. G. (2008). Beliefs about life-after-death, psychiatric symptomology and cognitive theories of psychopathology. *Journal of Psychology & Theology, 36*, 94–103.
32. Dantzer, R. (2005). Somatization: A psychoneuroimmune perspective. *Psychoneuroendocrinology, 30*(10), 947–952.
33. Proctor, M. T., Miner, M., McLean, L. D., Devenish, S., & Bonab, B. G. (2009). Exploring Christians' explicit attachment to God representations: The development of a template for assessing attachment to God experiences. *Journal of Psychology and Theology, 37*(4), 245–264.
34. Miner, M. H. (2007). Back to the basics in attachment to God: Revisiting theory in light of theology. *Journal of Psychology & Theology, 35*(2), 112–122.
35. Pollner, M. (1989). Divine relations, social relations and well-being. *Journal of Health and Social Behavior, 30*(March), 92–104.
36. Ellison, C. G. (1991). Religious involvement and subjective well-being. *Journal of Health and Social Behavior, 32*(1), 80–99.
37. Pargament, K. I., Kennell, J., Hathaway, W., Grevengoed, N., Newman, J., & Jones, W. (1988). Religion and the problem-solving process: Three styles of coping. *Journal for the Scientific Study of Religion, 27*(1), 90–104.
38. Fabricatore, A. N., Handal, P. J., Rubio, D. M., & Gilner, F. H. (2004). Stress, religion, and mental health: Religious coping in mediating and moderating roles. *International Journal for the Psychology of Religion, 14*(2), 91–108.
39. Krause, N. (2010). The social milieu of the church and religious coping responses: A longitudinal investigation of older Whites and older Blacks. *International Journal for the Psychology of Religion, 20*(2), 109–129.
40. Krause, N., & Hayward, D. (2013). Older Mexican Americans and God-mediated control: Exploring the influence of Pentecostal/Evangelical affiliation. *Mental Health, Religion & Culture, 16*(3), 319–333.
41. Krause, N. (2005). God-mediated control and psychological well-being in late life. *Research on Aging, 27*(2), 136–164.
42. Krause, N. M. (2007). Social involvement in religious institutions and God-mediated control beliefs: A longitudinal investigation. *Journal for the Scientific Study of Religion, 46*(4), 519–537.
43. Krause, N. (2010). God-mediated control and change in self-rated health. *International Journal for the Psychology of Religion, 20*(4), 267–287.
44. Hayward, R. D., & Krause, N. (2013). Trajectories of late-life change in God-mediated control. *Journals of Gerontology. Series B, Psychological Sciences and Social Sciences, 68*(1), 49–58.

45. Krause, N. (2002). Church-based social support and health in old age: Exploring variations by race. *Journal of Gerontology, 57B*(6), S332–S347.
46. Pargament, K. I. (1997). *The psychology of religion and coping: Theory, research, practice.* New York: Guilford Press.
47. Pargament, K. I., Smith, B. W., Koenig, H. G., & Perez, L. (1998). Patterns of positive and negative religious coping with major life stressors. *Journal for the Scientific Study of Religion, 37*(4), 710–724.
48. Harrison, M. O., Koenig, H. G., Hays, J. C., Eme-Akwari, A. G., & Pargament, K. I. (2001). The epidemiology of religious coping: A review of recent literature. *International Review of Psychiatry, 13*(2), 86–93.
49. Pargament, K. I., Koenig, H. G., & Perez, L. M. (2000). The many methods of religious coping: Development and initial validation of the RCOPE. *Journal of Clinical Psychology, 56*(4), 519–543.
50. Pargament, K. I., Zinnbauer, B. J., Scott, A. B., Butter, E. M., Zerowin, J., & Stanik, P. (1998). Red flags and religious coping: Identifying some religious warning signs among people in crisis. *Journal of Clinical Psychology, 54*(1), 77–89.
51. Ellison, C. G., Roalson, L. A., Guillory, J. M., Flannelly, K. J., & Marcum, J. P. (2010). Religious resources, spiritual struggles, and mental health in a nationwide sample of PCUSA clergy. *Pastoral Psychology, 59*(3), 287–304.
52. Ellison, C. G., Fang, Q., Flannelly, K. J., & Steckler, R. A. (2013). Spiritual struggles and mental health: Exploring the moderating effects of religious identity. *International Journal for the Psychology of Religion, 23*, 214–229.
53. McConnell, K. M., Pargament, K. I., Ellison, C. G., & Flannelly, K. J. (2006). Examining the links between spiritual struggles and symptoms of psychopathology in a national sample. *Journal of Clinical Psychology, 62*(12), 1469–1484.
54. Bowlby, J. (1969). *Attachment and loss: Volume 1. Attachment.* New York: Basic Books.
55. Bowlby, J. (1980). *Attachment and Loss: Volume 3. Loss.* New York: Basic Books.
56. Bowlby, J. (1973). *Attachment and loss: Volume 2. Separation: Anxiety and anger.* New York: Basic Books.
57. Bretherton, I. (1992). The origins of attachment theory: John Bowlby and Mary Ainsworth. *Developmental Psychology, 28*(5), 759–775.
58. Ainsworth, M. S. (1979). Infant–mother attachment. *American Psychologist, 34*(10), 932–937.
59. Ainsworth, M. D. S. (1985). Patterns of infant-mother attachments: Antecedents and effects on development. *Bulletin of the New York Academy of Medicine, 61*(9), 771–791.
60. Kirkpatrick, L. A., & Shaver, P. R. (1990). Attachment theory and religion: Childhood attachments, religious beliefs, and conversations. *Journal for the Scientific Study of Religion, 29*(3), 315–334.
61. Radin, P. (1957). *Primitive religion: Its nature and origin.* New York: Dover Press.
62. Thouless, R. (1971). *An introduction to the psychology of religion* (3 ed.). Cambridge: Cambridge University Press.
63. Kirkpatrick, L. A., & Shaver, P. R. (1992). An attachment-theoretical approach to romantic love and religious belief. *Personality and Social Psychology Bulletin, 18*(3), 266–275.
64. Kirkpatrick, L. A. (1992). An attachment-theory approach to the psychology of religion. *International Journal for the Psychology of Religion, 2*(1), 3–28.
65. Kirkpatrick, L. A., Shillto, D. J., & Kellas, S. L. (1999). Loneliness, social support, and perceived relationships with God. *Journal of Social and Personal Relationships, 16*(4), 513–522.
66. Wei, M., Ku, T. Y., Chen, H. J., Wade, N., Liao, K. Y. H., & Guo, G. J. (2012). Chinese Christians in America: Attachment to God, stress, and well-being. *Counseling and Values, 57*(2), 162–180.
67. Freeze, T. A., & Di Tommaso, E. (2015). Attachment to God and church family: Predictors of spiritual and psychological well-being. *Journal of Psychology and Christianity, 34*(1), 60–72.

68. Homan, K. J. (2014). A mediation model linking attachment to God, self-compassion, and mental health. *Mental Health, Religion & Culture, 17*(10), 977–989.
69. Bradshaw, M., Ellison, C. G., & Marcum, J. P. (2010). Attachment to God, images of God, and psychological distress in a nationwide sample of Presbyterians. *International Journal for the Psychology of Religion, 20*(2), 130–147.
70. Ellison, C., Bradshaw, M., Kuyel, N., & Marcum, J. (2012). Attachment to God, stressful life events, and changes in psychological distress. *Review of Religious Research, 53*(4), 493–511.
71. Arndt, J., Routledge, C., Cox, C. R., & Goldenberg, J. L. (2005). The worm at the core: A terror management perspective on the roots of psychological dysfunction. *Applied and Preventive Psychology, 11*(3), 191.
72. Dechesne, M., Arndt, J., Ransom, S., Sheldon, K. M., Pyszczynski, T., Van Knippenberg, A., et al. (2003). Literal and symbolic immortality: The effect of evidence of literal immortality on self-esteem striving in response to mortality salience. *Journal of Personality & Social Psychology, 84*(4), 722–737.
73. Pyszczynsi, T., Greenberg, J., Solomon, S., Arndt, J., & Schimel, J. (2004). Why do people need self-esteem? A theoretical and empirical review. *Psychological Bulletin, 130*(3), 435–468.

Chapter 30
Belief in Meaning, Other Religious Beliefs, Religious Doubt, and Mental Health

Abstract This chapter highlights the most important findings from Chaps. 22, 23, and 24, including the association of mental health with belief in (a) meaning in life, (b) forgiveness from God, (c) Satan, (d) human evil, and (e) biblical literalism, as well as (f) the association of mental health with religious doubt. For example, the belief that there is meaning and purpose in life and the belief that one has been forgiven by God have salubrious associations with mental health, and psychiatric symptomology, in particular. Belief in Satan and human evil, on the other hand, have pernicious associations with psychiatric symptoms, especially paranoid ideation. My own analysis of data from the 2010 Baylor Religion Survey found that believing the Bible is literally true is associated with paranoid ideation. Moreover, the chapter describes how belief in Biblical literalism appears to affect the utilization of mental-health services. In addition, the chapter discusses how doubts about one's religious beliefs have a pernicious effect on psychological well-being and psychiatric symptoms, which is more pronounced for individuals who have a stronger religious commitment than for other individuals. The findings are interpreted within the framework of ETAS Theory.

Keywords Biblical literalism • Divine forgiveness • Evil • Forgiveness • Meaning in life • Psychiatric symptoms • Psychological well-being • Religious doubt • Satan

30.1 Belief in Meaning and Purpose in Life and Mental Health

30.1.1 Background

Many social scientists believe that one of the major psychological benefits of religion is that it provides a sense of meaning and purpose in life. The American psychologist Roy Baumeister classified the belief that life has meaning into four categories. They are the belief that: (1) one's life has purpose; (2) one is able to meet challenges and achieve goals; (3) one is a worthy person with desirable characteristics; and (4) one's actions are good and justified [1]. Though individuals find meaning in life in many ways [2, 3], religion is unique in providing answers to existential

K.J. Flannelly, *Religious Beliefs, Evolutionary Psychiatry, and Mental Health in America*, Religion, Spirituality and Health: A Social Scientific Approach 1,
DOI 10.1007/978-3-319-52488-7_30

questions that we all have [4–6]. Some psychologists suggest that the need to believe one's life has meaning and purpose is so universal that it must be an evolutionary adaptation [7–9]. While few U.S. studies have explored the relationship between religion and believing that life has meaning and purpose, several U.K. studies have reported significant positive relationships between various measures of religion and the belief that life has meaning and purpose [10–15].

30.1.2 Belief in Meaning and Mental Health

A review of research in the U.S. and elsewhere showed that there is a consistent positive association between mental-health outcomes and belief in meaning and purpose in life [16]. Cross-sectional studies, mainly of U.S. college students, have shown that belief in meaning and purpose in life is positively correlated with hope [17, 18], personal growth [19], and positive affect [20–22], and negatively correlated with negative affect [21, 22] and depression [17, 18]. Moreover, a large national study found that believing life has meaning predicts lower levels of affective and somatic symptoms of depression [23]. Another large study of older Christian Americans found that finding religious meaning in life was associated with three measures of psychological well-being (i.e., life satisfaction, optimism, and self-esteem) [24].

30.2 Religious Doubt and Mental Health

30.2.1 Background

Although religious beliefs can provide a sense of meaning in life, some people do not find the explanation of life events that religion provides to be satisfactory at an intellectual or emotional level, which may lead them to doubt their religious beliefs [25]. For some people, religious doubts arise because of the conflict between the belief that God is good and omnipotent and the existence of evil in the world [26]. For other people, religious doubts arise because of the disparate explanations of nature offered by religion and science [27].

30.2.2 Religious Doubt and Mental Health

Studies of convenience samples of religious Americans indicate that there is a pernicious association between religious doubt and psychological well-being, including self-esteem, trait anxiety, negative mood [28], life satisfaction [29], and optimism

[30]. National studies of the U.S. general population provide even stronger evidence for a pernicious association between religious doubt and psychological well-being [31–36].

In addition, several large-scale studies of mainly Christian samples have found a pernicious association between religious doubt and symptoms of depression [37–39]. Related research has found that this pernicious association is particularly profound among congregants who are more involved in their church. This finding has been interpreted in terms of Identity Theory [40–42], in that congregants who are more invested in their personal/social roles in their church community are especially threatened when these roles are undermined; in this case, by their own religious doubt [33, 43]. A 2015 study by Galek et al. extended the findings of earlier studies [33, 39, 43] in showing that religious doubt (i.e., doubting that life has meaning) had a pernicious association with mental health, and that it had a more pronounced effect in persons who had a strong religious commitment [44].

Based on Identity Theory, Galek et al. suggested that believing life lacks meaning exacerbates psychiatric symptoms among people who have a strong religious commitment because it "threatens their social role within the religious community" (p. 8) [44], which is consistent with ETAS Theory. Moreover, they suggested, from the perspective of ETAS Theory, that such a threat to one's identity represented a direct threat to one's self-esteem, which is one of Baumeister's four basic needs for meaning [1].

30.3 Belief in Divine Forgiveness and Human Evil and Mental Health

30.3.1 Background

Much of Chap. 24 is devoted to a discussion of belief in Divine forgiveness, belief in human evil, and their interaction on mental health, particularly a 2016 study by Jeremy Uecker et al. that examined all three of these topics in relation to psychiatric symptoms [45]. Thus, I will focus on that study in this section.

It is notable that extensive research has documented a salubrious association between forgiveness and mental health, but very little of this research has examined belief in Divine forgiveness. Nevertheless, a series of studies published in 1988 reported consistent negative correlations between symptoms of depression and belief in Divine forgiveness of sin among U.S. university students [46–48]. Forgiveness of sin is an important theological concept with psychological implications. Human evil is subsumed under the concept of sin in Judeo-Christian theology [49, 50], and Sigmund Freud [51, 52] and others have argued that belief in sin leads to guilt, which in turn, leads to anxiety [53]. Christian writers have countered that the guilt associated with sin does not automatically lead to psychological disturbances because of the Christian belief that God forgives sinners, and that the beneficial effects of this belief can offset the adverse effects of guilt on psychological well-being [46].

30.3.2 Findings on Belief in Divine Forgiveness and Human Evil and Psychiatric Symptoms

The findings of the Uecker et al. study [45] address all three of the areas just mentioned; the association of belief in Divine forgiveness on psychiatric symptoms; the association of belief in human evil (or sin) on psychiatric symptoms, and the interaction of these beliefs on psychiatric symptoms. First, the study found that belief in Divine forgiveness had significant salubrious associations with agoraphobia, depression, general anxiety, and obsessive-compulsive disorder (OCD). Second, the study found that believing that human nature is basically evil had a significant pernicious association with agoraphobia, depression, general anxiety, OCD, and paranoia. Belief in human evil had the strongest association with paranoid ideation, which might be expected on a priori grounds, as paranoia is essentially a distrust of people. Third, the study found that belief in Divine forgiveness interacted with belief in human evil, such that belief in Divine forgiveness significantly off-set the pernicious effects of belief in human evil on agoraphobia, general anxiety, and paranoid ideation.

30.4 Belief in Satan and Psychiatric Symptoms

Christianity, Judaism, and other world religions traditionally recognize two sources of evil in the world, human beings and malevolent supernatural beings [54–59]. The major source of supernatural evil in the Christian theology is Satan, who is the personification of evil, tempting people to commit sins that destroy themselves spiritually, physically harm others, and aid Satan in his battle against God [58, 60]. Although Catholicism and liberal Protestant denominations have down-played Satan's role in the world [61–63], many Americans believe in the existence of Satan. For example, the 2005 Baylor Religion Survey found that 58% of American adults "absolutely" believed that Satan exists and another 17% believed he "probably" exists [64].

People who believe in Satan should also believe in the danger he poses, so we would expect belief in Satan to be associated with greater psychiatric symptomology. My analysis of data from the 2010 Baylor Religion Survey found that belief in Satan had a significant pernicious association with general anxiety, social anxiety, compulsion, obsession, and paranoid ideation. However, the strongest association was with paranoid ideation, probably because Satan acts through people.

30.5 Belief in Biblical Literalism and Seeking Help for Mental-Health Problems

I think it is natural that people who are more religious are more likely to seek help from clergy for mental-health problems [65]. A 2006 study by Chris Ellison, me, and other colleagues found that several aspects of religion influence the likelihood of seeking mental-health assistance from clergy [66]. Individuals who attended religious services more often were significantly more likely to recommend clergy as a primary source of mental-health assistance, but this effect varied by religious denomination. Catholics were more likely to recommend clergy as a primary source of assistance than were all other survey respondents, except Protestants. Moreover, Conservative Protestants were more likely than other Protestants to recommend clergy. After controlling for church attendance and denomination, people who believed that the Bible was literally true were more likely than other people to recommend clergy as a primary a source of assistance for mental-health problems.

30.6 Belief in Biblical Literalism and Psychiatric Symptoms

I do not know of any published study that has specifically investigated the association between belief in Biblical literalism and mental health. So, I decided to test the net effects of belief in Biblical literalism on the major measures of psychiatric symptoms contained in the 2010 Baylor Religion Survey (anxiety, obsession, compulsion, social anxiety, and paranoia), using a regression model that controlled for age, gender, race, and frequency of private prayer and attending religious services. Belief in Biblical literalism was found to have a significant pernicious association with paranoid ideation, but not any of the other measures of psychiatric symptoms. I suspect that the higher level of paranoia among persons who believe the Bible is literally true may be attributable to the threats posed to their religious beliefs and values by science and various aspects of modern American culture [67–72]. I think the response to these threats is expressed as paranoia because the source of the threats is personified as evil people from outside their religious group.

30.7 Conclusions

30.7.1 Religion, Meaning and Mental Health

Religion has a positive association with believing that life has meaning and purpose, and believing that life has meaning and purpose is associated with psychological well-being among Christians. Belief in meaning and purpose in life may partly bolster mental health by instilling the belief, especially among religious people, that one's life is part of a Divine plan, which reduces fears about life's uncertainties and vicissitudes. Since the amygdala treats uncertainty as a threat, reducing uncertainty reduces anxiety, according to ETAS Theory.

30.7.2 Religious Doubt and Mental Health

Research has shown that religious doubt has a pernicious association with psychological well-being. In keeping with ETAS Theory, these pernicious effects may be attributed to the fact: (1) that doubts undermine the sense of meaning and security provided by religious faith; (2) that uncertainty about one's beliefs increases anxiety, just as uncertainty about the future increases anxiety; (3) that people fear their fellow congregants will become aware of their lack of faith; and (4) that doubts create a fear of retribution from God for having religious doubts.

Related research has shown the pernicious effects of religious doubt on mental health are particularly troubling for persons who have a strong religious commitment. This effect is probably due to the fact that religious doubt undermines the social identity and threatens the self-esteem of individuals with a strong commitment to their religion and their religious community. A threat to self-esteem has a two-pronged effect on mental health because it has a primary effect of undermining psychological well-being and a secondary effect resulting from the fact that lowered self-esteem makes one feel less safe, which makes a person more vulnerable to psychological distress from other sources of threat.

30.7.3 Belief in Divine Forgiveness, Evil, and Mental Health

The major findings related to ETAS Theory are the association of psychiatric symptoms with belief in (a) Divine forgiveness, (b) human evil, (c) Satan, and (d) the interaction of belief in human evil and Divine forgiveness. From the perspective of ETAS Theory, I think believing one has been forgiven by God has a salubrious association with psychiatric symptomology because this implies the beliefs that one has a good relationship with God and that God is involved your life, both of which provide a sense of safety, which lowers psychiatric symptoms. Obtaining forgiveness from God also is a form of protection, since God chose to forgive you rather than to punish you. The finding that belief in evil interacts with belief in forgiveness by God is consistent with the ETAS proposition that beliefs interact with one another in their effects on psychiatric symptoms.

The findings that belief in Satan and belief in human evil have pernicious associations with psychiatric symptoms are consistent with ETAS Theory in that people who believe in Satan and human evil should also believe that Satan and evil people pose direct threats of harm. Paranoia had the strongest association with both belief in Satan and human evil probably because: (1) Satan causes harm by working through people, and (2) belief in human evil implies there are evil people who intend to do you harm

30.7.4 Belief in Biblical Literalism and Mental Health

My analyses of the association between belief in Biblical literalism and psychiatric symptoms found that it only had a pernicious association with paranoia. I think this can be explained, in light of ETAS Theory, by the fact that science poses a direct threat to belief in Biblical literalism, and aspects of modern American culture pose a threat to other religious and cultural beliefs of people who believe the Bible is literally true. Because the source of these threats is personified as evil outsiders, the reaction to the threats is paranoia.

An equally important finding, which is not directly related to ETAS Theory, is that belief in Biblical literalism influences personal attitudes about whom one should seek for help for psychological problems. Individuals who believe the Bible is literally true are inclined to seek help for psychological problems from clergy rather than from mental health professionals.

References

1. Baumeister, R.F. (1991). *Meaning of life*. New York: Guilford Press.
2. Wong, P.T.P. (2012). From logotherapy to meaning-centered counseling. In P.T.P. Wong (Ed.), *The human quest for meaning: Theories, research, and application* (2nd ed., pp. 619–647). New York: Routledge/Taylor & Francis.
3. Wong, P.T.P. (Ed.). (2012). *The human quest for meaning: Theories, research, and application* (2nd ed.). New York: Routledge/Taylor & Francis.
4. Wong, P.T.P. (1998). Spirituality, meaning, and successful aging. In P.T.P. Wong (Ed.), *The human quest for meaning: A handbook of psychological research and clinical applications* (pp. 359–394). Mahwah: Erlbaum.
5. Pargament, K.I. (1997). The psychology of religion and coping: Theory, research, and practice. New York: Guilford Press.
6. Park, C.L. (2005). Religion as a meaning-making framework in coping with life stress. *Journal of Social Issues, 61*(4), 707–729.
7. King, L.A., & Hicks, J.A. (2012). Positive affect and meaning in life. The intersection of hedonism and eudiamonia. In P.T.P. Wong (Ed.), *The human quest for meaning: Theories, research, and application* (2nd ed., pp. 125–142). New York: Routledge/Taylor & Francis.
8. Klinger, E. (2012). The search for meaning in evolutionary goal-theory perspective and its clinical implications. In P.T.P. Wong (Ed.), *The human quest for meaning: Theories, research, and application* (2nd ed., pp. 23–56). New York: Routledge/Taylor & Francis.
9. Sommer, K.L., Baumeister, R.F., & Stillman, T.F. (2012). The construction of meaning from life events: Empirical studies of personal narratives. In P.T.P. Wong (Ed.), *The human quest for meaning: Theories, research, and application* (2nd ed., pp. 297–314). New York: Routledge/Taylor & Francis.

10. Robbins, M., & Francis, L.J. (2000). Religion, personality, and well-being: The relationship between church attendance and purpose in life. *Journal of Research on Christian Education, 9*(2), 223–238.
11. Francis, L.J. (2000). The relationship between bible reading and purpose in life among 13–15-year-olds. *Mental Health, Religion & Culture, 3*(1), 27–36.
12. Francis, L.J., & Burton, L. (1994). The influence of personal prayer on purpose in life among Catholic adolescents. Journal of Beliefs and Values, *15*(2), 6–9.
13. Francis, L.J., & Evans, T.E. (1996). The relationship between personal prayer and purpose in life among churchgoing and non-churchgoing twelve-to-fifteen year-olds in the UK. *Religious Education, 91*(1), 9–18.
14. Francis, L.J., Jewell, A., & Robbins, M. (2010). The relationship between religious orientation, personality, and purpose in life among an older Methodist sample. *Mental Health, Religion & Culture, 13*(7–8), 777–791.
15. Francis, L.J., & Robbins, M. (2009). Prayer, purpose in life, and attitudes toward substances: A study among 13- to 15-year-olds in England and Wales. *Counselling and Spirituality/ Counseling et Spiritualité, 28*(2), 83–104.
16. Steger, M.F. (2012). Making meaning in life. *Psychological Inquiry, 23*(4), 381–385.
17. Mascaro, N., & Rosen, D.H. (2008). Assessment of existential meaning of and its longitudinal relations with depressive symptoms. *Journal of Social & Clinical Psychology, 27*(6), 576–599.
18. Mascaro, N.D.H. (2005). Existential meaning's role in the enhancement of hope and prevention of depressive symptoms. *Journal of Personality, 73*(4), 985–1014.
19. Ryff, C.D., & Keyes, C.L.M. (1995). The structure of psychological well-being revisited. *Journal of Personality and Social Psychology, 69*(4), 719–727.
20. Hicks, J.A., Cicero, D.C., Trent, J., Burton, C.M., & King, L.A. (2010). Positive affect, intuition, and feelings of meaning. *Journal of Personality and Social Psychology, 98*(6), 967–979.
21. King, L.A., Hicks, J.A., Krull, J.L., & Del Gaiso, A.K. (2006). Positive affect and the experience of meaning in life. *Journal of Personality and Social Psychology, 90*(1), 179–196.
22. Hicks, J.A., Trent, J., Davis, W.E., & King, L.A. (2012). Positive affect, meaning in life, and future time perspective: An application of socioemotional selectivity theory. *Psychology and Aging, 27*(1), 181–189.
23. Krause, N. (2007). Evaluating the stress-buffering function of meaning in life among older people. *Journal of Aging and Health, 19*(5), 792–812.
24. Krause, N. (2003). Religious meaning and subjective well-being in late life. *Journals of Gerontology. Series B, Psychological Sciences and Social Sciences, 58*(3), S160-S170.
25. Exline, J.J. (2002). Stumbling blocks on the religious road: Fractured relationships, nagging vices, and the inner struggle to believe. *Psychological Inquiry, 13*(3), 182–189.
26. Thang Moe, D. (2015). Sin and evil in Christian and Buddhist perspectives: A quest for theodicy. *Asia Journal of Theology, 29*(1), 22–46.
27. Allport, G.W. (1956). *The individual and his religion: A psychological interpretation.* New York: Macmillan.
28. Pargament, K.I., Zinnbauer, B.J., Scott, A.B., Butter, E.M., Zerowin, J., & Stanik, P. (1998). Red flags and religious coping: Identifying some religious warning signs among people in crisis. *Journal of Clinical Psychology, 54*(1), 77–89.
29. Gauthier, K.J., Christopher, A.N., Walter, M.I., Mourad, R., & Marek, P. (2006). Religiosity, religious doubt, and the need for cognition: Their interactive relationship with life satisfaction. *Journal of Happiness Studies, 7*(2), 139–154.
30. Hunsberger, B., Pratt, M., & Pancer, S.M. (2002). A longitudinal study of religious doubts in high school and beyond: Relationships, stability, and searching for answers. *Journal for the Scientific Study of Religion, 41*(2), 255–266.
31. Ellison, C.G. (1991). Religious involvement and subjective well-being. *Journal of Health and Social Behavior, 32*(1), 80–99.

32. Ellison, C.G., Roalson, L.A., Guillory, J.M., Flannelly, K.J., & Marcum, J.P. (2010). Religious resources, spiritual struggles, and mental health in a nationwide sample of PCUSA clergy. *Pastoral Psychology, 59*(3), 287–304.
33. Ellison, C.G., & Lee, J. (2010). Spiritual struggles and psychological distress: Is there a dark side of religion? *Social Indicators Research, 98*(3), 501–517.
34. Krause, N., Ingersoll-Dayton, B., Ellison, C.G., & Wulff, K.M. (1999). Aging, religious doubt, and psychological well-being. *The Gerontologist, 39*(5), 525–533.
35. Ellison, C.G., Bradshaw, M., Storch, J., Marcum, J.P., & Hill, T.D. (2011). Religious doubts and sleep quality: Findings from a nationwide study of Presbyterians. *Review of Religious Research, 53*(2), 119–136.
36. Krause, N. (2006). Religious doubt and psychological well-being: A longitudinal investigation. *Review of Religious Research, 50*(Special Issue), 94–110.
37. Krause, N. (2012). Religious doubt, financial strain, and depressive symptoms among older Mexican Americans. *Mental Health, Religion & Culture, 15*(4), 335–348.
38. Krause, N. (2003). A preliminary assessment of race differences in the relationship between religious doubt and depressive symptoms. *Review of Religious Research, 45*(2), 93–115.
39. Krause, N., & Wulff, K.M. (2004). Religious doubt and health: Exploring the potential dark side of religion. *Sociology of Religion, 65*(1), 35–56.
40. Stets, J.E., & Burke, P.J. (2000). Identity theory and social identity theory. *Social Psychology Quarterly, 63*(3), 224–237.
41. Burke, P.J. (1991). Identity process and social stress. *American Sociological Review, 56*, 836–849.
42. Thoits, P.A. (1991). On merging identity theory and stress research. *Social Psychology Quarterly, 54*, 101–112.
43. Ellison, C.G., Fang, Q., Flannelly, K.J., & Steckler, R.A. (2013). Spiritual struggles and mental health: Exploring the moderating effects of religious identity. *International Journal for the Psychology of Religion, 23*, 214–229.
44. Galek, K., Flannelly, K.J., Ellison, C.G., Silton, N.R., & Jankowski, K.R.B. (2015). Religion, meaning and purpose, and mental health. *Psychology of Religion and Spirituality, 7*(1), 1–12.
45. Uecker, J.E., Ellison, C.G., Flannelly, K.J., & Burdette, A.M. (2015). Belief in human sinfulness, belief in experiencing divine forgiveness, and psychiatric symptoms. *Review of Religious Research 58*(1), 1–26.
46. Watson, P.J., Morris, R.J., & Hood, R.W. (1988). Sin and self-functioning: I. Grace, guilt, and self-consciousness. *Journal of Psychology & Theology, 16*, 254–269.
47. Watson, P.J., Morris, R.J., & Hood, R.W. (1988). Sin and self-functioning: II. Grace, guilt, and psychological adjustment. *Journal of Psychology & Theology, 16*, 270–281.
48. Watson, P.J., Morris, R.J., & Hood, R.W. (1988). Sin and self-functioning: III. The psychology and ideology of irrational beliefs. *Journal of Psychology & Theology, 16*, 348–361.
49. Richardson, A., & Bowden, J. (Eds.). (1983). *The Westminister dictionary of Christian theology*. Philadelphia: The Westminister Press.
50. Lotker, M. (2004). *A Christian's guide to Judaism*. Mahwah: Paulist Press.
51. Freud, S. (1939). *Moses and monotheism*. London: The Hogarth Press.
52. Freud, S. (1939/1962). *Civilization and its discontents*. New York: W.W. Norton & Company.
53. Ellis, A. (1962). *Reason and emotion in psychotherapy*. Secaucus: Lyle Stuart.
54. Kolakowski, L. (2004). Leibniz & Job: The metaphysics of evil and the experience of evil. *The New Criterion, 22*(5), 18–23.
55. Buchholz, E.S., & Mandel, J.K. (2000). Reaching for virtue, stumbling on sin: Concepts of good and evil in a postmodern era. *Journal of Religion &* Health, *39*(2), 123.
56. Martinez, B. (2013). Is evil good for religion? The link between supernatural evil and religious commitment. *Review of Religious Research, 55*(2), 319–338.
57. Pagels, E. (1991). The social history of Satan, the "intimate enemy": A preliminary sketch. *Harvard Theological Review, 84*(2), 105–128.
58. Perry, M. (1990). Taking Satan seriously. *The Expository Times, 101*(4), 105–112.

59. Atran, S., & Norenzayan, A. (2004). Religion's evolutionary landscape: Counterintuition, commitment, compassion, communion. *Behavioral and Brain Sciences, 27*(6), 713–730.
60. Russell, J.B. (1977). *The devil: Perceptions of evil from antiquity to primitive Christianity*. Ithaca: Cornell University Press.
61. Camille, A. (2003). Where have all the demons gone?. *U.S. Catholic, 68*(2), 45–47.
62. Mallowe, M. (1995). Is evil just the devil in disguise?. *U.S. Catholic, 60*, 6–13.
63. Quay, P.M. (1981). Angels and demons: The teaching of IV Lateran. *Theological Studies, 42*(1), 20–45.
64. Baker, J. (2008). Who believes in religious evil? An investigation of sociological patterns of belief in Satan, hell, and demons. *Review of Religious Research, 50*(2), 206–220.
65. Abe-Kim, J., Gong, F., & Takeuchi, D. (2004). Religiosity, spirituality, and help-seeking among Filipino Americans: Religious clergy or mental health professionals? *Journal of Community Psychology, 32*(6), 675–689.
66. Ellison, C.G., Vaaler, M.L., Flannelly, K.J., & Weaver, A.J. (2006). The clergy as a source of mental health assistance: What Americans believe. *Review of Religious Research, 48*(2), 190–211.
67. Evans, J.H. (2011). Epistemological and moral conflict between religion and science. *Journal for the Scientific Study of Religion, 50*(2), 707–727.
68. Evans, J.H. (2013). The growing social and moral conflict between conservative Protestantism and science. *Journal for the Scientific Study of Religion, 52*(2), 368–385.
69. Sherkat, D. E., & Ellison, C. G. (1997). The cognitive structure of a moral crusade: Conservative Protestantism and opposition to pornography. *Social Forces, 75*(3), 957–980.
70. Bartkowski, J.P., & Ellison, C.G. (1995). Divergent models of childrearing in popular manuals: Conservative Protestants vs. the mainstream experts. *Sociology of Religion, 56*(1), 21–34.
71. Ellison, C.G., & Musick, M.A. (1995). Conservative Protestantism and public opinion toward science. *Review of Religious Research, 36*(3), 245.
72. Ellison, C.G., & Nybroten, K.A. (1999). Conservative Protestantism and opposition to state-sponsored lotteries: Evidence from the 1997 Texas poll. *Social Science Quarterly, 80*(2), 356–369.

Chapter 31
Directions for Future Research on ETAS Theory and Mental Health

Abstract This chapter proposes future research related to ETAS Theory's four levels of analysis. Research at the behavioral level (Level I), particularly, psychological and sociological research, is proposed to test behavioral predictions from ETAS Theory about the association between mental health and beliefs, threats, and safety. Future Level I research should examine more beliefs and more classes of psychiatric symptoms, as well as their lifetime prevalence. The chapter notes that much more cognitive-affective neuroscience research (Level II) is needed to determine the association of many classes of psychiatric symptoms with brain structure and function, and the relationship between beliefs, brain function, and psychiatric symptoms, to test ETAS Theory predictions at this level of analysis. One section of the chapter describes the design of three experiments to test the effects of different religious beliefs on psychiatric symptoms and the activity of the ventromedial prefrontal cortex, the amygdala, and other brain structures implicated by ETAS Theory to be involved in processing beliefs and the threat assessments that underlie psychiatric symptoms. The studies contrast the effects of beliefs that should enhance or reduce the perceptions of threat. Level III involves detailed neuro-anatomical and neuro-physiological analyses to define the specific neural circuits or networks that comprise different ETAS and determine how they operate. Level IV is an evolutionary level of analysis that uses the methodology of comparative anatomy and comparative behavior to understand the evolutionary origins of psychiatric disorders as well as beliefs.

Keywords Amygdala • Anxiety • ETAS theory • Cognitive-affective neuroscience • Comparative research • Defense • Evolution • Fear • Galvanic skin response • God • Levels of analysis • Optogenetic research • Neural circuits • Prevalence • Self-esteem • Social support • Proximate mechanisms • Psychiatric symptoms • Satan • Threat

K.J. Flannelly, *Religious Beliefs, Evolutionary Psychiatry, and Mental Health in America*, Religion, Spirituality and Health: A Social Scientific Approach 1,
DOI 10.1007/978-3-319-52488-7_31

31.1 Background

As discussed in Chap. 1, Evolutionary Threat Assessment Systems Theory (ETAS Theory) encompasses four perspectives or levels of analysis and these levels of analysis are associated with different research methodologies. Level I encompasses psychological and sociological research methods to test behavioral predictions from ETAS Theory. Level II entails research methods in cognitive-affective neuroscience to confirm the association between psychiatric symptoms and brain structures that are implicated by ETAS Theory. Level III must be investigated using detailed neuro-anatomical and neuro-physiological research methods that can define specific ETAS and can determine their operation at different levels of neural organization (e.g. neurons, neural clusters, and neural circuits). Level IV requires comparative anatomical and comparative behavioral methods to investigate the evolutionary origin of psychiatric symptoms, as proposed by ETAS Theory. This chapter makes research recommendations to address these different perspectives of ETAS Theory.

31.2 Research on Level I of ETAS Theory: Survey Research on Beliefs and Psychiatric Symptoms

31.2.1 General Comments

The Level I analysis of ETAS Theory entails testing behavioral predictions from ETAS Theory. As the focus of this book is on religious beliefs, I will concentrate on those predictions that involve religious beliefs. However, comparable studies could be conducted on the association between mental health and beliefs that lie outside the bounds of religion, especially: (a) beliefs that imply the world is dangerous; (b) beliefs that convey a sense of safety; and (c) the interaction of such beliefs. Studies of different religious beliefs, secular beliefs, and mental-health outcomes should be conducted, and more studies are needed that include representative samples.

To test ETAS Theory, it is also important to investigate specific psychiatric symptoms that may be influenced more or less by cognition, and therefore by beliefs. We tried to do this by studying somatization, with some success, and separately analyzing the effects of beliefs on obsessions (cognitions) and compulsions (behaviors) without success. Hence, I think it would be worthwhile to see if different beliefs differentially affect specific types of phobias. I also think more refined and detailed measures are needed to differentiate between subtypes of various classes of psychiatric symptomology, such as subtypes of obsessive-compulsive disorder (OCD) and social anxiety, persecutory and jealousy delusions in paranoid ideation, and the specific symptoms of panic attack and agoraphobia.

31.2.2 Belief in a Protective God and Anxiety

My colleagues and I published two studies that attempted to determine the salutary effect of a benevolent God on psychiatric symptoms [1, 2]. Though the results were in the predicted direction, our operational definition of a benevolent God fell far short of conveying belief in an involved and protective God, which I think is a more suitable for testing ETAS Theory. My colleagues Holly Gaudette and Kathy Jankowski [3] introduced a six-item scale that I think is good for studying beliefs about one's relationship with God because it is better at capturing a sense of protection from God than any existing scales. The six items are: (1) I believe God protects me from harm; (2) I believe God is punishing me; (3) I believe God is involved in my life; (4) I believe God has abandoned me; (5) I believe God loves and care for me; and (6) I believe my life and death follow a plan from God. Obviously, items 2 and 4 are reversed scored to provide a measure of a protective God.

31.2.3 Social Support, Self-Esteem, and ETAS Theory

We usually think of social support in the context of ongoing social relationships in which people provide emotional support and tangible support to each other, both of which have been found to be indirectly associated with better physical and mental health. However, the actual social support provided by others has cognitive and affective components, which are represented in the brain, and the brain mechanisms that symbolically represent social support in cognitive and affective terms are likely to have a direct effect on mental health. One way in which these mechanisms are likely to affect mental health directly is by providing a sense of safety, as Paul Gilbert has proposed [4]. Some survey research has found that perceived social support is more beneficial than tangible support, and I think a finer analysis of perceived social support should be able to determine the degree to which it reflects a sense of safety and security, and the association of this sense of safety and security with mental health, especially psychiatric symptoms.

Studies also should be conducted to determine the degree to which self-esteem contributes to a sense of security, and thereby reduces anxiety. Theoretically, Terror Management Theory (TM Theory) considers self-esteem to be an evolved mechanism that buffers against anxiety about death and other forms of anxiety that the terror of death creates [5–7]. It is more likely, however, that self-esteem evolved in primates, long before our ancestors became aware of their own mortality, as a cognitive mechanism to assess one's relative status within a dominance hierarchy. It is not immediately obvious to me how these theoretical differences can be resolved at the behavioral level (Level I) of ETAS Theory, but it would be useful to do so. Self-esteem clearly makes a contribution to psychological well-being, and there is evidence that it is related to mother-infant attachment. Self-esteem is a particularly interesting phenomenon from the perspective of ETAS Theory because it presumably decreases anxiety by providing a sense of security [8–10]; yet threats to self-esteem increase anxiety [11–14], presumably by reducing this sense of security. I can imagine several lines of research based on these premises, including studies on the mediating and moderating of effects of self-esteem on positive and negative religious beliefs and mental health, particularly psychiatric symptoms. In addition, research should be conducted on the related concept of self-efficacy because it provides a sense of safety according to ETAS Theory.

31.2.4 ETAS Theory Versus Terror Management Theory

Some of our research on belief in an afterlife indicates that ETAS Theory provides a more reasonable interpretation of the association between beliefs about life-after-death and mental health than TM Theory does. In particular, the 2014 study by Ellison et al. [15], which was described in Chap. 18 undermines TM Theory's major premise that being made aware of one's own mortality (i.e., mortality salience) inevitably increases anxiety. Though some advocates of TM Theory claim that anxiety disorders result from an inability to quell one's fear of death [5], they do not explain how fear of death is translated into the many different types of anxiety disorders that exist. In contrast, ETAS Theory, which incorporates the theoretical work of Randolph Nesse, explains how each anxiety disorder represents the action of proximate brain mechanisms that protect us from specific types of threat of harm [16–19]. Although I do not have specific studies in mind, I think future research may be able to differentiate between predictions from TM Theory and ETAS Theory about the underlying causes of anxiety disorders.

31.3 Research on Level I of ETAS Theory: Surveys of the Lifetime Prevalence of Psychiatric Symptoms

If is also important, from the perspective of ETAS Theory, to continue to conduct epidemiological studies on the lifetime prevalence of sub-clinical cases of psychiatric disorders in the general U.S. population. Of the ten psychiatric disorders I discussed as probable evolutionary adaptations, there are reasonable lifetime prevalence estimates of sub-clinical cases of these disorders for just four of them: small-animal phobia, acrophobia, panic attack, and OCD. Even though we have good estimates of the prevalence rates of generalized anxiety disorder (GAD), social anxiety disorder (SAD), and major depressive disorder (MDD), the rate of sub-clinical cases of GAD, SAD, and MDD are not known. It is worth noting that even the incidence rate of clinical cases of GAD is very sensitive to relatively minor changes in diagnostic criteria. I do not know of any U.S. data on the prevalence rates of clinical cases or sub-clinical cases of agoraphobia, separate from panic attack, or non-psychotic paranoid ideation.

31.4 Research on Level II of ETAS Theory: Cognitive-Affective Neuroscience Studies

31.4.1 Correlational Research on Psychiatric Symptoms

Further brain research is still necessary to clarify the roles of the PFC, the limbic system, the basal ganglia and the brain stem in psychiatric symptoms. Although the involvement of these brain regions is fairly well established for some psychiatric disorders, far less is known about the involvement of specific structures within these regions in different classes of psychiatric symptoms. Moreover, there are many disorders in which information about their involvement is fragmentary, at best. Surprisingly, though the bed nucleus of the limbic system[1] is thought to play a key role in anxiety [20, 21], I could only find one functional magnetic resonance imaging (fMRI) study that identified its involvement in any psychiatric disorder (i.e., spider phobia) [22]. The role of the "aversive amplification circuit,"[2] which has been found to enhance amygdala activity in generalized anxiety disorder [23], also needs to be examined in other anxiety disorders.

I think existing research has provided good evidence of the involvement of the PFC, the limbic system, and the basal ganglia in four of the ten psychiatric disorders I discussed as possible proximate mechanisms that protect us from harm: panic attack, social anxiety, major depression, and paranoid ideation. However, the possible role of the brain stem in these disorders has yet to be determined one way or the other. Furthermore, the role of specific parts of these structures is not definitive. Even though the research conducted to date on the brain areas involved in OCD seem to suggest that the amygdala is not involved in OCD, their possible role should be investigated further using more refined brain imaging techniques.

Though current research suggests that the basal ganglia and the brain stem are not active in general anxiety or animal phobia, more research is needed to clarify if they are involved so or not. Unfortunately, there are so few studies on acrophobia, agoraphobia (without panic attack), and somatization that the existing evidence is insufficient to determine what brain regions may be involved in them. Future studies on these and other psychiatric disorders should use functional instead of structural measures, and whenever possible, employ experimental manipulations that activate the associated symptoms.

---

[1] Technically, its name is the bed nucleus of the stria terminalis.

[2] The "aversive amplification circuit" consists of the dorsomedial prefrontal cortex, anterior cingulated gyrus, and the amygdala.

31.4.2 Experimental Research on Religious Beliefs and Psychiatric Symptoms

I am sure there are many experiments that could be done to test neural cognitive-affective predictions from ETAS Theory, but I will only suggest three possibilities. I think they can be conducted with relatively few participants who are selected from a pool of college students. Based on previous research showing that the inhibition of anxiety partly depends on the capacity of the ventromedial prefrontal cortex (vmPFC) to modulate negative emotional responses [24–27] by modulating amygdala activity [28, 29], the three studies would measure vmPFC and amygdala activity. All three studies would measure vmPFC and amygdala activity under conditions designed to decrease or increase anxiety, measured by brain imaging. A peripheral nervous system measure of anxiety should be recorded during all the experiments: i.e., galvanic skin response (GSR). The three studies would extend our knowledge of the neural bases of psychiatric symptoms, as well as the role of beliefs in modulating psychiatric symptoms. My hypotheses mainly pertain to the amygdala and the vmPFC, but as the three studies include cognitive manipulations, I would expect the anterior cingulate cortex (ACC), the insula, and other parts of the PFC would be activated by them.

The first study would compare the neuro-physiological correlates of belief in a protective God or a deistic God (or higher power) on social anxiety. The students would be screened simultaneously for moderate-high levels of social anxiety and strength of belief in a deistic and a protective active God, using relevant instruments. I hypothesize that participants who believe in a protective God will have higher vmPFC activity and lower amygdala activity when presented with stimuli designed to elevate social anxiety, than will participants who believe in a deistic God. The stimuli would be pictures or verbal descriptions of situations that evoke social anxiety. A more complicated design would include another experimental group that would prime thoughts about a protective God, presumably by having participants read statements about the protection God provides. Other variants of the study could investigate other religious beliefs that should provide a sense of protection, such as beliefs in guardian angels.

From the perspective of ETAS Theory, I think belief in a protective God reduces anxiety because this belief provides a sense of protection from harm. In contrast, belief in a deistic God should not reduce anxiety because it does not provide a sense of protection.

I chose social anxiety for the first experiment for several reasons. It is fairly common in the general population, its onset is usually in the teens and twenties, [30, 31], and I think it would be relatively easy to elicit fear from the amygdala in individuals with social anxiety. Moreover, there is good evidence that the amygdala, the ACC and the insula (of the limbic system) and the vmPFC are involved in social anxiety. There is some evidence that the basal ganglia and possibly the brain stem also are involved in social anxiety, but what specific parts of these brain structures are involved is not clear. This study could help to clarify the specific areas of those structures that are active in social anxiety.

The second experiment would explore the neural correlates of the paranoid ideation associated with belief in Satan, as my analysis of the 2010 Baylor Religion Survey data found that belief in Satan had a larger net effect on paranoid ideation than it did on other psychiatric symptoms. Participants would be preselected for high or low belief in Satan and randomly assigned to control and experimental conditions. Measures of paranoid ideation would be taken before and after the experimental procedures, and galvanic skin response (GSR) would be measured in conjunction with brain imaging. The experimental condition would consist of demonic images accompanied by a narrative about Satan. The main hypotheses would be that images of Satan (with an accompanying narrative) will increase paranoia, amygdala activity, and GSR in participants with a strong belief in Satan. Here too, another experimental group could be added to see if belief in a protective God counters the effects of the demonic images among the participants with a strong belief in Satan. Based on ETAS Theory, I expect that images of Satan will increase amygdala activity and GSR in participants who strongly believe in Satan because Satan poses a threat of harm. I would expect an experimental manipulation about a protective God would off-set the effects of the Satan manipulation, especially in those participants who strongly believe in Satan, because most people that believe in Satan also believe in God. Another variant of the study could examine other religious beliefs that would be expected to heighten anxiety, such as wrathful and punishing God, instead of Satan. Still another obvious variation of the study could investigate whether belief in guardian angels counters the effects of belief in Satan.

The third experiment would specifically test the effects of pleasant and unpleasant beliefs about life-after-death on amygdala activity, GSR, and vmPFC activity, by having participants read short phrases of what the afterlife could be. The participants would be pretested to select individuals who believed in an afterlife and to see the extent to which they held specific beliefs about the afterlife. The design would include three conditions: descriptions about a pleasant afterlife, descriptions about an unpleasant afterlife, and neutral statements unrelated to the afterlife (the control condition). Participants would be asked to indicate if they agreed or disagreed with the descriptions. The study would directly test predictions from ETAS Theory and TM Theory. ETAS Theory predicts that pleasant afterlife beliefs should decrease anxiety and that unpleasant afterlife beliefs should increase anxiety relative to each other and the control condition. TM Theory's mortality salience hypothesis predicts that both pleasant and unpleasant afterlife beliefs should increase anxiety relative to the control condition because enhancing the salience of one's death should increase anxiety.

Finally, since ETAS Theory applies to all beliefs, not just religious beliefs, I think it would be valuable to design experiments to examine whether secular beliefs about safety and danger modulate amygdala activity through the vmPFC or other parts of the PFC. It would also be worthwhile to test whether different types of secular beliefs have cumulative or interactive effects. Research also is needed to identify the functional brain activity associated with a perceived social support and self-esteem, and their relationship to anxiety and other psychiatric symptoms. Recent research has implicated parts of the PFC in social cognition and self-esteem, including the orbitofrontal PFC and the vmPFC [32, 33].

31.5 Research on Level III of ETAS Theory: Neural Organization and Functioning of ETAS

Level III involves research to provide more detailed analysis of the neural organization of ETAS and their neural processing. Functional connectivity studies using fMRI have helped to establish the neural circuits underlying several psychiatric disorders at a gross level of analysis like those illustrated in Figs. 14.3, 14.4, and 14.5 of Chap. 14 including major depression [34], general anxiety [35, 36], social anxiety [37], and obsessive-compulsive disorder [38, 39]. However, a finer level of analysis is required to determine the specific neural circuits that form the proximate mechanisms that underlie classes and subtypes of psychiatric symptoms, which I call evolutionary threat assessment systems (ETAS). A 2014 article in *The Lancet Psychiatry* proposed that further advances in mapping the specific neural networks involved in different classes of psychiatric symptoms would require a combination of molecular imaging using positron emission tomography of the human brain and optogenetic research on animal models of psychiatric disorders [40]. Optogenetic research entails inserting light-sensitive proteins involved in neural transmission into a part of the brain, activating its neurons with an optic fiber, and electrically recording their activity *in vivo* [41, 42]. This technique has been used to define a neural circuit involved in fear conditioning in rats that includes the central and lateral regions of the amygdala, the periaqueductal gray of the brain stem, and the ACC [43]. The amygdala consists of a dozen or more regions [44] that may be involved in assessing different types of threats that underlie psychiatric symptoms in humans, such a fear of heights, insects, predators, and conspecifics (members of one's own species). Oliver Robinson and his colleagues at the National Institute of Mental Health have said, "A detailed understanding of the relationship between neural circuitry and … core anxiety symptoms is, we argue, a perquisite for more targeted diagnosis and treatment" (p. 301) [23].

More refined neuro-physiological research is also needed to determine how neural decision-making about sensory stimuli [45–47] operates in the context of threat assessments by different brain structures. All key brain structures involved in ETAS are thought to make decisions about what constitutes a threat, but we do not know how they do this. Nor do we know how multiple threat assessments from different structures are combined to make a single decision about whether a stimulus poses a threat of harm. Some researchers suggest that the vmPFC assigns emotional values or valences to stimuli [48], but how it that done?

I have said that the vmPFC sets the threshold of what constitutes a threat, but that is an analogy. It may be that some beliefs make the vmPFC or other areas of the PFC, such as the dmPFC, more sensitive (the equivalent of a lower threshold) or less sensitive (the equivalent of a higher lower threshold) to threat stimuli. In any case, I do not know how ETAS actually work or how beliefs actually affect them. Nor do I have sufficient knowledge of neuro-physiological methodology to offer detailed research proposals.

31.6 Research on Level IV of ETAS Theory: Comparative Research on the Evolution of Fear and Defense

In my opinion, far more comparative research needs to be done to expand upon Paul MacLean's work on the evolutionary roots of human emotions and psychiatric symptoms. Although the research of Joseph LeDoux and his colleagues has done much to establish the neuro-anatomical basis of fear, this and related research is mainly based on fear-conditioning [44, 49–51]. More animal research on fear and anxiety needs to be done using ethological models like those developed by Caroline and Robert Blanchard [52–54]. Certain strains of domesticated or "laboratory" rats, for example, show high levels of agonistic behavior (aggressive and defensive behaviors) [55, 56], which allows researchers to study fear-related reactions to the threats posed by a conspecific (i.e., another rat). They also exhibit freezing in the presence of a predator, which is an innate fear response to hide from predators [57]. Wild Norway rats (*Rattus norvegicus*, the ancestor of the laboratory rat) exhibit a systematic pattern of species-typical defensive reactions to predators (not exhibited by their domesticated cousins) in which different behaviors are exhibited depending on the proximity of the predator and the possibility of escape. Their defensive repertoire includes freezing to avoid detection, escape from a predator, and defensive attack when a predator is too close to try to escape. The last two of behaviors are classic examples of the "fight or flight reaction" [54]. The entire defensive repertoire of rats reflects the response flexibility that emotions (in this case, fear) provide for addressing environmental challenges, which I mentioned in Chaps. 9 and 10. Limited research has already been conducted on the brain structures involved in these defensive behaviors in wild rats [58], but given the difficulty of working with wild rats, the first generation of the mating of Long-Evans with and wild *Rattus norvegicus* might make it easier for brain researchers to study this pattern of behavioral reactions to threat.

In addition, Long-Evans rats, and presumably other domesticated rats, engage in a very distinctive, but seemingly trivial behavior, which traditionally has been called the "stretched attention posture" [59]. It recently has come to be called "risk assessment" behavior because it is thought to be akin to the kind of vigilance behavior associated general anxiety in humans [53]. Similar behaviors in laboratory mice (risk assessment, freezing, escape, and defensive attack) have been used as animal models of anxiety and panic attack in pharmacological research [52, 53].

Further research should be done on rat and mouse models of psychiatric symptoms, such as anxiety and panic attack. In addition, more neuro-anatomical and pharmacological research on repetitive behaviors in laboratory rats and mice, such as digging and grooming [60–64], should provide insights into OCD in humans [65, 66].

However, comparative research should not be restricted to studies of laboratory rats and mice. I think it should also be conducted with reptiles and fish. Surprisingly little research seems to have been done on the neural control of threat displays in lizards [67–69] since Paul MacLean's research [70]; an extensive literature search identified only one study related to neural mechanisms related to defensive responses to threats in lizards [71].

Research on fish conducted in the 1990s provided evidence for a neural pathway controlling specific threat displays [72], and brain neurotransmitter systems involved in intra-specific agonistic behaviors [73, 74]; these systems, which evolved in fish hundreds of millions years ago are also involved in the agonistic behavior of reptiles and mammals [67, 73]. Other older studies examined the neural control of the startle response in fish, which is a basic reaction to potential threats of harm [20, 75, 76]. Comparative research on the startle response would be particularly useful for studying the evolution of fear and anxiety because it is ubiquitous in the vertebrates [20]. Equally important, the bed nucleus of the limbic system (or its ancestral homologue), which controls the startle response [20], has been identified in fish, amphibians, reptiles, birds, and mammals [77, 78].

On the upper end of the evolutionary tree, research could explore the existence of beliefs in non-human primates and how, if they exist, they affect decisions such as threat assessments. Research, to date, has not settled the question whether monkeys or apes develop beliefs based on their observations (or perceptions). However, it has been suggested that monkeys have beliefs and there is some evidence that monkeys and apes can develop expectations about the behavior of other members of their own species based on their observations [79, 80]. The evolutionary biologist Lewis Wolpert has argued that the cognitive demands of the tool-making process, rather than the cognitive demands of primate social processes, led to the evolution of strong causal beliefs, which appear to be unique to humans [81, 82]. Nevertheless, it certainly would be worth the effort to: (a) examine the extent to which social and other possible forms of beliefs may have contributed to the development of the strong causal beliefs, and (b) to more fully investigate the degree to which other primates have a primitive form of causal beliefs.

Collectively, this research should help to demonstrate the underlying similarities between animal defensive behaviors and human psychiatric symptoms. In doing so, they might also confirm the evolutionary origins and adaptive functions and psychiatric symptoms, as well as beliefs.

References

1. Flannelly, K.J., Galek, K., Ellison, C.G., & Koenig, H.G. (2010). Beliefs about God, psychiatric symptoms, and evolutionary psychiatry. *Journal of Religion & Health,* 49(2), 246–261.
2. Silton, N.R., Flannelly, K.J., Galek, K., & Ellison, C.G. (2014). Beliefs about God and mental health among American adults. *Journal of Religion and Health,* 53(5), 1285–1296.
3. Gaudette, H., & Jankowski, K.R. (2013). Spiritual coping and anxiety in palliative care patients: A pilot study. *Journal of Health Care Chaplaincy,* 19(4), 131–139.
4. Gilbert, P. (1993). Defence and safety: Their function in social behaviour and psychopathology. *British Journal of Clinical Psychology,* 32(Pt 2), 131–153.
5. Arndt, J., Routledge, C., Cox, C.R., & Goldenberg, J.L. (2005). The worm at the core: A terror management perspective on the roots of psychological dysfunction. *Applied & Preventive Psychology,* 11(3), 191.
6. Dechesne, M., Arndt, J., Ransom, S., Sheldon, K.M., Pyszczynski, T., Van Knippenberg, A., et al. (2003). Literal and symbolic immortality: The effect of evidence of literal immortality on

self-esteem striving in response to mortality salience. *Journal of Personality & Social Psychology,* 84(4), 722–737.
7. Pyszczynsi, T., Greenberg, J., Solomon, S., Arndt, J., & Schimel, J. (2004). Why do people need self-esteem? A theoretical and empirical review. *Psychological Bulletin,* 130(3), 435–468.
8. Martens, A., Greenberg, J., & Allen, J.J.B. (2008). Self-esteem and autonomic physiology: Parallels between self-esteem and cardiac vagal tone as buffers of threat. *Personality and Social Psychology Review,* 12(4), 370–389.
9. Baldwin, M.W., & Wesley, R. (1996). Effects of existential anxiety and self-esteem on the perception of others. *Basic and Applied Social Psychology,* 18(1), 75–94.
10. Karademas, E.C., Kafetsios, K., & Sideridis, G.D. (2007). Optimism, self-efficacy and information processing of threat- and well-being-related stimuli. *Stress and Health,* 23(5), 285–294.
11. Gruenewald, T.L., Aziz, N., Fahey, J.L., & Kemeny, M.E. (2004). Acute threat to the social self: Shame, social self-esteem, and cortisol activity. *Psychosomatic Medicine,* 66(6), 915–924.
12. Houston, B.K., Olson, M., & Botkin, A. (1972). Trait anxiety and beliefs regarding danger and threat to self-esteem. *Journal of Consulting and Clinical Psychology,* 38(1), 152.
13. van Dellen, M.R., Campbell, W.K., Hoyle, R.H., & Bradfield, E.K. (2001). Compensating, resisting, and breaking: A meta-analytic examination of reactions to self-esteem threat. *Personality and Social Psychology Review,* 15(1), 51–74.
14. Leary, M.R., Barnes, B.D., & Griebel, C. (1986). Cognitive, affective, and attributional effects of potential threats to self-esteem. *Journal of Social & Clinical Psychology,* 4(4), 461.
15. Elllison, C.G., Flannelly, K.J., & Barrie, C.K. (2014, November 1). *Do afterlife beliefs moderate the association between recent serious illness and symptoms of anxiety-related disorders?* Paper presented at the National Meeting of the Society for the Scientific Study of Religion, Indianapolis, IN.
16. Nesse, R. (1998). Emotional disorders in evolutionary perspective. *British Journal of Medical Psychology,* 71(4), 397–415.
17. Nesse, R.M. (1984). An evolutionary perspective on psychiatry. *Comprehensive Psychiatry,* 25(6), 575–580.
18. Nesse, R.M. (1987). An evolutionary perspective on panic disorder and agoraphobia. *Ethology & Sociobiology,* 8, 73S–83S.
19. Nesse, R.M. (1990). Evolutionary explanations of emotions. *Human Nature,* 1(3), 261–289.
20. Grillon, C. (2008). Models and mechanisms of anxiety: Evidence from startle studies. *Psychopharmacology,* 199(3), 421–437.
21. Walker, D.L., Toufexis, D.J., & Davis, M. (2003). Role of the bed nucleus of the stria terminalis versus the amygdala in fear, stress, and anxiety. *European Journal of Pharmacology,* 463(1), 199–216.
22. Munsterkotter, A.L., Notzon, S., Redlich, R., Grotegerd, D., Dohm, K., Arolt, V., et al. (2015). Spider or no spider? Neural correlates of sustained and phasic fear in spider phobia. *Depression and Anxiety,* 32(9), 656–663.
23. Robinson, O.J., Krimsky, M., Lieberman, L., Allen, P., Vytal, K., & Grillon, C. (2014). Towards a mechanistic understanding of pathological anxiety: The dorsal medial prefrontal-amygdala "aversive amplification" circuit in unmedicated generalized and social anxiety disorders. *The Lancet. Psychiatry,* 1(4), 294.
24. Ochsner, K.N., Bunge, S.A., Gross, J.J., & Gabrieli, J.D. (2002). Rethinking feelings: An fMRI study of the cognitive regulation of emotion. *Journal of Cognitive Neuroscience,* 14(8), 1215–1229.
25. Ochsner, K.N., & Gross, J.J. (2005). The cognitive control of emotion. *Trends in Cognitive Science,* 9(5), 242–249.

26. Ochsner, K.N., Knierim, K., Ludlow, D.H., Hanelin, J., Ramachandran, T., Glover, G., et al. (2004). Reflecting upon feelings: An fMRI study of neural systems supporting the attribution of emotion to self and other. *Journal of Cognitive Neuroscience,* 16(10), 1746–1772.
27. Ochsner, K.N., Ray, R.D., Cooper, J.C., Robertson, E.R., Chopra, S., Gabrieli, J.D., et al. (2004). For better or for worse: Neural systems supporting the cognitive down- and up-regulation of negative emotion. *Neuroimage,* 23(2), 483–499.
28. Greenberg, T., Carlson, J.M., Cha, J., Hajcak, G., & Mujica-Parodi, L.R. (2013). Ventromedial prefrontal cortex reactivity is altered in generalized anxiety disorder during fear generalization. *Depression and Anxiety,* 30(3), 242–250.
29. Motzkin, J.C., Philippi, C.L., Wolf, R.C., Koenigs, M., & Baskaya, M.K. (2015). Ventromedial prefrontal cortex is critical for the regulation of amygdala activity in humans. *Biological Psychiatry,* 77(3), 276–284.
30. Magee, W.J., Eaton, W.W., Wittchen, H.U., McGonagle, K.A., & Kessler, R.C. (1996). Agoraphobia, simple phobia, and social phobia in the national comorbidity survey. *Archives of General Psychiatry,* 53, 159–168.
31. Kessler, R.C., McGonagle, K.A., Zhao, S., Nelson, C.B., Hughes, M., Eshleman, S., et al. (1994). Lifetime and 12-month prevalence of DSM-III-R psychiatric disorders in the United States: Results from the National Comorbidity Study. *Archives of General Psychiatry,* 51(1), 8–19.
32. Yang, J., Xu, X., Chen, Y., Shi, Z., & Han, S. (2016). Trait self-esteem and neural activities related to self-evaluation and social feedback. *Scientific Reports,* 6. Retrieved from: http://www.ncbi.nlm.nih.gov/pmc/articles/PMC4740758/pdf/srep20274.pdf
33. Pan, W., Liu, C., Yang, Q., Gu, Y., Yin, S., & Chen, A. (2016). The neural basis of trait self-esteem revealed by the amplitude of low-frequency fluctuations and resting state functional connectivity. *Social Cognitive and Affective Neuroscience*, nsv119. Retrieved from http://scan.oxfordjournals.org/content/11/3/367.short
34. Mulders, P.C., van Eijndhoven, P.F., Schene, A.H., Beckmann, C.F., & Tendolkar, I. (2015). Resting-state functional connectivity in major depressive disorder: A review. *Neuroscience & Biobehavioral Reviews,* 56, 330–344.
35. Mochcovitch, M.D., da Rocha Freire, R.C., Garcia, R.F., & Nardi, A.E. (2014). A systematic review of fMRI studies in generalized anxiety disorder: Evaluating its neural and cognitive basis. *Journal of Affective Disorders,* 167, 336–342.
36. Hilbert, K., Lueken, U., & Beesdo-Baum, K. (2014). Neural structures, functioning and connectivity in Generalized Anxiety Disorder and interaction with neuroendocrine systems: A systematic review. *Journal of Affective Disorders,* 158, 114–126.
37. Bruhl, A.B., Delsignore, A., Komossa, K., & Weidt, S. (2014). Neuroimaging in social anxiety disorder – A meta-analytic review resulting in a new neurofunctional model. *Neuroscience & Biobehavioral Reviews,* 47, 260–280.
38. Jang, J.H., Kim, J.-H., Jung, W.H., Choi, J.-S., Jung, M.H., Lee, J.-M., et al. (2010). Functional connectivity in fronto-subcortical circuitry during the resting state in obsessive-compulsive disorder. *Neuroscience Letters,* 474(3), 158–162.
39. Harrison, B.J., Soriano-Mas, C., Pujol, J., Ortiz, H., Lopez-Sola, M., Hernández-Ribas, R., et al. (2009). Altered corticostriatal functional connectivity in obsessive-compulsive disorder. *Archives of General Psychiatry,* 66(11), 1189–1200.
40. Kasper, S., Gryglewski, G., & Lanzenberger, R. (2014). Imaging brain circuits in anxiety disorders. *The Lancet Psychiatry,* 1(4), 251–252.
41. Fiala, A., Suska, A., & Schluter, O.M. (2010). Optogenetic approaches in neuroscience. *Current Biology,* 20(20), R897-R903.
42. Kravitz, A.V., & Kreitzer, A.C. (2011). Optogenetic manipulation of neural circuitry in vivo. *Current Opinion in Neurobiology,* 21(3), 433–439.
43. Johansen, J.P., Wolff, S.B.E., Luthi, A., & LeDoux, J.E. (2012). Controlling the elements: An optogenetic approach to understanding the neural circuits of fear. *Biological Psychiatry,* 71(12), 1053–1060.

44. LeDoux, J.E. (2000). Emotion circuits in the brain. *Annual Review of Neuroscience, 23*(1), 155–184.
45. Gold, J.I., & Shadlen, M.N. (2007). The neural basis of decision making. *Annual Review of Neuroscience, 30*, 535–574.
46. Gold, J.I., & Shadlen, M.N. (2001). Neural computations that underlie decisions about sensory stimuli. *Trends in Cognitive Sciences, 5*(1), 10–16.
47. Averbeck, B.B., & Lee, D. (2004). Coding and transmission of information by neural ensembles. *Trends in Neuroscience, 27*(4), 225–230.
48. Winecoff, A., Clithero, J.A., Carter, R.M., Bergman, S.R., Wang, L.H., & Huettel, S.A. (2013). Ventromedial prefrontal cortex encodes emotional value. *Journal of Neuroscience, 33*(27), 11032–11039.
49. Fellous, J.-M., Armony, J.L., & LeDoux, J.E. (2002). Emotional circuits and computational neuroscience. In M.A. Arbib (Ed.), *The handbook of brain theory and neural networks*. 2nd ed.). Cambridge, MA: MIT press.
50. LeDoux, J.E. (1995). Emotion: Clues from the brain. *Annual Review of Psychology, 46*, 209–235.
51. Phelps, E. A., & LeDoux, J. E. (2005). Contributions of the amygdala to emotion processing: From animal models to human behavior. Neuron, 48, 175–187.
52. Blanchard, D.C., Griebel, G., & Blanchard, R.J. (2001). Mouse defensive behaviors: Pharamacological and behavioral assays for anxiety and panic. *Neuroscience and Behavioral Reviews, 25*, 205–218.
53. Blanchard, D.C., Griebel, G., & Blanchard, R.J. (2003). The mouse defense test battery: Pharmacological and behavioral assays for anxiety and panic. *European Journal of Pharmacology, 463*(1), 97–116.
54. Blanchard, R.J., Flannelly, K.J., & Blanchard, D.C. (1986). Defensive behaviors of laboratory and wild Rattus norvegicus. *Journal of Comparative Psychology, 100*(2), 101–107.
55. Flannelly, K., & Lore, R. (1977). The influence of females upon aggression in domesticated male rats (Rattus norvegicus). *Animal Behaviour, 25*, 654–659.
56. Flannelly, K.J., & Thor, D.H. (1978). Territorial aggression of the rat to males castrated at various ages. *Physiology & Behavior, 20*(6), 785–789.
57. Blanchard, R.J., Kleinschmidt, C.K., Flannelly, K.J., & Blanchard, D.C. (1984). Fear and aggression in the rat. *Aggressive Behavior, 10*(4), 309–315.
58. Blanchard, D.C., Williams, G., Lee, E.M.C., & Blanchard, R.J. (1981). Taming of wild Rattus norvegicus by lesions of the mesencephalic central gray. *Physiological Psychology, 9*(2), 157–163.
59. Grant, E.C., & Mackintosh, J.H. (1963). A comparison of the social postures of some common laboratory rodents. *Behaviour, 21*(3), 246–259.
60. Liu, C., & Cerny, V. (1976). Release of grooming responses in basal ganglia and thalamic cats. Anatomical Record, 184(3), 464.
61. Strazielle, C., Lefevre, A., Jacquelin, C., & Lalonde, R. (2012). Abnormal grooming activity in Dab1 scm (scrambler) mutant mice. *Behavioural Brain Research, 233*(1), 24–28.
62. Cromwell, H.C., & Berridge, K.C. (1996). Implementation of action sequences by a neostriatal site: A lesion mapping study of grooming syntax. *Journal of Neuroscience, 16*(10), 3444–3458.
63. Thompson, R., Huestis, P.W., Shea, C.N., Crinella, F.M., & Yu, Y. (1990). Brain structures important for solving a sawdust-digging problem in the rat. *Physiology & Behavior, 48*(1), 107–111.
64. Aldridge, J.W., Berridge, K.C., & Rosen, A.R. (2004). Basal ganglia neural mechanisms of natural movement sequences. *Canadian Journal of Physiological Pharmacology, 82*, 732–739.
65. Langen, M., Durston, S., Kas, M.J.H., van Engeland, H., & Staal, W.G. (2010). The neurobiology of repetitive behavior: And men. *Neuroscience & Biobehavioral Reviews, 35*(3), 356–365.

66. Langen, M., Kas, M.J.H., Staal, W.G., van Engeland, H., & Durston, S. (2010). The neurobiology of repetitive behavior: Of mice. *Neuroscience & Biobehavioral Reviews,* 35(3), 345–355.
67. Baxter Jr, L.R., Clark, E.C., Ackermann, R.F., Lacan, G., & Melega, W.P. (2001). Brain mediation of Anolis social dominance displays. *Brain, Behavior and Evolution,* 57(4), 184–201.
68. Baxter, L.R. (2003). Basal ganglia systems in ritualistic social displays: Reptiles and humans; function and illness. *Physiology & Behavior,* 79, 451–460.
69. Baxter, L.R., Jr., Ackermann, R.F., Clark, E.C., & Baxter, J.E. (2001). Brain mediation of Anolis social dominance displays. I. Differential basal ganglia activation. *Brain, Behavior and Evolution,* 57(4), 169–183.
70. MacLean, P.D. (1977). The Triune brain in conflict. *Psychotherapy and Psychosomatics,* 28, 207–220.
71. Baxter Jr, L.R. (2001). Brain mediation of Anolis social dominance displays: III. Differential forebrain (3) H-sumatriptan binding to dominant vs. submissive males. *Brain, Behavior and Evolution,* 57(4), 202–213.
72. Gorlick, D.L. (1990). Neural pathway for aggressive display in Betta splendens: Midbrain and hindbrain control of gill-cover erection display. *Brain, Behavior and Evolution,* 36(4), 227–236.
73. Winberg, S., & Nilsson, G.E. (1993). Roles of brain monoamine neurotransmitters in agonistic behaviour and stress reactions, with particular reference to fish. *Comparative Biochemistry and Physiology Part C: Pharmacology, Toxicology and Endocrinology,* 106(3), 597–614.
74. Winberg, S., Myrberg Jr, A.A., & Nilsson, G.E. (1996). Agonistic interactions affect brain serotonergic activity in an acanthopterygiian fish: The bicolor damselfish (Pomacentrus partitus). *Brain, Behavior and Evolution,* 48(4), 213–220.
75. Anderson, J.J. (1988). A neural model for visual activation of startle behavior in fish. *Journal of Theoretical Biology,* 131(3), 279–288.
76. Yasargil, G.M., & Diamond, J. (1968). Startle-response in teleost fish: An elementary circuit for neural discrimination. *Nature,* 220(October 18), 241–243.
77. Goodson, J.L. (2005). The vertebrate social behavior network: Evolutionary themes and variations. *Hormones and Behavior,* 48(1), 11–22.
78. Maximino, C., Lima, M.G., Oliveira, K.R.M., de Batista, E.J.O., & Herculano, A.M. (2013). "Limbic associative" and "autonomic" amygdala in teleosts: A review of the evidence. *Journal of Chemical Neuroanatomy,* 48, 1–13.
79. Martin, A., & Santos, L.R. (2014). The origins of belief representation: Monkeys fail to automatically represent others' beliefs. *Cognition,* 130(3), 300–308.
80. Povinelli, D.J., & Giambrone, S. (2001). Reasoning about beliefs: A human specialization? *Child Development,* 72(3), 691–695.
81. Wolpert, L. (2007). *Six impossible things before breakfast: The evolutionary origins of beliefs.* New York: W.W. Norton & Co.
82. Flannelly, K.J. (2008). Review of the book *Six impossible things before breakfast: The evolutionary origins of beliefs* by L. Wolpert. *Journal of Nervous & Mental Disease*, 196(7), 581–582.

Index

K.J. Flannelly, *Religious Beliefs, Evolutionary Psychiatry, and Mental Health in America*, Religion, Spirituality and Health: A Social Scientific Approach 1,
DOI 10.1007/978-3-319-52488-7

MIX
Papier aus verantwortungsvollen Quellen
Paper from responsible sources
FSC® C105338

If you have any concerns about our products,
you can contact us on
ProductSafety@springernature.com

In case Publisher is established outside the EU,
the EU authorized representative is:
Springer Nature Customer Service Center GmbH
Europaplatz 3, 69115 Heidelberg, Germany

Printed by Libri Plureos GmbH
in Hamburg, Germany